A Time for Listening and Caring

A Time for Listening and Caring

Spirituality and the Care of the Chronically Ill and Dying

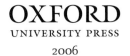

CHRISTINA M. PUCHALSKI

OXFORD

UNIVERSITY PRESS

2006

OXFORD
UNIVERSITY PRESS

Oxford University Press, Inc., publishes works that further
Oxford University's objective of excellence
in research, scholarship, and education.

Oxford New York
Auckland   Cape Town   Dar es Salaam   Hong Kong   Karachi
Kuala Lumpur   Madrid   Melbourne   Mexico City   Nairobi
New Delhi   Shanghai   Taipei   Toronto

With offices in
Argentina   Austria   Brazil   Chile   Czech Republic   France   Greece
Guatamala   Hungary   Italy   Japan   Poland   Portugal   Singapore
South Korea   Switzerland   Thailand   Turkey   Ukraine   Vietnam

Copyright © 2006 by Oxford University Press, Inc.

Published by Oxford University Press, Inc.
198 Madison Avenue, New York, New York 10016
www.oup.com

Oxford is a registered trademark of Oxford University Press

Library of Congress Cataloging-in-Publication Data
A time for listening and caring : spirituality and the care of the
chronically ill and dying / edited by Christina M. Puchalski.
p. ; cm.
Includes bibliographical references and index.
ISBN-13: 978-0-19-531178-5
ISBN-13: 978-0-19-514682-0 (pbk.)
1. Palliative treatment—Religious aspects.   2. Terminal care—Religious aspects.   3. Medical care—Religious aspects.
4. Chronically ill—Religious aspects.   5. Terminally ill—Religious life.   6. Spirituality—Health aspects.
I. Puchalski, Christina M.   II. Title: Spirituality and the care of the chronically ill and dying.
[DNLM: 1. Palliative care   2. Caregivers—psychology.   3. Religion and Medicine.
4. Spirituality.   5. Terminal Care.   6. Terminally ill—psychology.
WB 310 T583 2005]
R726.8.T56 2005
616'.029—dc22
2005017930

5 7 9 8 6
Printed in the United States of America
on acid-free paper

To my parents, Anthony and Krystyna Puchalski, who loved me unconditionally, accepted me fully, and supported me in pursuing my dreams. They shared their spiritual wisdom with me and guided me to a life of service to others.

To Ed O'Donnell, my best friend and soulmate, who taught me how to find hope and to live in the midst of life's challenges. In his presence to me, he taught me how to be present to others.

To Terry Van Vliet, my teacher, who taught me the importance of finding meaning in life and living life with passion.

And to my patients, who teach me how to live life to the fullest, with honesty, integrity, and with grace.

Foreword

In the practice of healing, a kind heart is as valuable as medical training, because it is the source of happiness for both oneself and others. Not only do other people respond to kindness even when medicine is ineffective, but cultivating a kind heart is a cause of our own good health.

When people are overwhelmed by illness, we must give them physical relief, but it is equally important to encourage the spirit through a constant show of love and compassion. It is shameful how often we fail to see that what people desperately require is human affection. Deprived of human warmth and a sense of value, other forms of treatment prove less effective. Real care of the sick does not begin with costly procedures, but with the simple gifts of affection, love, and concern.

As living beings, we all wish for happiness and seek to avoid suffering. Our basic attitude toward suffering makes a great difference to the way in which we experience it. Similarly, the way to prepare for death, whether we are approaching our own or caring for someone who is, is to train the mind. On one level this means cultivating a sincere, compassionate motivation and performing positive actions, serving other sentient beings. At another level it means calming and controlling the mind, which is a more profound way of preparing for the future. Identifying negative states of mind like anger, hatred, jealousy, and pride, we can work to eliminate them. At the same time we can cultivate positive attitudes like compassion and love, tolerance and contentment. Training the mind in this way is both useful and realistic.

Death is a form of suffering. It is an experience we would rather avoid, and yet it is something that will inevitably befall each and every one of us. Nevertheless, it is possible to adopt a course of action such that when we face this undesirable suffering we can do so without fear.

In many parts of the world the circumstances of death are changing. Many people can no longer rely on their family's being able to care for them as they die. With advances in medicine some people, who would previously have died, but in great pain, can have the process delayed and made more comfortable. The advice and experience contained in this book, *A Time for Listening and Caring*, reflect the widespread growth of interest in helping people to die in peace with dignity, such as we find in the hospice movement, which is very encouraging. There is no greater way of repaying the kindness that each and every one of us has received at different stages of our lives, than to offer help and comfort to those who are no longer able to help themselves. This is the true expression of compassion, and I am always encouraged when people take practical steps like this to put such positive motivation into effect. Such conduct vividly demonstrates that love and kindness are not a luxury, but a necessary source of health and happiness for others and ourselves.

THE DALAI LAMA

January 4, 2005

Preface

Why write a book on spirituality and the care of chronically or terminally ill and dying people? Certainly thousands of years have passed with people acknowledging the importance of the spiritual dimension of human existence. Billions of sermons and homilies have been preached about dying, redemption, suffering, the divine, and coping with loss. There are hundreds of self-help books on finding and exploring the spiritual path. Yet, in the clinical setting, there has been a noticeable separation between things of the spirit and things of the body.

How We Face Dying

People have an instinctual drive to live and to overcome adversity. In the United States, we strive to look younger, to think younger, and to live forever. Illness is seen as an aberration in an otherwise healthy and functional life. There is an avoidance of facing the ultimate fact that all of us will die. As a result, people who have chronic or terminal illness often express to me the feeling that they are useless and no longer a part of society. They feel undervalued and less of a person than they were before their illness. Some of my patients who are elderly or disabled feel afraid to ride the subway or to use escalators because younger, healthier, and more able-bodied people might overrun them. Some of my patients have become virtually homebound because of this fear. As a medical student, I remember feeling deeply saddened when I saw dying patients moved from rooms near the nurses' station to rooms at the end of the hall, because these patients were "less time-intensive." On intern sign-outs (at the end of day, sign-outs on all patients are given to cross-covering interns), dying patients were given the notation NTD, "Nothing To Do." Yet, there is so much that needs to be done for and with the ill and dying.

Medicine has made magnificent advances in the last 60 years with the discovery and development of antibiotics, transplants, insulin, chemotherapy, advanced radiological procedures, and sophisticated diagnostic tests. These advances offered people the promise and hope of curative treatments and longer life, and that did happen. People's life expectancy was increased from an average life span of 50 years at the end of the nineteenth century to the current life expectancy of over 80 years of age. Many illnesses are treated effectively and even cured. There are new advances now on the horizon that may extend our lives even longer; some of these, such as cloning, border on promising immortality. Quantity of life is being addressed, but quality of life tends to be forgotten. People are living longer, but with chronic illness. What has been ignored is that no matter how much we study, research, and develop, there is an inherent mystery to life that has yet to be answered. People still die, people still suffer, some get cured, and others don't. In spite of all the advances in science and technology, as I face my patients who ask me, "Why me?" and "Why now?" I don't have any answers.

Spiritual Questions

The inherent mystery of life triggers spiritual questions and experiences. We all search for some meaning and purpose for our lives here on earth, for ourselves in the midst of living, and for answers to the mystery of life. That search is something that binds all of us, regardless of our race, gender, health status, cultural background, religious and spiritual beliefs, age, education, or social status. Chronic illness, death, stress, and loss of relationships can all provoke challenges to the very things we thought gave us meaning in life. These challenges can be ignored or suppressed, or they can be faced. When facing them, we are embarking on a spiritual journey that will last our whole life, a journey of questions, new intimacies with the divine and with others, and new discoveries—as well as painful moments of darkness and isolation.

By giving credence to this important dimension in our lives, we open ourselves up to a type of healing that, while not necessarily curative, does restore us to a wholeness that is perhaps more significant than the cure of a physical illness. This is why I believe it is so critical that our healthcare system not only recognize the spiritual dimension of people's lives but also recognize that the field of medicine is itself spiritual. Integral to my professional life, as well as to the professional lives of all my colleagues and the contributors to this book, and also those who care for people who are ill, is the call of service to others. We all place the needs of those for whom we care above our needs, even in times when our need and our pain may be great. Our work is grounded in love for others. The relationships we form with our patients, clients, and colleagues are born out of a compassionate connection and call to service. From this connection and call comes forth the healing that is so necessary in all of our lives, whether we are currently ill or not. We are not mechanics, taking care of people's broken parts. We are partners with our patients in a therapeutic relationship from which springs forth the potential for healing. That healing may manifest itself as peacefulness, acceptance, better coping, happiness, or contentment. In the end, a life that may be shattered from illness and stress becomes whole again. By our presence, we serve others and walk with them in the midst of suffering and joy. This is why spirituality is essential to health care.

Each year, I teach medical students about issues faced by chronically ill and dying patients. Most of the students are apprehensive about a potentially depressing topic. As we discuss hope, many wonder how hope and dying can coexist. As one of my patients, Marilyn, who was dying of breast cancer, told my students, "It's all about hope ... the hope of new meaning and relationships, finishing important goals, living life to the fullest and having a peaceful death."

Source of Deep Concern

I became passionate about this area of medicine for a number of different reasons. My parents were and continue to be examples of people for whom spirituality is central to their lives. Both of my parents experienced huge losses and suffering while living in Poland during World War II. While they survived, they also had many dreams and hopes dashed by the atrocities of war and violence. Their stories of their experience and the way they live their lives reflect their strong faith and resilience, especially in the face of adversity. They were able to grasp onto faint rays of hope in the midst of total darkness. They were able to see the richness of life in the midst of impoverished isolation. They have lived and continue to live a life rooted in faith, hope, and love. They live compassionately and in service to others, to each other, and to their children. Their lessons to me have formed the basis of not only what I do but also who I am.

In my own life, my fiancé and friend, Eric, died of leukemia. I felt shattered and totally bereft of any sense of connection or hope. Through the help of my family and friends, I grabbed onto my spiritual path and eventually trusted that all would work out. When I was hopeless, my friend Ed helped me find hope; when I ached with sorrow, my mother listened and shared her pain and the lessons she learned, helping me realize that I, too, could survive as she had. My father was there constantly, reminding me of faith, purpose, and welcoming of mystery as an opportunity for growth. Friends, spiritual support groups, and time helped me heal.

While caring for Eric, I was thrust into the middle of a dysfunctional medical system, a system that dealt well with people who got better but which was unable to care for the dying. Eric spent months in a hospital and died in the midst of aggressive chemotherapy. His care was focused on curative approaches; his suffering and spiritual questions were never addressed or supported. I struggled to find a chaplain, but there was no spiritual care department. So Eric and I cared for each other, alone amidst the suffering, uncertainty, and pain. I remember feeling as though I was on a moving walkway that had no direction and which I had no ability to slow down. In retrospect, I would have loved to have had many of the resources described in this book for both Eric and me.

These personal and professional experiences fueled my desire to work toward creating a more compassionate system of care for people, especially those coping with chronic illness and dying. While there have been many changes, and the care of ill and dying people and their caregivers is improving, there are also many more improvements that are needed. In these times of economic and political pressure, which are threatening an already fragile healthcare system, it is especially important for all of us, whether healthcare professionals, patients, or administrators, to reclaim the spiritual roots of our profession of medicine.

Outline of the Book

This book is a compilation of lessons learned from all of our patients, from research, and from clinical work. It is rooted not only in scholarly study but also in each of our experiences as clinicians, chaplains, clergy, caregivers, and educators. It is a practical guide for clinicians, clergy, patients, and family alike, as well as educators. My colleagues were chosen for their commitment to the care of patients, their reputation as leaders in their areas of expertise, for their openness about their own spiritual journeys, and for their love and compassion for others. The authors represent a diverse group of physicians, theologians, ethicists, medical educators, counselors, and artists. They are all highly esteemed members of their professions. It was a tremendous privilege to work with each and every one of these colleagues. I continue to learn from them and feel proud to be part of such a special group.

This book is divided into four parts. The first part describes general principles about the role of spirituality in the healthcare of adults and children, ethical aspects of integrating spirituality into the care of patients, the role of the chaplain, and the spirituality of the caregiver. It explores themes of being a compassionate presence to another, of the healing power of relationship-centered care, and of the spiritual issues that the ill and dying face. The second part describes the theological implications of spiritual care at the end of life and in serious illness from the perspective of several different religious and cultural traditions. The third part describes practical tools, including spiritual histories, honoring the patient's stories, grief, and bereavement, and the role of art, music, and dance. The arts help our spirits continue to grow and are important resources for patients, family, and clinicians. In the final part, two of my patients speak from their experience in facing serious illness. In the closing chapter, I share the lessons I have learned personally from all my patients, and I offer challenges for all of us as we advocate to make healthcare systems more healing environments. In the appendices you will find some general resources, a religious and spiritual beliefs and practices chart, and advanced directives for several of the religious traditions presented in the following chapters.

While the title of this book focuses on the spirituality in the lives of people with serious and chronic illness and in end-of-life care, the principles apply to all people at any stage in their lives. It is intended for patients as well as professional and personal caregivers. Spirituality is what makes us human and therefore is integral to how we live our lives, as well as how we all face our dying and the dying of others.

Acknowledgments

I am very grateful to and wish to thank each individual for his or her part in helping this book become a reality. To my contributors, I thank you for your effort and the gift of yourselves. You are very much appreciated and respected by me and by the staff at the George Washington Institute for Spirituality and Health (GWish). To the editorial staff at Oxford University Press, especially Jennifer Rappaport and Carrie Pederson, I thank you for your guidance and assistance and mostly for your patience. To my parents, thank you for all your love, support, guidance, and wisdom. To my friend, Ed O'Donnell, thank you for your love, support, and for sharing your wisdom about the spiritual life. I also thank you for your advice and expertise in spiritual and theological issues. Without your guidance, editorial assistance, dedication, and support, this book would have never been published. To Nina Fry, I thank you for shepherding this project to completion. Your persistence in keeping track of all of us authors, in spite of our busy schedules, was a challenge, and I am grateful for your flexibility. And to the rest of the GWish staff, fellows, and volunteers, especially Beverly Lunsford, DNSc, RN, Janet Wade, Michele Zwolinski, Barbara Markwood, and Cybilline Aclan, thank you for your support and assistance. I, of course, am indebted to each and every one of my patients and those of my colleagues—the patients who have died, those struggling with suffering now, and those patients to come. Your stories and experiences create the woven thread that runs throughout this whole book.

In writing this book, my colleagues and I wanted to convey the hopeful side of dying and living. Illness, dying, and loss give all of us the opportunity to explore ourselves, what we perceive of as the divine or sacred, and to live in a way that is filled with richness, not just struggle. Jeff, my patient who died last year of AIDS, told me that in his last three years he thanked God for his illness, as it drew him closer to his family, to others, and eventually to God. As he died he told me that he loved himself and others in a way he never thought possible. Rhonda called her cancer a "blessing." Are we so different from the Jeffs and Rhondas of the world? We, too, are dying. In the end what matters is not how we die but how we lived our lives, with the reality of our dying present in every day of our lives. That is what our patients and loved ones do every day. As you read this book, I hope you will find this a helpful resource, whether you are a healthcare professional caring for patients, a family member or loved one of a dying person, someone who is struggling with illness and/or dying, or just any of us who search for hope and meaning in our lives.

Contents

Contributors

Christina M. Puchalski, MD, OCDS
Associate Professor of Departments of
  Medicine and Health Sciences
The George Washington University
  School of Medicine and Health
  Sciences
Associate Professor of Health Services
  Management and Leadership
The George Washington University
  School of Public Health
Director and Founder
The George Washington University
  Institute of Spirituality and Health
  (GWish)
2131 K Street NW, Suite 510
Washington, DC 20037
E-mail: hcsmp@gwumc.edu

The Reverend Natalia Vonnegut Beck
Christ Church Cathedral
55 Monument Circle
Indianapolis, IN 46204
Office Phone: (317) 636-4577
E-mail: tanyabeck@sbcglobal.net

Cornelius Bennhold, PhD
Professor of Physics
The George Washington University
Department of Physics
725 21st Street
Washington, DC 20052
E-mail: bennhold@gwu.edu

William Breitbart, MD
Memorial Sloan-Kettering Cancer
  Center
Department of Psychiatry and
  Behavioral Sciences
1275 York Avenue
New York, NY 10021-6007
E-mail: breitbaw@mskcc.org

BetheAnne DeLuca-Verley, MD
KidsDreams2
Behavioral Pediatric & Adolescent
  Medicine with Creative Clay
  Works
78 Ave de Pezenas
34320 Roujan, France
E-mail: BADVdream2@aol.com

John D. Engel, PhD
Senior Founding Fellow
Institute for Professionalism Inquiry
Summa Health System
Professor Emeritus
Northeastern Ohio Universities College
  of Medicine
4209 State Route 44
PO Box 95
Rootstown, OH 44272
E-mail: jengel@neoucom.edu

Pat Fosarelli, MD, DMin
Assistant Professor of Pediatrics
Professor of Spirituality and Practical
  Theology
The Ecumenical Institute of Theology
  at St. Mary's Seminary and
  University
5400 Roland Avenue
Baltimore, MD 21210-1929
E-mail: pfosarelli@stmarys.edu

Nina Fry, BA
Program Manager
The George Washington Institute for
  Spirituality and Health
2131 K Street NW, Suite 510
Washington, DC 20037
E-mail: hcsnaf@gwumc.edu

Christopher Gibson, PhD
Department of Psychiatry
Memorial Sloan-Kettering Cancer
  Center
1242 Second Avenue
New York, NY 10021-6007
E-mail: gibsonc@mskcc.org

Yusuf Hasan, BCC
Staff Chaplain
Memorial Sloan Kettering Cancer
  Center
1275 York Avenue
New York, NY 10021-6007
E-mail: hasani@mskcc.org

Gary Malkin
Co-Founder
Wisdom of the World, Inc.
PO Box 2528
Novato, CA 94948-2528
E-mail: gary@wisdomoftheworld.com
Web: www.wisdomoftheworld.com

The Reverend Stephen Mann, MDiv,
  BCC
12270-F Green Meadow Drive
Columbia, MD 21044
(410) 370-0202
E-mail: stephen_mann2@comcast.net

Uma Mysorekar, MD, FACOG
Hindu Temple Society of North
  America
4557 Browne Street
Flushing, NY 11355
E-mail: nytemple@aol.com

Laurence J. O'Connell, PhD, STD
President and Chief Executive Officer
The Park Ridge Center for the Study of
  Health, Faith, and Ethics
205 West Touhy Avenue, Suite 203
Park Ridge, IL 60068-4202
E-mail: Laurence.o'connell@
  advocatehealth.com

Mary Lou O'Gorman, MDiv
E-mail: MOGORMAN@stthomas.org

Rhonda Oziel (1949-2001)

Dennis Oziel

Robert Chi-Noodin Palmer, MD
Director of Behavioral Health
The American Indian Health and
    Services, Santa Barbara
1995 La Lomita Way
San Luis Obispo, CA 93401
E-mail: robertcpalmermd@aol.com

Marianne Leslie Palmer, MA

Lura Pethtel, MEd
Research Coordinator
Institute for Professionalism Inquiry
Summa Health System
55 Arch Street, Suite G4
Akron, OH 44304
E-mail: llp@neoucom.edu

Lobsang Rapgay, PhD
Assistant Clinical Professor of
    Psychiatry and Director
University of California, Los Angeles
Behavioral Medicine Clinic and
    Program
300 Medical Plaza, #2331
Westwood, CA 90024
E-mail: LRapgay@mednet.ucla.edu

Janet Lynn Roseman, PhD
Clinical Instructor
Brown University Medical School
21731 Arriba Real, #27B
Boca Raton, FL 33433
E-mail: Dancejan@aol.com

Yusef Salaam
Author and Teacher
New York, NY

Michael Stillwater-Korns
Co-Founder
Companion Arts
PO Box 2528
Novato, CA 94948-2528
E-mail: music@innerharmony.com
Web: www.careforthejourney.net

Daniel P. Sulmasy, OFM, MD, PhD
Sisters of Charity Chair in Ethics
SVCMC, Saint Vincent's Hospital
    Manhattan
Professor of Medicine and Director
Bioethics Institute of New York Medical
    College
153 West 11th Street
New York, NY 10011
E-mail: Daniel_sulmasy@nymc.edu

Rabbi Bonita E. Taylor, MA, BCC
Associate Director
The Center for Clinical Pastoral
    Education (CPE)
ACPE Supervisor, Pastoral Care
    Educator
The HealthCare Chaplaincy
307 East 60th Street
New York, NY 10022-1505
E-mail:
    btaylor@healthcarechaplaincy.org

Alexis Tomarken, MSW
Research Coordinator
Memorial Sloan Kettering
Adjunct Professor
Long Island University
E-mail: tomarkea@mskcc.org

Paul F. Tschudi, MA, LPC
Director
End-of-Life Care Program
The George Washington University
GWU Hospital, Suite 6168
900 23rd Street, NW
Washington, DC 20037
E-mail: paultsch@gwu.edu

Joseph Zarconi, MD
Professor of Clinical Internal Medicine
    (NEOUCOM)
Vice President for Medical Education
    and Research, and Founding Director
Institute for Professionalism Inquiry
Summa Health System
55 Arch Street, Suite G4
Akron, OH 44304
E-mail: zarconi@summa-health.org

Rabbi David J. Zucker, PhD, BCC
Chaplain/Director of Spiritual Care
Shalom Park
14800 East Belleview Drive
Aurora, CO 80015-2258
E-mail: djzucker@juno.com

A Time for Listening and Caring

PART I

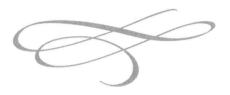

Spirituality, Beliefs, Ethics, Presence, and Relationship

I

The Role of Spirituality in the Care of Seriously Ill, Chronically Ill, and Dying Patients

CHRISTINA M. PUCHALSKI

Medicine is both an art and a science. We weave scientific data with the expe-
riences of the patient and the healthcare professional, with the way each un-
derstands illness and health, and with the worldview of each person, to create
a tapestry that approximates the reality. The fabric of this tapestry is the
spiritual connection we form with each other. The science is only a piece of
the whole picture. Faith, spirituality, intuition, and love play a vital role in
understanding the patient and ourselves, and ultimately in healing.

Christina M. Puchalski

Dying is a normal part of life. In today's society, however, dying is still treated as an illness. All too often people die in hospitals or nursing homes, alone and burdened with unnecessary treatments. In many cases, treatment choices would be different if patients were given the chance to talk about their desires with their physicians long before the deathbed scene. Dying people are not always listened to—their wishes, their dreams, and their fears go unheeded. They want to share these with us. In our culture, dying has become something to avoid. We strive to live forever, no matter what the cost. I have patients who have depleted their financial resources to search for cures that have a low probability of working. Families of dying patients are reluctant to talk with their loved one about dying because it might depress that person. Yet, the patient wonders why people are not mentioning the proverbial elephant in the room. Many patients feel isolated when their families, friends, and healthcare providers won't discuss what is obviously happening. Medical residents often say that they are reluctant to break "bad news" to their patients. The reasons I hear are "she is too nice," and "I can't be the one to upset him." I have worked with clergy who have avoided the topic for fear it was too depressing and would result in church members not returning to services.

The reasons for avoiding this topic, however, may have more to do with our own basic discomfort with dying, rather than with a motive to avoid hurting the dying person. Talking about death and dying touches people in very profound ways. It has the potential to open the door to deep personal and intimate interactions. Questions about self worth, meaning, and purpose in one's life, as well as the reason for suffering and loss, can be triggered as a result of talking about dying. One can experience a profound awareness of loneliness and isolation. Feelings of anticipatory grief, death anxiety, and sadness can come up. Ultimately, there is a sense of how little we can control and how much uncertainty there is in life. A desire to run from intimate connections with others, from the often unanswerable questions, from the feelings, and from the uncertainty can prevent us from talking with our patients and loved ones about dying. Therefore, in order to be with a dying person and to talk about dying, we need to confront our own awareness that we too will die. This process is inherently spiritual, as we ask the very existential questions of who we are, why we are here on earth, and why we die.

The task of dying, therefore, is not just spiritual for the patient or loved one who is dying, but also for all of us who have connections to others who die and ultimately for ourselves as we die. There is a natural tendency for us to separate people into the "ill and dying" or the "healthy and living." The differences lie in the type of illness someone has, the details of his or her life, his or her treatment, and how she or he approaches living and dying. But at the very core of who we all are, we are not that different. We all struggle with issues of loss, meaning and purpose, suffering, and eventual dying. In that struggle there is communion between all of us on earth. In that communion, the relationships and connections we form are the basis for partnership, help, and healing. One of the most important lessons I have learned from my patients is that I am not so different from them. We have a lot in common, for we are all in the process of living with dying. The time of death and the circumstances of death may differ, but not the journey.

Science and Technology

During the past century, there have been significant changes in healthcare. At the turn of the twentieth century, physicians were visiting patients in their homes. People died in their homes. The focus of care was patient- and family-centered. Physicians were on call 7 days a week, 24 hours per day. Physicians were committed to caring for their patients until the "end," (i.e., when the person died). In the 1950s and 1960s we saw the advent of huge technological and scientific advances. This caused, in part, the growth of specialization of medicine, because this increased knowledge and ways to treat patients expanded the specialties of medicine. Oncology, pulmonology, cardiology, infectious disease, and many other fields grew. There was a shift away from the primary care doctor to the specialist in order to treat illnesses. House calls greatly diminished, for many practical reasons; as the population expanded and cities grew in size, it was not practical to drive long distances to see patients. There were more treatments that physicians could offer to patients, and much of that treatment was delivered in a hospital-based setting. And so care became more outpatient and hospital based.

These advances also affected the cost of healthcare. Today we are facing questions about who should pay for the high cost of healthcare. Insurance companies have stepped in and developed guidelines for what is appropriate for doctors to order and what will be covered under certain plans. The primary care physician returned as the gatekeeper of services, in part to control the amount of money spent on specialty care. Places of employment change plans frequently to keep the cost at a minimum and still provide healthcare benefits. As a result, often people can no longer stay with the same physician, because insurance plans change frequently. The culture of staying with your family doctor until the end has changed to one where patients see numerous physicians. This is not conducive to forming long-term relationships—relationship building today has to be done in a compressed time situation.

People also did not live as long as they do now. At the turn of the nineteenth century, an average American's life expectancy was 50 years. Now, 73% of deaths are among people at least 65 years old and 24% of deaths are among those at least 85 years old. The causes of deaths in 1900 were influenza, tuberculosis, diphtheria, heart disease, cancer, and stroke. Today, heart disease is the number one cause of death, followed by cancer and stroke.[1] Infection usually was not treatable in the early 1900s, and people frequently died quickly from these causes. The time frame for dying from heart disease, cancer, and stroke is much longer. In effect, modern medicine has increased the period of time over which a chronically ill patient dies.

As stated previously, as technological and scientific advances occurred, and cures for illness became possible, people started living longer. Thus, people's sources of hope focused on science and science's ability to cure illness and delay death. Healing became synonymous with cure. When chemotherapy no longer worked, people started talking about losing their battle with cancer and having nowhere else to turn. Physicians explained this as "There is nothing more I can do for you." Science had failed and had opened the door to a seemingly desolate darkness. This is one reason I think physicians have a hard time talking with patients about their dying. A study by the American Board of Internal Medicine found that the majority of residents in internal medicine are very uncomfortable talking with patients about dying.[2] Medical education focuses on our ability to diagnose, fix, and cure, but until recently, little attention has been given to the concept of being present to another in the midst of their suffering and uncertainty.

Rachel Naomi Remen, MD, challenges us to think about medicine as service rather than as simply fixing.[3] Most of our work as physicians and healers comes from the partnership that arises from the service nature of our work. In that model, there is no room for "There is nothing more I can do." In fact, there is always more we can do. We can be present as our patients find healing, even in the midst of no cure and in the face of dying. There is always room for healing, even when cure is no longer possible. In Greek mythology, Asklepios was a physician, half-god and half-man, who cured illness and alleviated suffering. He was a compassionate healer who cared so much for humanity that he was willing to risk death to alleviate the suffering of those he encountered. Over the years this myth gave rise to the sixteenth-century adage, "To cure sometimes, to relieve often, and to comfort always."[4]

Living with Dying

The end of life can now last several years. Because the end of life can last so long, the question arises as to how to live with dying. Some people choose to live fighting their illness to the end, with much of their focus on the fight. Others focus their attention on other aspects of their lives: work, family, hobbies. Still others pursue a mix of these approaches. Each person's way of handling dying is often reflective of who that person is, what is important to him or her, and how he or she faces crisis. One needs to remember that there is no set map for living with dying. Each individual patient creates his or her own path and approach. I would argue that spirituality is the foundation of the path that people take and should therefore have a central part in the systems of care that care for chronically ill and dying people.

In the last decade, the United States has seen tremendous changes in the way death and dying are viewed by the medical professionals and by society itself. In 1995, the *Journal of the American Medical Association* published the results of a Study to Understand Prognosis and Preferences for Outcomes and Risks of Treatment (SUPPORT), a landmark study in end-of-life care.[5] SUPPORT concluded that most people in the United States die in pain; their wishes about resuscitation and other aggressive interventions are not known, or, if known, they are not respected. They also found that people die alone in hospitals, even when death at home is desirable. Much of the pain these people suffered at the end of life was spiritual.[6]

This data was so startling to professionals and lay people alike that it stimulated numerous initiatives to improve care at the end of life. One of these initiatives was LAST ACTS, a multimillion-dollar national campaign to improve care near and at the end of life. LAST ACTS has developed research, education, and policy initiatives for the professional and consumer groups, as well as policy makers. As a result, we have seen remarkable improvements in the area of end-of-life care, from better symptom management to improved communication between professionals and their patients and patients' families, to increased support for and legitimization of hospices. However, the attention to spiritual issues is still minimal and needs to form the basis of care.

Hospice and Palliative Care

Hospice and palliative care recognize the importance of the spiritual dimension in the care of dying patients. When Dame Cicely Saunders started St. Christopher's Hospice in London, she listed as one of the goals the relief of "total pain," including the physical, emotional, social, economic, and spiritual.[7] The basic tenets of this field are rooted in patient-centered care: attention to all these dimensions of a patient—physical, emotional, social, and spiritual. Most hospice and palliative care teams include a chaplain, and spiritual assessments are done on many patients. However, even in this ideal setting, spirituality is still neglected. In a recent report in *State Initiatives in End of Life Care*, a hospice consult is proposed, giving attending physicians authority to organize a series of consults with a team of palliative care experts.[8] While this is an excellent idea, the chaplain is missing from the proposed consult team, which includes the physician, nurse, and social worker. My hope is that as new models of care are proposed, the spiritual dimension will be actively included and chaplains will become integral members of all care teams.

The holistic approach to the treatment of the dying is one of the strengths of hospice. The patient is seen not as a physical entity with symptoms but as a whole person with physical, emotional, social, and spiritual components of healthcare. Of all the systems of care that we have in this country—hospitals, nursing homes, and outpatient clinics—hospice is the one where spiritual care is integrated. In spite of this, there is evidence that hospice overemphasizes medical care. One indication is the predominant use of nurses to deliver hospice care. In a study of home hospice patients, nurses visited patients five times as often as social workers and seven times as often as clergy.[9] A nationwide survey found that nurses felt overburdened by heavy caseloads and wanted help.[10] Furthermore, social workers and clergy report that psychosocial and spiritual needs are viewed as secondary.[11]

There are many reasons for this medical approach, including the need for skilled nursing care at home visits and issues related to cost and staffing. However, there is an opportunity to improve holistic care, and some hospices that I have worked with are implementing interventions that can help: routine spiritual assessment by all staff members, and increased referral to chaplains; increased literature and resources available to patients and their families and friends; and a greater awareness of the spiritual aspects of all the interdisciplinary team members' work, and how better to support that work among the staff. Ultimately, economic considerations take a lead role. So, to make changes in these systems requires both data and policy changes in which values such as a spiritual foundation to healthcare, especially in the care of the chronically ill and dying, can be valued and supported by administrators. Furthermore, while those in hospices have a chance to have their spiritual needs met, those with chronic illness treated outside of a hospice, or those who are not in hospice programs, are not in systems of care where the care is holistic and spiritual needs are attended to. Thus, any change must also involve a systemic change in the care of all patients, whether actively dying or not. There are two main areas where change with regard to spirituality in the healthcare setting is occurring. One has to do with increased research in the field, looking at healthcare outcomes as well as quality of life. The second has to do with the training of physicians.

Research in Spirituality and Health

There has been increased attention to the role of spirituality and religion in health over the last 15 years. There is a growing body of data studying the role of religious variables on physical and mental health outcomes. In more recent years, spiritual variables have also been studied. However, most of these studies have been mostly survey or associational studies. The exact aspect of a person's religion or spirituality that has an association to health benefits has not been determined, although this is an active area of research. Furthermore, there are no studies that show a causal relationship of a particular religious or spiritual variable to a particular health outcome. Part of the difficulty in researching this area is that the definition of religion and spirituality is different for different people. Generally, spirituality can be seen as a broader, more inclusive term than religion, one that relates to meaning-making or the search for the sacred or divine. One can have specific spiritual beliefs, rituals, and practices, or not. Spiritual does not imply any belief in a supreme being. Religion refers to beliefs, practices, and rituals within the context of a specific system of beliefs. Religion is defined in Webster's Dictionary as a "belief in and reverence for a supernatural power accepted as the creator and governor of the universe; a specific unified system of belief."[12] Religion is an objective and often codified expression of the deep spiritual beliefs of a specific group of people.

John Hardwig uses the term spiritual to mean "concerns about the ultimate meaning and values in life. It has to do with our deepest sense of who we are and what life is all about."[13] Balfour Mount similarly talks of spirituality, writing that it is "a deep connection to place, to family, to teachers, to things we have created and accomplished and to art, poetry and music."[14] He further talks about how spirituality might affect the caregivers: "These connections can help us confront our own death and the deaths of others." James Ellor (1997) defines spiritual well-being as "being 'healthy' in the very core of the person."[15] The term "spiritual well-being" was introduced into the nomenclature by the 1971 White House Conference on Aging. The goal was to introduce a term that would allow religious dialogue but in an interfaith, nondenominational context. The leadership of the National Interfaith Coalition on Aging defined spiritual well-being as "the affirmation of life in relationship with God, self, community, and environment that nurtures and celebrates wholeness."[16]

In 1999, a consensus group on developing guidelines for teaching courses on spirituality and medicine in medical education described spirituality as "a factor that contributes to health in many persons. The concept of spirituality is found in all cultures and societies. It is expressed in an individual's search for ultimate meaning through participation in religion and/or God, family, naturalism, rationalism, humanism, and the arts. All of these factors can influence how patients and healthcare professionals perceive health and illness and how they interact with one another."[17] The key elements of this definition are that spirituality is common to all people. It is the core of our humanity. Viktor Frankl writes, "The spiritual dimension cannot be ignored, for it is what makes us human."[18] Secondly, how our patients or loved ones understand and live their spirituality varies from person to person. Some people express it in religious terms; others, in more general terms. A religious person may or may not find meaning in his or her religion; meaning may come from relationship with others or God. Finally, spirituality is not just about the patient's spirituality, but also about the professional's or family's or friend's spirituality as well. It is the foundation of the relationship we have with each other: how we connect to one another and how we help each other in times of stress and serious illness, particularly dying. It is out of these caring relationships that healing is possible.

In 1994, the Fetzer Institute, with the National Institutes of Health (NIH), convened a group of researchers to develop a multidimensional approach to measuring the complex construct of spirituality and religiousness.[19] The result is a general survey that is being currently used in studies. Some of the constructs are meaning and purpose in life, forgiveness, religious coping, and daily spiritual experience.

Relative to other variables that are often studied, such as social support, gender, and economic status, spirituality is still an under-studied variable. Most fields of medicine have neglected to address the spiritual dimensions of health and well-being in their published research.[20] In the major journals of most fields of medicine

(1% of medicine, 1% of psychiatry, 2.5% of family medicine, and 3.5% of geriatrics) only 1–3% of the studies include quantitative measures of spirituality or religion.[21] The field of palliative care is slightly better. In a recent systematic review of the leading journals in palliative care, 6.3% of the articles surveyed use some quantitative spirituality and/or religion variables.[22] Thus, it appears that in the field of palliative medicine there is a greater recognition of the importance of spirituality than in many other areas of medical care.

The reason we evaluated the literature for quantitative methods is that much of medical treatment and reimbursement is based on quantitative data. Evidence-based medicine (EBM), which is based on population studies, now forms the basis of medical decision making. However, it has its limitations. Medical decision making is multifactorial. It includes scientific data and data from clinical trials (EBM), as well as the clinical experience of the physician. Intuition plays a large part in how physicians are able to elicit information from a patient. Both the patient and physician bring their beliefs and values to the relationship, and those beliefs and values impact decision making.[23] Trying to fit spirituality into the medical scientific model has its limitations. Spirituality is so personal to each individual that evidence-based medicine may not, therefore, be the best venue to study spirituality as a clinical intervention in medicine. Pat Boston and her colleagues suggest that spirituality is such a complex and personal construct that perhaps it cannot be adequately studied with quantitative methodology.[24] Spirituality, meaning, and inner life are subject to personal interpretation and are therefore difficult to define quantitatively. Qualitative research allows rigorous exploration of the subjective experience while at the same time allowing for its complexity and individual interpretation.

In spite of the paucity of solid data relative to other fields, there is still convincing evidence to suggest that spirituality and religion are important aspects of people's lives that potentially could affect both health outcomes and coping with illness and dying. It is also important to remember that spirituality and health is a relatively new field. It is a fast-growing area where new research is being conducted. I suspect that over the next 5 to 10 years there will be a large body of data in this area.

The Importance of Spirituality in Patients' Lives

That spirituality is central to the dying person is well recognized by many experts, the most important of which are our patients. Several national surveys have documented our patients' desire to have spiritual concerns addressed by their physicians. A 1990 Gallup poll showed that religion, as one expression of spirituality, plays a central role in the lives of many Americans.[25] A more recent Gallup survey showed that

94% of Americans surveyed profess a belief in God or a higher power; 6 out of 10 Americans surveyed say that religion is very important in their lives, and another 3 out of 10 say it is fairly important. About two-thirds of Americans polled claim to be a member of a church or synagogue. Additionally, when asked to state their religious preference, only 9% of the public say "none."[26]

Reed (1987) found that hospitalized terminally ill adults indicated a greater spirituality than both hospitalized nonterminally ill as well as healthy adults.[27] These findings support other research in which terminally ill outpatients, facing the end of their lives, indicated a significantly greater degree of spirituality than did a matched group of healthy adults who did not perceive their death as being close.[28] Similarly, critically ill hospitalized patients reported a greater sense of purpose in life than either a noncritically ill hospitalized or a healthy group.[29] In a study of women with gynecological cancers, 49% noted becoming more spiritual after their diagnosis. These data suggest that confronting one's inevitable mortality triggers questions of a spiritual nature for many people.[30]

The need for attentiveness to the spiritual concerns of dying patients has been well recognized by many researchers.[31] A survey conducted in 1997 by the George H. Gallup International Institute showed that people overwhelmingly want their spiritual needs addressed when they are close to death. In the preface to the survey report, George H. Gallup, Jr., wrote, "The overarching message that emerges from this study is that the American people want to reclaim and reassert the spiritual dimensions in dying."[32] In the study, survey respondents said they wanted to have warm relationships with their providers, to be listened to, to have someone to share their fears and concerns with, to have someone with them when they are dying, to be able to pray and have others pray for them, and to have a chance to say good-bye to loved ones. When asked what would worry them, they said not being forgiven by God or others or having continued emotional and spiritual suffering. When asked about what would bring them comfort, they said they wanted to believe that death is a normal part of the life cycle and that they would live on, either through their relationships, their accomplishments, or their good works. They also wanted to believe that they had done their best in their life and that they will be in the presence of a loving God or Higher Power. It is as important for healthcare providers and other caretakers to talk with patients about these issues as it is to address the medical/technical side of care. This same study found that the majority of people would first turn to friends for spiritual care—clergy, physicians, and nurses were lower on the list. This certainly is a wake-up call for all of us in the service professions to reflect on how we can better meet the spiritual needs of our patients and congregants. Interestingly, the Gallup Institute also found that "many survey respondents want a closer relationship with their doctor, and that as many as 40 percent would like to be spiritually in tune with their doctors."[33] The Gallup report concludes, "Medical professionals need to understand more fully that dying is not only a discussion between them and the patient about medical care. It involves other dimensions that define human beings. . . . They need to understand and integrate into their own thinking about the patient and the spiritual beliefs that guide their patient."[34]

The 1990 Gallup survey found that 75% of Americans said that religion is central to their lives; a majority felt that their spiritual faith could help them recover from their illness.[35] Additionally, it was found that 63% of patients surveyed believed it is good for doctors to talk to patients about spiritual beliefs.[36] Ehman and colleagues (1999) found that 94% of patients with religious beliefs agreed that physicians should ask them about their spiritual beliefs if they became gravely ill; 45% of patients who denied having any religious beliefs still agreed that physicians should ask their patients about their spiritual beliefs.[37] In this survey, 68% of patients said they would welcome a spiritual question in a medical history; only 15% said they recalled being asked by their physicians whether spiritual or religious beliefs would influence their decisions. A study surveying more that 200 hospital inpatients found that 77% said physicians should consider patients' spiritual needs. Furthermore, 37% wanted their physician to discuss spiritual beliefs with them more frequently, and 48% wanted their physicians to pray with them.[38] A Time/CNN poll found that 65% of people surveyed want their physicians to address their spiritual issues.[39] In a *USA Today Weekend* health survey, the majority of people polled felt that doctors should talk with their patients about spiritual concerns, yet only 10% reported that their doctors had discussed such issues with them.[40] This statistic is understandable because, until recently, spirituality has been overlooked in medical school curricula and in the standards of medical care.

Spiritual Beliefs and Illness

There is a growing body of evidence documenting the relationship between patients' religious and spiritual lives and their experiences of illness and disease.[41] In addition to surveys that demonstrate that spirituality is important to people and that a significant percentage of patients would like their physicians to discuss their spiritual beliefs with them, a number of studies show that having spiritual beliefs is beneficial to patients, particularly those with serious illnesses. Reviews of the literature indicate potential relationships between measures of religious commitment and health indicators, including morbidity and mortality, in studies of many diseases.[42] Research suggests that mortality is reduced following cardiac surgery among those who receive comfort and support from religion.[43]

TABLE I.I

Pain Questionnaire by American Pain Society to Hospitalized Patients

Most Commonly Used Method for Pain Management	
Pain pills	82%
Prayer	76%
Pain IV med	66%
Pain injections	62%
Relaxation	33%
Touch	19%
Massage	9%

Spirituality has been found to be an important factor in bereavement. It has been reported that parents who have lost a child have found much support in their spiritual beliefs following their child's death.[44] Spirituality is important in coping with pain and with dying. Ninety-three percent of patients with gynecologic cancers noted that their spiritual beliefs helped them cope with their cancer.[45] Patients with advanced cancer who found comfort from their spiritual beliefs were more satisfied with their lives, were happier, and had diminished pain.[46] In a questionnaire sent out by the American Pain Society (1998), prayer was the second most common method of pain management after oral pain medications, and was the most common nondrug method of pain management (Table I.I).[47]

In a study of patients with HIV, those who were spiritually active had less fear of death and less guilt about their illness. Fear of death was more likely among the 26% of religious patients who felt their illness was a punishment from God. Fear of death diminished among patients who had regular spiritual practices or who stated that God was central to their lives. Patients who believed in God's forgiveness were more likely to engage in discussions about advance directives.[48]

In a current study of the effect of spirituality on the will to live in HIV patients, we are finding that spirituality and nonorganized religious measures (relationship with God) have a positive impact on patients' feeling that their life is better after diagnosis than before. Organized religious measures (church attendance, frequency of prayer) have no effect (Table 1.2).[49]

This study supports what I have observed in my clinical practice: Spirituality has a strong influence on how patients come to understand their suffering and illness.

Quality-of-life instruments used in end-of-life care try to measure an existential domain that addresses purpose, meaning in life, and capacity for self-transcendence. In studies with one such instrument, three items correlate with good quality of life for patients with advanced disease: if the patient's personal existence is meaningful,

TABLE I.2
Spirituality and the Will to Live in HIV Patients

Patients with HIV who said life was better after their diagnosis also had increased:
- Spirituality
- Nonorganized religious activity
- Optimism

TABLE I.3
Spirituality and the Will to Live in Patients with Advanced Illness

Patients with advanced illness had good quality of life if they:
- Had meaningful personal existence
- Had fulfillment in achieving life goals
- Found life worthwhile

if the patient finds fulfillment in achieving life goals, and if life to this point has been meaningful (see Table 1.3).[50]

This study demonstrates the importance of addressing meaning and purpose in a dying person's life.

Writings on addiction also have supported the importance of finding meaning. The 12-step program of Alcoholics Anonymous, one of the best-known programs in the treatment of addiction, lists as one of the 12 steps (which were described by some of the earliest members of the group) as: "[We] came to believe that a power greater than ourselves could restore us to sanity."[51] In this view, addicts see their drug of choice as central in their lives; recovery hinges on one's ability to find a meaning and purpose outside of oneself and one's illness.

Spirituality and Caregiving

Spirituality is important not just for the patient but also for those caring for the patient: family, friends, and professional caregivers. Caring for loved ones or patients who have a chronic or serious illness or disability can be one of the most challenging times in a personal or professional caregiver's life. The experience is filled with many challenging events, which can result in emotional, physical, social, and spiritual changes, not only in the patient but also in those who care for the patient. These changes can create considerable problems for those involved in the caring process, as well as offer an opportunity for growth, fulfillment, and deepening of relationships.[52] Caring for an ill person presents numerous challenges. Caregivers may feel unprepared to handle the challenges as they arise. This can result in stress for the caregivers, with resultant physiological and psychological responses.[53] Spirituality may help caregivers deal with the stress in more effective ways.

Folkman and colleagues (1994) showed that increased stress motivated the engagement of religious coping in caregivers.[54] Cupertino (1998) showed that caregivers who felt closer to God and prayed frequently believed religion to be important and were better able to cope and experienced less stress with caregiving demands. They felt more useful, found new meaning in life, experienced strengthened relationships, and were more able to appreciate life.[55] Jivanjee (1994) did a descriptive study of caregivers of patients with Alzheimer's disease.[56] Spiritual support was consistently mentioned by all but 2 of the 18 participants in the study as being central to their sense of well-being, as well as giving them the strength to cope with the demands of caregiving.

In another study, Wyatt (1999) found that caregivers of patients with cancer had more depressive symptoms than the general public.[57] Depression was passively correlated with negative thinking and inversely correlated with positive outlook and with spirituality. Caregivers endorsed the following spiritual items:

- I believe in a power greater than myself;
- I know what is important in life;
- My values and beliefs help me meet daily challenges;
- I accept the mysteries of life and death.

Positive attitudes, therefore, as well as an acceptance of the unknown and an ability to deal with the inevitable uncertainty of life, helped caregivers.

Kaye and Robinson (1993) suggest that caregiving results in increased feelings of depression and need for social support. Spirituality was shown to improve depression and enhance social support among caregiving wives.[58] Robinson and Kaye further described spiritual practices that caregivers utilized, which included:

- Talking with friends and family about spiritual matters;
- Reading spiritually related material;
- Engaging in private prayer;
- Seeking spiritual guidance.

Caregivers further described spirituality as important in everyday life, forgiveness as an important part of spirituality, and feeling close to God or a higher power in prayer, worship, or important moments in life.

Chang and colleagues (1998), in a study examining the factors that influence and are influenced by religious/spiritual coping among those providing care for disabled adults, showed that religious/spiritual coping reduces symptoms of depression and role submersion.[59] This effect is due to higher relationship quality. The authors hypothesize that religion and spirituality may play a role in sustaining human relationships, which are often strained by the necessities of providing care for others. This study speaks to the relational aspects of spirituality.

Studies also support the observations noted in patient stories[60] and in the writings of Foglio and Brody[61] that illness can cause people to question their lives, their identities, and what gives their life meaning. For example, in a study of 108 women undergoing treatment for gynecological cancer, 49% noted becoming more spiritual after their diagnosis.[62] In a study of parents who had a child who died of cancer, 40% of those parents reported a strengthening of their own spiritual commitment over the course of the year prior to their child's death.[63] Illness, or facing one's mortality, is an opportunity for new experience, self-awareness, and meaning in life.

Religion and religious beliefs can play an important role in how patients understand their illness. In a study asking older adults about God's role in health and illness, many respondents saw health and illness as being partly attributable to God and, to some extent, God's interventions.[64] Prayer, in this study, appeared to complement medical care rather than compete with it. Meditation has been found to be a useful adjunct to conventional medical therapy for chronic conditions such as headaches, anxiety, depression, premenstrual syndrome, AIDS, and cancer.[65]

Mechanism of Action

How spiritual modalities contribute to health and recovery is unclear. Koenig and his colleagues (1997) propose an immune-related mechanism that might mediate the stress response.[66] In a study of 1,700 older adults, they found that those attending church were half as likely to have elevated levels of IL-6, an interleukin associated with stress and disease. The authors hypothesize that religious commitment and perhaps spiritual practices in general may improve stress control by establishing better coping mechanisms, richer social support, and strengthening of personal values and worldview.

Herbert Benson and his colleagues have studied the relaxation response and have shown it to be beneficial in a number of conditions, including hypertension,[67] cardiac arrhythmia,[68] chronic pain,[69] insomnia,[70] depression, and anxiety.[71] The postulated mechanism—the relaxation response—relates to the stress response and may counter the effects of stress. There has been plentiful anecdotal and research evidence of the physiological and emotional effects of stress on a person. Dr. Benson and others have demonstrated that stress can result in deleterious health effects, such as hypertension, cardiovascular disease, ulcers, insomnia, anxiety, depression, anger, and fatigue.[72] That the relaxation response improves outcomes in these conditions suggests a mechanism involving the stress response. In a more recent work, they propose a mechanism mediated through neural processes and their coupling to constitutive nitric oxide that could explain, on a biochemical and neurological basis, the beneficial effects seen with the relaxation response and, possibly, with spiritual beliefs.[73]

Pargament and colleagues (1990) have studied both positive and negative coping and have found that religious experiences and practices, such as seeking God's help or having a vision of God, extend the individual's coping resources and are associated with improvement in healthcare outcomes.[74] Patients showed less psychological distress if they sought control through a partnership with God or a higher power in a problem-solving way, if they asked God's forgiveness or were able to forgive others, if they reported finding strength and comfort from their spiritual beliefs, and if they found support in a spiritual community. Patients had more depression, poorer quality of life, and callousness toward others if they saw the crisis as a punishment from God, if they had excessive guilt, or if they had an absolute belief in prayer and a cure and an inability to resolve their anger if the cure did not occur. Pargament and his colleagues have also noted that sometimes patients refuse medical treatment based on religious beliefs.[75] People have the right to refuse medical treatment. However, refusal of treatment or acceptance of treatment should be done with the patient's informed consent. As a physician, I explain the possible medical outcomes if patients decline or accept a particular course of action. Chaplains similarly go over spiritual informed consent. Patient may misunderstand what their particular religion says about a course of action. Chaplains help clarify those misunderstandings but also help people reflect on their decision, so that whatever decision a person comes to is one that is freely and comfortably accepted and congruent with the person's beliefs.

Spiritual Coping

The data supports the role of spirituality in peoples' lives, particularly as people deal with illness and with dying. How does spirituality work to help people cope with their illness and with dying or with the illness and dying of their loved one? (Table 1.4).

One coping mechanism might be hope. Spirituality and religion offer people hope. It helps people find hope in the midst of the despair that often occurs in the course of serious illness and dying. Hope can change during the course of an illness. Early on, the person may hope for a cure; later, when a cure becomes unlikely, the per-

TABLE I.4
Spiritual Coping

- Hope: for a cure, for healing, for finishing important goals, for a peaceful death
- Sense of control
- Acceptance of the situation
- Strength to deal with the situation
- Meaning and purpose: in life, in the midst of suffering

---

son may hope for time to finish important projects or goals, travel, make peace with loved ones or with God, and have a peaceful death. This can result in a healing, which can be manifested as a restoration of one's relationships with others or one's sense of self. Often our society thinks in terms of cures. While cures may not always be possible, healing—the restoration of wholeness—may be possible to the very end of life.

Religious beliefs offer people a language for hope. For example, in Catholicism, hope in Jesus' promise of victory over death through resurrection and salvation gives Catholics hope in a life beyond death. In the funeral rites, it is stated, "I believe in the resurrection of the dead and the life of the world to come."[76] In the Protestant view, the concept of salvation in death gives hope. Jesus' dying and rising from the dead means that those who participate in His death no longer participate in sinful human nature.[77] In Eastern traditions, such as Buddhism and Hinduism, the hope of rebirth and a belief in karma offer people hope in the face of their mortality.[78] In Judaism, there are many diverse ways of viewing death. For some, hope is found in the living on through one's children. In the orthodox and conservative view, there is a belief in a resurrection, when the body arises to be united with the soul.[79] For patients without specific religious beliefs as well as for those with religious beliefs, there is a need to transcend death that also may be manifested by living on through one's relationships or one's accomplishments and deeds.[80] Irion (1993) suggests that humans may create abstractions by portraying a life after death.[81] For religious people, this may take the form of concepts found in their religious traditions. For others, life after death might be in terms of one's descendants. For some, it might be being immortalized in the memory of others or in the contributions one makes in life. Cultural beliefs and traditions can also contribute to how people find meaning and hope in the midst of despair.[82]

In addition to hope, spirituality can offer people a sense of control. Illness can disrupt life completely. Some people can find a sense of control by turning worries or a stressful situation over to a higher power or God.[83] Similarly, people can use their beliefs to help them accept their illness and find strength to deal with their situation.[84] Reconciliation may be an important aspect of a dying person's spiritual journey. Often people seek to forgive others or themselves as they review their life and their relationships. Finally, finding meaning and purpose in the midst of suffering, as discussed earlier, is integral to spirituality.

Suffering

As mentioned previously, much of the pain patients experience is not just physical pain, but also spiritual.[85] In fact, from my clinical experience with patients, I have found that spiritual suffering underlies most of the pain that patients and their families experience. Pain is multifactorial: physical, emotional, social, and spiritual. Any one of these can exacerbate the total experience of pain. One of my patients who has just had a recurrence of ovarian cancer is recovering from surgery for removal of the tumor. She is experiencing abdominal pain, which by tests and exams does not appear to be related to an obstruction or to the surgery itself. She is also anxious and often asks me why God would inflict this suffering on her. I suspect her pain is the result of some postoperative pain but is also part of the overwhelming existential crisis she is in as she faces the progression of her illness and the real possibility that she may die from the cancer.

What is suffering? Cassel (1982) writes of understanding suffering as a threat to our personhood. We suffer until the threat to our personhood is removed or until we can accept it and deal with it.[86] Medicine has for years been influenced by the Cartesian dualism of the separation of mind and body. In the Cartesian model, physical pain is relegated only to the physical domain. In this model, the patient's body is assigned to science and his mind to religion. This results in the longstanding justification for treating the disease separate from spiritual or existential suffering and what some refer to as the separation of religion and medicine. The result of this, however, is that suffering is only viewed as physical pain. The medical model, therefore, focuses only on objective laboratory data and not on the patient's stories or beliefs. The goal of physicians in communication emphasizes the gathering of objective data rather than compassionate, empathic listening to learn about the disease in the context of the patient's story: his or her beliefs, values, relationships, hopes, fears, and dreams. The patient's personhood, as Cassel writes,[87] is devalued. Only the body is of concern to medical professionals.

However, threat to one's physical body can also threaten the very nature of who we are and what gives us meaning, that is, what is often assigned to the mind. The lack of meaning and purpose can in turn lead to spiritual or existential suffering, which can affect physical pain and manifest as physical symptoms. Thus, the mind and body are connected. Medicine today is recognizing more and more the importance of the connection between the body and the mind. The human being is not dualistic. Body and mind are one; suffering stems from the whole—body *and* mind. There is not an artificial separation of the two domains. Recognizing suffering and helping people deal with it is part of spiritual care. Cassel writes, "The alleviation of suffering is the warrant of medicine and its test of adequacy. It is a test that contemporary medicine fails, despite the brilliance of its science and its awesome technological power."[88]

How can we understand another's suffering? Henri Nouwen's (1972) concept of the wounded healer is relevant to medical professional caregivers as well as to family and friends who care for a loved one.[89] We understand because we are also wounded by past hurts, disappointments, and losses. We, too, experience pain and suffering. From the understanding of our own suffering, we can understand and help others. When we can face our own mortality and pain, we can then help others as they face their mortality, pain, and suffering. Rachel Naomi Remen (1997) writes, "It is our woundedness that allows us to trust each other. I can trust another person only if I can sense that they, too, have woundedness . . . pain . . . fear."[90]

Viktor Frankl (2000) writes of the importance of finding meaning in the midst of suffering.[91] That may be one of the most important tasks of the spiritual journey. Meaning in one's life can be found in one's job and in relationships with others and/or God; it can also be experienced in art or music or nature. How one finds meaning may change as people encounter illness or dying. While the job may no longer hold the same meaning, relationships might take on greater importance. Some people find meaning in suffering, in terms of self-improvement or as a trigger for enlightenment. The Buddhist understands pain and suffering as part of life; resisting the inevitability of life's turmoil is what gives rise to suffering, whereas acceptance may relieve the suffering. Religions offer people an understanding of human suffering. Philosopher Robert Smith (1996) writes that "The religious experience of suffering—mediated through religion's own intellectual, ethical or experiential dimensions—opens the therapeutic encounter into very large and richly complex human worlds."[92] In the following chapters on different religious traditions, the concepts of suffering will be explored. From the perspective of the caregiver, it is important to listen and learn from the patients what their religious traditions or spiritual beliefs teach them about suffering and how they integrate those teachings into their lives.

Medical Education

The American College of Physicians has convened two consensus conferences and concluded that physicians are obligated to address all dimensions of suffering—the physical, psychosocial, spiritual, and existential.[93] The Joint Commission on Accreditation of Healthcare Organizations (JCAHO), which accredits hospitals, recognized that spiritual concerns are often important for patients and that hospitals should provide spiritual care.[94] As described previously, studies indicate that patients would like their spirituality addressed and integrated into their care, and some studies even indicate that a patient's spirituality may impact healthcare outcomes. Medical schools are now recognizing that spirituality can be important in patient care and in the well-being of physicians. In 1991, I initiated one of the first courses on spirituality and health in the United States at the George Washington University School of Medicine. This course has evolved into a required curriculum and has served as the basis for courses that are now held in over 60% of U.S. medical schools.[95] As director of an awards program sponsored by The John Templeton Foundation, I developed, with the help of many colleagues in medicine, a national program that gives competitive grants to medical schools for innovative curricula in spirituality and health.

The reason that medical schools have supported these courses has to do with a major change in medical schools, spearheaded by M. Brownell Anderson, MEd, of the Association of American Medical Colleges (AAMC). She led a major medical school initiative called the Medical School Objectives Project.[96] A group of leading academic faculty critically evaluated the needs of patients and their families and then proposed changes in the curricula to help meet those needs. Training compassionate and altruistic physicians is a top priority. Consequently, medical education is changing, to include more attention to ethical issues, patient-doctor communication issues, and professionalism. The courses in spirituality help meet the new requirements by assisting students in learning to communicate with patients about their hopes, fears, and beliefs. The courses teach students about suffering and how to address it, as well as how to understand and incorporate spirituality into the clinical setting. The consensus conference with AAMC,[97] which I chaired with Ms. Anderson, developed guidelines and learning objectives for the courses. The learning objectives are:

> *With regard to* spirituality *and* cultural *issues, before graduation students will have demonstrated to the satisfaction of the faculty:*

- The ability to elicit a spiritual history;
- The ability to obtain a cultural history that elicits the patient's cultural identity, experiences and explanations of illness, self-selected health practices, culturally relevant interpretations of social stress factors, and availability of culturally relevant support systems;
- An understanding that the spiritual dimension of people's lives is an avenue for compassionate caregiving;

- The ability to apply the understanding of a patient's spirituality and cultural beliefs and behaviors to appropriate clinical contexts (e.g., in prevention, case formulation, treatment planning, challenging clinical situations);
- Knowledge of research data on the impact of spirituality on health and on healthcare outcomes, and on the impact of patients' cultural identity, beliefs, and practices on their health, access to and interactions with healthcare providers, and health outcomes;
- An understanding of, and respect for, the role of clergy and other spiritual leaders and culturally based healers and care providers, and how to communicate and/or collaborate with them on behalf of patients' physical and/or spiritual needs;
- An understanding of their own spirituality and how it can be nurtured as part of their professional growth, promotion of their well-being, and the basis of their calling as a physician.

With regard to end-of-life care issues, before graduation students will have demonstrated to the satisfaction of the faculty:

- An understanding that death is a natural part of life, that suffering and loss are integral parts of the human life cycle, and that the physician's role encompasses the comprehensive care of the patient and his or her family during the entire transition between life and death;
- The ability to deliver difficult news about end-of-life issues to patients and their families in a caring and compassionate manner, to elicit patient's values and beliefs and preferences for treatment at the end of life, and to obtain advance directives and knowledge of surrogate issues;
- Recognize that when death becomes a likely possibility treatment, options may change depending on the risks and benefits of a particular treatment, the consequences of that treatment for the patient, and patient preference for type of care;
- An understanding that the concept of palliative care refers to all the dimensions of care (physical, emotional, social, and spiritual) that should be provided at the end of life;
- The ability to recognize the spectrum of the physical, emotional, sociocultural, and spiritual symptoms of distress patients may exhibit at the end of life and the appropriate ways to respond to them;
- The ability to work with and value a multidisciplinary team delivering end-of-life care and to communicate effectively, both orally and in writing, with colleagues and other healthcare providers in order to deliver appropriate care to patients at the end of life;

- The ability to access data on end-of-life issues and utilize these data in the case formulations and management plans of patients at the end of life.

The overall outcome is that students become aware of the need to address spirituality in the healthcare setting and in their patients' lives. They also learn to address all dimensions of a patient's and the patient's family's lives: their physical, emotional, social, and spiritual concerns and issues. Students should also address their own spirituality and how their spirituality affects not only those for whom they care but also affects themselves and how they interact with others on the interdisciplinary healthcare team. Thus, addressing one's own suffering and confronting one's own mortality becomes central to the training of physicians.

Spiritual Considerations

The definition of spirituality that we agreed would be most relevant in the clinical setting is cited earlier in this chapter.[98] The basis for this definition is spirituality as relevant in clinical settings; that is, how do patients present their spiritual issues in the context of their health and illness. From the clinical perspective, a patient's specific religious affiliation is relevant only in the context of specific beliefs that might affect healthcare decisions. But what gives people the source of their meaning, strength, and hope is relevant in terms of healing. Therefore, we need to be attentive to what is the source of meaning that can be expressed in religious or other terms and what are the beliefs or practices that might be relevant to the way a person copes with stress and illness. The final sentence of our definition reminds us that it is not just about our patients' spirituality but also about our own. All of us search for meaning in our lives; all of us search for that connection to another or to God. It is our spirituality that is the basis of who we all are as human beings, the basis of our calling to be physicians and other healthcare providers, and the basis of the practice of medicine as a spiritual practice. Service to others may be one of the highest of spiritual values, and that is what we do as physicians and caregivers. Sulmasy (1999) writes that "to heal a person, one must first be a person."[99] It is from our spiritual roots that we reach out to others, to connect, to help, and to heal. Medicine is very much a spiritual practice. Spirituality is the foundation for the relationship we have with each other, how we connect to one another, and how we help each other in times of stress and serious illness, particularly dying. It is out of these caring relationships that healing is possible.

We will all die one day. We may be fearful and anxious, but we can always push off the inevitable in the face of good health. People who are actively confronting their dying, either with chronic illness or active end-of-life care, face fears and anxieties on a daily basis. There are no obvious answers, no roadmaps for the journey. There is a lot of uncertainty and trepidation. Patients need doctors and other caregivers who are warm and willing to connect to them. They need doctors and other caregivers whose concern for them will be lifelong, even in the absence of curative treatments. They need doctors and other healthcare providers that can support and help patients and their families find a sense of hope, meaning, and purpose in the midst of suffering. Within the context of the connection we form with each other, the time we take to listen to fears, dreams, hopes, and grief, and the unselfish love we give to those who need us, healing is possible. It is then that I believe medicine will reclaim its spiritual roots.

2

Spirituality in Palliative Care
An Ethical Imperative

LAURENCE J. O'CONNELL

Although I am not a clinician, I have spent much time in the presence of dying patients. They have taught me to accept the mystery of life and to acknowledge hope as the source of life-giving confidence and the ultimate ground of peace-filled resignation as the inevitable approaches. A book title from the 1960s put it well: 'Broken Bones May Joy!'

Laurence J. O'Connell

Introduction

Spirituality is inextricably woven into the fabric of palliative care. "Palliative care is formally committed to holistic—that is, physical, social, psychological, and spiritual—care of the dying person and his or her family."[1] If spiritual concern is an essential part of palliative care, do medical caregivers have an ethical obligation to address the spirituality of their patients and families? What would be the scope and grounds of such a moral imperative?

Tony Walter (2002) has questioned what he considers "an assumption in palliative care literature, namely, that all patients have a spiritual dimension and that all staff can offer spiritual care."[2] Although Walter's understanding of spirituality and its role in personal and public life certainly is open to challenge, he does argue his way to a defensible practical point: "We might . . . be well advised to drop the assumption that any healthcare professional can offer spiritual care to any patient."[3] Walter feels that by abandoning the universalist assumption, individual caregivers escape a logic that requires them to personally, in a hands-on way, deliver spiritual care in each case. He wants to "reduce the likelihood of any one member of staff feeling spiritual care to be an unwelcome burden."[4]

Although Walter may have succeeded in relieving "each member of the team of the burden of feeling obliged to accompany each and every patient,"[5] he, at least, implicitly admits that the palliative care team and its individual members are obliged to address, or at very least accommodate, spiritual concerns. Absent clear prescriptions of who must accompany whom on the spiritual path, Walter is receptive to finding "someone who can accompany each patient at least a little of the way."[6] While protecting the sensibilities—the spiritual privacy—of individual caregivers, Walter does not explore the inherent, public promise of palliative care to acknowledge and act upon spiritual concern as an integral part of its philosophy and practice. How do individuals and institutions deal with the moral commitment to honor the promise of spiritual support? What are the ethical duties, moral challenges, and professional obligations of medical caregivers?

Before moving on, it should be noted that this discussion focuses narrowly on that point in the continuum of palliative care where end-of-life care is clearly in view. Palliative care, of course, embraces much more than end-of-life care, but it certainly encompasses and aspires to a good death.

Spirituality and Healthcare

Spirituality is one of those weasel words that escapes easy or succinct definition, but it does point to a dimension of human experience that is discrete and identifiable. Sidestepping an obsessional quest to define spirituality, John Shea (2000) has suggested an approach by which "spirituality would be characterized in ways that would be appropriate to its contexts and its ambitions."[7] He has crafted a very useful and highly pertinent approach to spirituality within the context of healthcare. His perspective is rooted in the firm conviction that spirituality and healthcare go hand in hand. "Healthcare is a world of practicalities that needs to be in touch with the inner world . . . lest it carry on its tasks in mechanical and dispirited ways. Spirituality points to the human capacity for transcendence and needs to be tested and tempered, in this case by the concrete and practical concerns of healthcare."[8]

Shea's strategy is powerful and effective, as evidenced by its direct and, as we shall soon see, arguably elegant applicability to the question at hand: Given the formal role of spirituality in palliative care, what ethical obligations must medical caregivers accept? If they are to preserve their own integrity and fulfill their promises to patients and families, how will they identify and address spiritual needs? How will they weigh the respective demands of a world of practicalities, on the one hand, with the human drive for transcendence, on the other hand, especially where palliative care is practiced within the context of end-of-life care?

Spiritual Interests, the Spiritual, and Spiritualities

Shea breaks up spirituality into three component parts—spiritual interests, the spiritual, and spiritualities. Interest in the spiritual is breaking out on many specific fronts as American culture becomes generally more attuned to the spiritual dimension of the human condition. For example, "interest in the spiritual is emerging in the corporate world; in the athletic sphere; in the areas of social justice; in the struggles of community organizing; in the ecological, feminist, and elder movements; and, of course, in healthcare."[9] Each area seems to be lifting up the spiritual, assessing its specific interest in this complementary side of our humanity, and striving to integrate it. Healthcare has certainly moved in this direction, and developments in palliative care are a singular example of emerging spiritual interests in healthcare.

Shea attempts to provide a working knowledge of the spiritual, especially as it relates to the context of healthcare. Here, Shea offers a very accessible primer on the spiritual itself as a foundation for the specific interest that healthcare is now taking in spirituality. Finally, Shea points to spiritualities, that is, the personal forms—beliefs, stories, and practices—that shape and direct the personal lives of individuals as they both seek and offer health and healing.

In three broad strokes, Shea provides a roadmap for describing key spiritual interests in healthcare, the source of those interests, and the way they find concrete expression in the lives of patients, their caregivers, and families, as well as the institutions that support them. It is within this masterful presentation that we can identify and clarify the moral warrants, that is, the scope and grounds of the ethical obligation to address spirituality in the palliative care setting, with special reference to end-of-life care.

Spiritual Interests

All ethical analysis involves weighing competing values and interests. Within the realm of spiritual interests in healthcare, one interest may be weighed against another interest(s). This kind of analysis is directed toward two general goals: understanding and guidance. We seek to understand our duties and find guidance in how we can most effectively meet the moral demands of a given situation. Each area of spiritual interest in healthcare must be weighed against the others as we seek an overall pattern of ethical engagement.

Although there are many potential spiritual interests in healthcare, Shea delineates six compelling interests that are particularly relevant to the task at hand. Each is charged with moral ramifications, each is a potent reservoir for ethical reflection and consequent action. More specifically, an analysis of Shea's catalogue of spiritual interests will likely deliver unique perspectives on the fundamental question addressed in this chapter: How do individuals and institutions deal with the moral commitment to honor the promise of spiritual support in palliative care, especially within the context of end-of-life care?

The moral weight of spiritual interests gains special prominence in the realm of palliative care that focuses upon end of life. Despite its positive and supportive thrust, end of life care does evoke a sense of limitation and inevitable loss. As the proximity of death becomes palpably more present, spiritual interests naturally come to the fore. The impulse to seek meaning and the need to envision some form of transcendence are no strangers to those who regularly encounter terminally ill persons.

The terminally ill and those who care for them make up a complex web of spiritual interests that are largely unexplored and thus often unconnected and poorly understood. By illuminating and conceptually aligning the spiritual interests that intersect within end-of-life care, we can better understand the moral obligations that crisscross this critical range of human relationships. Here, the implicit commitment to honor the promise of spiritual support will find explicit and practical guidance for shaping an ethical agenda of care. Absent this kind of understanding and practical guidance, healthcare ethics easily becomes little more than a jungle gym, where ill-informed yet undeniably often well-intentioned players perform dangerous contortions that swing between avoidance, on the one hand, and intrusiveness, on the other.

The six areas of spiritual interest delineated by Shea each illustrates important elements in an overall understanding of the ethical imperative to acknowledge and explicitly respond to spirituality in palliative care, especially as it is practiced near the end of life. Each category addresses aspects of the core ethical consideration in this context, namely, the moral quality of caring relationships. How do medical caregivers relate to the spiritual demands of their patients? And how do patients engage their caregivers around issues of spirituality? Each bears responsibility for the personal quality and moral tenor of their relationship, as well as the adequacy of the outcomes achieved.

The kind of relationship that lends itself to the effective integration of spirituality rests upon three critical tasks: (1) attending to personal expectations; (2) achieving some shared insight about the relative importance and role of spirituality in the context of care; and (3) committing to a consistent pattern of engagement around issues of spirituality. An examination of spiritual interests in healthcare will provide useful, concrete information relevant to the emergence of expectations, the achievement of shared insight, and the development of consistency.

1. *The Spiritual Interests of Patients:* Good healthcare focuses upon the experience of the patient—the full range of the suffering person's personal, social, and clinical

needs. The personal experience of the patient is the stone that hits the water and creates a ripple effect. The foundational spiritual interest in healthcare, then, emanates from the inner life of the patient. But the patient does not stand alone. As the spiritual interest of the patient is piqued and expands, other ranges of spiritual interest are activated, especially among family members and caregivers.

The patient confronts limitation and loss, and within the context of end-of-life care, loss unto death. The spiritual interest of the patient revolves around questions of meaning and a practical interest in responding to the demands of fresh insight into what it means to be alive and to confront death. Here patients must make decisions—that is, exercise moral agency. They are forced to make decisions about how to manage suffering, loss, and limit. "Patients are interested in the spiritual because it may hold the secret to how they can relate to their own leave-takings, even the leave-taking of death."[10] The patient who makes the turn to the spiritual—and most do—begins to generate expectations and create personal needs. To the degree possible in a vulnerable situation, the patient has an obligation to share those expectations and express those needs. By doing so, the patient opens the way for shared understanding and an effective pattern of communication with others that will enhance care and patient satisfaction. In short, patients bear some responsibility for ensuring attention to their own spiritual care. But the patient is inevitably embedded in a network of personal and professional relationships that also involve taking responsibility for spiritual care.

2. The Spiritual Interest of Caregivers in Patients: In recent years medical caregivers have exhibited a new openness to the role of spirituality in their practice. For example, more than 60% of American medical schools now teach required or elective courses on religion, spirituality, and medicine. Nursing, too, has expanded offerings in the area of spirituality. Harold G. Koenig, MD, explains why spirituality ought to be a routine part of patient care: "(1) religious beliefs and spiritual needs are common among medical patients and serve a distinct function; (2) religious beliefs influence medical decision making; (3) there is a relationship between religion and both mental and physical health; (4) many patients would like their doctors to address these issues; and (5) there is historical precedent for doing so."[11] The expansion of clinical practice to include at least sensitivity to, if not the complete embrace of, spiritual and religious concerns has ethical implications. Increasingly, caregivers cannot, in good conscience, neglect the expectation that the spiritual interests of their patients will be addressed. Here we confront the dilemma raised by Tony Walter as addressed in the opening paragraphs of this chapter: While protecting the sensibilities—spiritual privacy—of individual caregivers, how will the inherent public promise of palliative care to acknowledge and act upon spiritual interests be honored?

Increasing cultural interest in the spiritual has sensitized more patients to the potential advantages of attending to the spiritual dimension of their care, while changes in clinical education have alerted caregivers to their own responsibilities with reference to spiritual care. Yet many clinical caregivers tend to remain aloof or at least quite tentative about their involvement in the spiritual concerns of their patients. There are many reasons, both personal and professional, that account for this reluctance; over time, such hesitancy will probably dissipate, as spiritual interests are more routinely considered. In the meantime, however, the ethical imperative rooted in the inherent nature of palliative care must be universally respected. Clinical caregivers have positive ethical responsibilities, and thus they cannot engage in embarrassed avoidance or arrogant disdain for the relevance of spiritual interests.

Although they may not—or in some cases cannot—personally engage the spiritual interests of their patients, caregivers must acknowledge the legitimacy of those interests. They have a duty to inquire about the expectations of their patients with reference to the role of spirituality in the context of care. A level of shared understanding must be achieved, and the caregiver must commit to helping—even if indirectly—their patients meet their spiritual needs. As empirical studies increasingly substantiate the clinical advantages of addressing spiritual concerns, the moral warrant for addressing the spiritual interests of patients becomes stronger and stronger.

3. The Spiritual Interest of Caregivers in Themselves: Caregiving is, of course, not unidirectional; it moves in a variety of ways. Caregivers, like their patients, have spiritual interests that deserve attention. The world of caregiving today is complex, fast paced, and often exhausting. As healthcare delivery continues to evolve in ways that seriously stress caregivers, patients, and families, spirituality has become an area of public discussion among many clinicians, as they seek to ground their vocation and to honor deeply engrained professional commitments.

Caregivers must consider their own spiritual interests as they engage the spiritual needs of patients and families. They, too, need to develop a set of expectations that will help them set appropriate boundaries around spiritual involvement, establish shared understandings of what is or is not possible for them in a particular clinical context, and develop reasonable patterns of engagement around issues of spirituality. Their moral duty to acknowledge and address the spiritual needs of patients and families must be weighed against their own legitimate need for spiritual space and personal integrity. The spiritual values of a particular patient may run contrary to the spiritual perspective of the caregiver. In such cases, shared understandings around the nature and role of spirituality, as well as an agreed-upon modus operandi for addressing spiritual issues, become critical. The moral duty to attend to the spiritual needs of the patient does not encompass doing violence to one's own spiritual convictions and fundamental beliefs.

For example, the spiritual path of a terminally ill patient might ultimately include a request for physician-assisted suicide. Many physicians simply cannot identify with the spiritual reasoning that may lie behind such a request. Here significant divergent values relieve the caregiver of responsibility for accompanying the patient along the chosen path. This does not, of course, imply desertion by the caregiver. If the tasks of attending to personal expectations, achieving shared insight, and committing to a consistent approach have been well done, the parting will take place quite naturally. The patient will seek, and the initial caregiver may well solicit, an alternate caregiver who can identify with the values and spiritual preferences of the patient.

Finally, caregivers must respect boundaries in the spiritual realm. Some patients will be initially reluctant to consider spirituality, and others will reject outright the introduction of spiritual concerns. Even when there is clear evidence of spiritual issues in such a case, the caregiver must exercise caution. An opening for the expression of spiritual concerns and its relevance to the clinical situation may be offered, but if the overture is clearly rebuffed, the caregiver has no further moral obligation to pursue the spiritual dimension. In fact, unwelcome intrusion at this point would be unethical, even if the caregiver is convinced that spirituality could be helpful.

4. *The Spiritual Interests of Chaplains:* The involvement of chaplains in spiritual care may seem self-evident, but their responsibilities are nonetheless far-reaching and ethically charged. Today, due to the overall heightened interest in spirituality, chaplains are called upon to address spirituality on several levels. Of course, the chaplain's primary responsibility within the healthcare setting is the care of patients and their families, but more than ever chaplains are called to respond to the spiritual concerns of other caregivers (physicians, nurses, social workers, etc.). And beyond personal involvement with patients, families, and other caregivers, chaplains are assuming more and more responsibility for the spiritual and ethical character of the organizations they serve.

On every level the chaplain helps elicit and define the personal expectations that contribute to shaping the kind of shared insight about spiritual concerns among patients, caregivers, families, and healthcare institutions that encourage respect and consistency in addressing particular spiritual needs. The contemporary chaplain offers a blend of spiritual depth and psychological competence that is attuned to spiritual needs in a time of crisis. Chaplains have a moral duty to understand the limits of their competence as well as the appropriate range of their interventions. They must be prepared to help patients differentiate between personal expectations surrounding spiritual care that can be reasonably met within a particular healthcare setting and demands that are more appropriately met elsewhere. Returning again to the issue of physician-assisted suicide, the chaplain may expect to be called upon to mediate between patient and physician. Although the patient may be part of a spiritual or religious tradition that accepts euthanasia, the physician and/or hospital may not be prepared to provide it. Without condemning the patient's preferences or dismissing his or her theological convictions, the chaplain has the duty to broker a shared understanding that will lend itself to a morally consistent approach. Perhaps the chaplain may even help make alternative institutional arrangements.

In the realm of spiritual care, chaplains also have a special responsibility for identifying morbid tendencies that often masquerade as expressions of spirituality, especially in end-of-life care. These tendencies usually signal clinical depression rather than spiritual depth. In these cases the chaplain should seriously consider deferring to a representative of the patient's own religious or spiritual tradition who might better understand the specific sources of the patient's spiritual disorientation. Ideally, personal perspectives and expectations can be adjusted, and the course of spiritual care can resume.

Chaplains increasingly express their spiritual interests within the context of organizational life. Today, chaplains are among the leading proponents of the emerging palliative care movement. Recognizing that spiritual concern is an essential part of genuine palliative care, chaplains have begun to assertively champion the advantages of a comprehensive palliative care program to the institutions they serve. Given their own core identity, many chaplains have rightfully assumed their own moral responsibility for promoting the ethical imperative to fully incorporate spirituality into end-of-life care. Given their critical position within healthcare organizations, vigilance in this respect has now arguably risen to the level of a personal moral duty and a professional obligation.

5. The Spiritual Interest in Organizational Life: Organizations are moral agents; that is, they engage in corporate choices that are either ethically consistent with their stated values or they are not. When a healthcare organization claims to embrace holistic care, which encompasses physical, mental, social, and spiritual care, it is making a moral commitment. The authenticity of organizational life will be judged in light of the expectations engendered by such a public commitment.

There are consequences. For example, "it would be contradictory to try to deliver spiritual care in a spiritually uncaring environment, to try to give to others what has not been given to you."[12] Healthcare organizations that claim to value a spiritually sensitive environment are thus obliged to embody spirituality in concrete organizational structures and specific programs. This is especially true of faith-based healthcare organizations that trace their fundamental intentions to spiritual motivations.

The moral consequence of the foregoing line of reasoning is clear: Healthcare organizations that claim to be holistic and thus responsive to spiritual concerns— whether they are faith-based or not—are ethically bound to address spirituality in end-of-life care. Within the contemporary context of palliative care, this duty to provide specifically spiritual care exceeds the mere provision of pastoral care to chronically and terminally ill patients. The duty to provide a spiritually responsive environment extends to the entire organization, including administrative, clinical, and support staff. As the saying goes: "You can't give what you don't have." Just as the entire staff is to some degree familiar with the demands of the physical, mental, and social identity of the institution and is more or less prepared to respond, so too should it be acquainted in a general way with the demands of a spiritually vibrant organization. This does not mean that staff members are compelled to embrace any particular religious or spiritual perspective, but that they should recognize spiritual attentiveness as a defining feature of the workplace. Organizational structures and specific programs should be in place to support the ethical imperative to provide spiritual care, especially within the context of end-of-life care. Failure to exhibit such concrete attentiveness to spiritual care smacks of hypocrisy, or at least gives evidence of a failure to understand that holistic claims impose specific moral obligations.

6. The Spiritual Interest of Ethics: Shea characterizes the spiritual interest of ethics as "a concern for the spiritual basis of ethical decision making, and as a concern for the inner state of the ethically acting person."[13] So far we have addressed the participants (patients, clinicians, chaplains, and organizations) and their ethical responsibilities vis-à-vis their spiritual interests as they relate to palliative care, especially where palliative care is practiced within the context of end-of-life care. In addressing the spiritual interests of ethics, we are brought full circle, returning to Harold Koenig's point (2002), namely, that spiritual beliefs and religious convictions influence decision making.[14] Shea puts it somewhat differently: "Ethics and spirituality are partners in the development of the whole person who acts."[15]

Throughout this chapter, ethics is defending its partner's rightful place within end-of-life care by pointing to the need for a broader moral context. In those precarious situations where death is in view, ethics privileges spiritual insight and provides a wide berth, giving spirituality space to work in the decision-making process. Doing the right thing cannot be severed from the spiritual basis for choosing one course of action over another.

Emerging Spiritual Interests: An Example

It may be helpful to illustrate briefly how spiritual interests arise within palliative care, especially near the end of life. In Madlyn's story, spiritual interests emerged with rare clarity. Each of the six areas of spiritual interest came to the fore, explicitly and in ways that highlighted the moral imperative to respond to spiritual concerns.

Madlyn was an 80-year-old woman, twice widowed and the mother of three children. She had lived a full life and was enjoying her time at an adult retirement village when she was suddenly diagnosed with metastatic cancer. After she had absorbed the shock and came to the realization that she would die soon, she called her nephew, who was a professor of theology. She wanted to discuss the spiritual side of dying. She told her nephew that something spiritual inside her "was pushing for the light of day." Here we see confirmation that the foundational spiritual interest in healthcare emanates from the inner life of the patient. Madlyn's initial conversation with her nephew signaled the emergence of spiritual interest and set the stage for each area of spiritual concern to make its entry. Madlyn used several meetings with her nephew to spell out her personal expectations and set her own course for engaging issues of spirituality as her death neared.

When Madlyn returned to her physician's office, she told him about that "something pushing for the light of day." She wanted to know if it had anything to do with the physical or psychological effect of her coming to terms with death. Her physician deflected the question with an almost embarrassed shrug. The resident who had accompanied Madlyn's attending physician looked a bit puzzled by the physician's noncommittal response but said nothing. When Madlyn and her daughter left the examining room, the resident followed them. She offered to discuss Madlyn's concerns about the link between spirituality and her clinical condition. Madlyn's daughter asked the young physician why she wanted to pursue the question. The resident explained that she had taken particular interest in the spirituality course offered in medical school, so she felt comfortable with the idea of integrating spirituality into her practice. Madlyn's office visit underscored how some physicians are uncomfortable with spiritual issues, while others have begun to understand that spiritual concerns are deeply relevant to their work and important to their patients. As noted earlier, physicians may not feel comfortable or especially competent in discussing spiritual concerns, but they do bear some responsibility for helping their patients as they inevitably confront spiritual concerns.

As Madlyn and her daughter sat down for a cup of coffee with the resident, they began to understand that her interest in Madlyn's spiritual needs was associated with her own spiritual interest. The young resident told Madlyn that she understood what Madlyn meant when she spoke about "something inside her pushing for the light of day." It led them into a discussion of meaning and how meaning—especially spiritual meaning—takes shape in life's situations where persons confront the unavoidable implications of loss, diminishment, and imminent death. Madlyn left the hospital that day with something she had been looking for, and the young resident had both given and received the gift of spiritual insight.

The remaining three areas of spiritual interest—spiritual interests of chaplains, organizations, and ethics—all came together in a perfect storm of conflicting moral values: Madlyn's request for physician-assisted suicide (PAS).

For several weeks, Madlyn had participated in a residential hospice care program at a leading Catholic hospital. Madlyn had followed the extended discussions of PAS during the Kevorkian trial. She had also read several articles discussing the philosophical and theological issues associated with PAS. In a conversation with her nephew, she explained that she wanted to request "an early exit." Her nephew was surprised, but he did not find her point of view out of character or simply the result of the increasing pain she had been experiencing. Typically, she wanted to control situations. She had a deep-seated need for dignity and decorum which, in her opinion, could not be guaranteed if she let nature take its course.

Madlyn's nephew asked the resident chaplain to join him and his aunt as they talked through the implications of her request. Father Kelly was an elderly Roman Catholic priest who served as the hospital's chief of chaplaincy services. He was widely respected for his ecumenical insight and pastoral competence.

Fr. Kelly said he knew that some Christian traditions did in fact approve of active voluntary euthanasia and that there were physicians who were willing to assist patients who chose to end their own lives. Fr. Kelly explained, though, that PAS was not condoned by the Roman Catholic Church and, therefore, would not be available to Madlyn in a Catholic institution. Fr. Kelly also told Madlyn that he could not personally support her decision, but he would assist her in making arrangements to be moved elsewhere if she insisted upon pursuing PAS. Madlyn ultimately decided against PAS, not because she thought it was immoral, but because she felt it would adversely affect her nephew and other members of the family. Fr. Kelly promised Madlyn that he and the clinical staff at the hospice would do everything in their power to protect her dignity as her death approached.

Madlyn's request for PAS triggered the spiritual interests of the chaplain and the Catholic healthcare organization that he represented. Although neither the chaplain nor the institution was willing to help Madlyn fulfill her wish, they did respond to her need in a positive, supportive manner. Most importantly, they promised to redouble their efforts to protect her interests and yet not compromise their own. Here the spiritual interests of ethics itself was clearly served. The spiritual bases of ethical decision making by Madlyn, Fr. Kelly, the resident, and the Catholic institution were all ultimately acknowledged and respected.

Viewing Madlyn's story from the perspective of spiritual interest highlights concretely how spirituality emerges within the context of palliative care, especially at the end of life. Circumstances surrounding end-of-life care are suffused with spiritual content. It need only be recognized, acknowledged, and thoughtfully integrated to do justice to the true nature of palliative care and the promise it holds.

⌐⌐ Conclusion

The partnership between spirituality and the way people approach end-of-life questions and make practical decisions about caring anchors the ethical obligation to acknowledge and act upon spiritual concerns. Palliative care at the end of life carries an implicit, and oftentimes explicit, promise to integrate spirituality into the care plan. How this promise is fulfilled depends upon the patient, the care team, and what is practically achievable in specific circumstances, but certain fundamental issues should be addressed whenever possible. Personal expectations should be surfaced, examined, and factored into any care plan. At the same time, the patient and each member of the care team has a responsibility to ensure the success of the chosen path by establishing a clear set of mutual expectations and committing to a consistent pattern of engagement around issues of spirituality.

To frustrate spiritual impulses in the face of death invites a disembodied form of ethics that skates upon the surface of human experience. A fully informed healthcare ethics will do justice to the whole person, body and soul, heart and conscience, mind and will. Spirituality, then, must be acknowledged, appreciated, and included. It may not be the law, but it is the ethically appropriate course of action.

3

Spiritual Care
Compassion and Service to Others

CHRISTINA M. PUCHALSKI

My patients, who face serious illness or dying, learn to value and live fully in the present moment. While driving to work one day, I spent the time worrying about job pressures, a proposal that was rejected, and whether I would get a promotion. I arrived in the clinic tense, filled with anticipatory anxiety about the day's stresses. My first patient, Rhonda, was in the midst of chemotherapy for recurrent ovarian cancer. As I entered her room, I saw a pale, thin woman, her balding head covered with a turban. Her radiant smile, however, lit up the room. Rhonda, in her upbeat tone, asked, "Dr. P, did you see the sunrise this morning? Wasn't it the most spectacular display of colors and brilliance?" In that moment, I realized that I had not even noticed if the sun was shining or not, in the midst of my own now-irrelevant preoccupations. In Rhonda's memory, I continue to cherish every sunrise and every sunset fully and to be present to the moment.

Christina M. Puchalski

Introduction

While on call one weekend, I was privileged to help two people face the dying of their loved ones. In one case, it was the son, John, who faced, for the first time, the terminal illness of his father, Miles. In another, it was my friend, Meredith, who decided to euthanize her cat Itny, her beloved companion of 20 years. No matter who is dying—a relative, a friend, or even a pet—the prospect of loss can paralyze, with fear, anxiety, and deep distress, not only the patient but also those who love the dying one. The basis of spiritual care is the connection we, the caregivers, form with the dying and their loved ones through the process of illness and death. People have used many words to describe that connection. Some are: love; compassion; the spirit; the essence of being; God; divine energy; and one-ness.

Which word is used is not as important as what happens between people and living beings. Spiritual care is the practice of compassionate presence. It is the ability to love another without judgment, prejudice, or a preconceived expectation of something in return. It is the act of sitting with the ill and dying in moments of deep and profound sadness and grief, sharing the pain with them. His Holiness, The Dalai Lama (1999), writes that compassion is "understood mainly in terms of empathy—our ability to enter into and, to some extent, share others' suffering."[1] It is the ability to be fully present—physically, emotionally, and spiritually—with a person in the midst of his or her pain.

Miles

Miles is 85 years old. He has had prostate cancer for 15 years; it has now metastisized to the bones. He lives in an independent-living facility and can no longer care for himself. I met Miles when I was on call for geriatrics at The George Washington University Hospital. It became apparent to me that Miles was at the end stage of his life and that hospice would be an appropriate referral. I spoke with Miles about this, but, because of his dementia, he was unable to fully comprehend the situation. Unfortunately, Miles had alienated all of his family members because he had abandoned his family when the children were all quite young. I was therefore unable to reach any next of kin to help with the decision process. Miles was deeply saddened by this. He was not able to verbalize a lot about his emotions, but he was able to tell me that he felt empty. Since Miles was unable to show much emotion, my only clue to Miles's pain was his deep, penetrating stare into empty space with wet, tear-covered eyes. I sat next to his bed in silence, sharing his pain and fighting my own anger at life's complications. One day he broke the silence by saying, as if understanding my own sadness for him, "Don't worry, my kids will show up before it is too late."

Miles was right. Fortunately, after 2 weeks in the hospital, his youngest son, John, showed up, without remorse, to care for his dad. In an emotion-filled conversation with me, John talked of his anger at the father who had abandoned him and forgiveness for the father who lay dying in the bed. Tears were shed, angry feelings rekindled, sadness for the lost years revealed as John shared story after story of his experiences with his father. There were gentle pauses of silence as we both reverenced the sacredness of what was shared. I offered a gentle but reassuring touch when appropriate and answered questions as they came up. Most of his questions were unanswerable: Why now? Why do we not have the time to get to know him better? These questions became the doors for more stories and more accounts of who Miles was and who he is. As John talked and I listened, his despair began to give way to hope. He began to see some value in his father's life. He began to see that perhaps this was, as I suggested to him, a new phase of discovery and reconciliation with his father. In the midst of darkness and confusion, John was able to find some light for himself to guide him over the next several months. At the end of our conversation John committed himself to being his father's durable proxy for healthcare and to help him on his final journey.

Itny

The next day my friend Meredith called to tell me that her beloved cat Itny was barely breathing. He had been gradually dying over the last year of old age and the infirmities that accompany aging. She and I discussed his end-of-life care during the year, avoiding aggressive, unnecessary treatment interventions. For many people, myself included, animals are spiritual beings and very important companions on life's journey. Itny was one such being, and his death was hard for my friend and for me. There had been similar calls over the last few months, but instinctively I knew this was the one. As much as I believe in natural deaths for all beings, I knew that hospice was not yet an alternative for animals and that the best way to alleviate Itny's pain was euthanasia. My friend Ed and I drove Meredith and Itny to the veterinary hospital to euthanize Itny. When we arrived, the entire staff responded with love and compassion. An aide helped us bypass the registration desk and gave us a room to spend the last moments with Itny in peace. Itny lay almost breathless in Meredith's arms, without any movement, until Ed led a prayer. As if sensing the spiritual energy, Itny, who was deaf, turned his head toward the prayer. The three of us honored the holiness of life and death in that moment. The veterinarian came in and quietly dimmed the lights as he, too, honored our grief. He gently explained the process, but only after listening to Itny's story: born in Sudan and adopted by Meredith when she was there on her tour of duty with USAID. We talked of his character, how he brought joy to Meredith's life, and how he will be missed. When it came time to let Itny die, the veterinarian became part of the circle of love that surrounded Meredith and Itny. His presence led the process but also reverenced the mystery that was occurring. He knew when to touch Meredith, offering support and understanding; he knew when to tell her it was time to let go. Itny's dying was grace-filled, loving, and holy.

Elements of Spiritual Care

Experiences such as the aforementioned describe moments of spiritual care. Some elements of spiritual care include:

- Compassionate presence and love for another
- Healing as partnership
- Reverence for mystery
- Self-care of the caregiver; having a spiritual practice

Compassionate Presence and Love for Another

Compassion comes from two Latin words: from the Latin *cum*, which means with, and *pati*, which means to suffer.[2] So the act of compassion is to suffer with another. The Dalai Lama talks of compassion as "defined in terms of a state of mind that is nonviolent, nonharming, and nonaggressive. It is a mental attitude based on the wish for others to be free of their suffering and is associated with a sense of commitment, responsibility, and respect towards the other."[3]

In being compassionate with others, we, in essence, love them unselfishly and without demand or expectation. We love them for who they are at their very core. Many of my patients suffer deeply, and often, in the midst of that suffering, they feel alone and unloved. By loving them, I see myself as holding them in a type of love that eventually allows them to heal and to see themselves as loving beings in the midst of their brokenness. It is then that they can see how others in their lives love them. They can then be open to healing the spiritual woundedness that they feel, by finding some hope in the midst of despair.[4] Compassionate care involves the caregiver's ability to share the patient's pain and suffering without becoming overwhelmed and disabled by that suffering. This love stems from an intimacy in which boundaries are respected for both the patient and the caregiver—an intimacy with formality. The caregiver feels the pain and suffering of the other by being empathic, is able to help the other by understanding this suffering at an intuitive and felt level, but then is able to detach enough to be able to help guide the patient toward a self-healing of that suffering.

Estelle

One weekend when I was on call, I was conducting rounds on patients in the hospital. One patient, Estelle, who had advanced breast cancer with metastases to the brain, was described to me by the residents as "not much to do; she is pretty out of it and won't talk." The sign-out from the previous attending noted that she was all squared away for discharge. I was running late that morning and wanted to be able to enjoy part of the weekend for myself. So, part of me felt relieved that this patient might not take quite as long as the others I had seen that morning. When I entered Estelle's room, I found a woman lying motionless in bed, propped up by several disorganized pillows, two of which were falling off the bed. Her left arm was dangling, and the sheets were tangled up around her legs. I felt a deep pang of sadness, an ache for the loneliness this woman must have felt. Some voice inside me told me to let go of my need to rush out and instead to just spend time with this woman. I approached her bed and asked her how she was. She opened her large brown eyes with a vacant stare. She did not answer. I asked if she was in pain; again, no response. I picked her head up gently in my arms and arranged the pillows to help prop her up more comfortably. I then straightened out her sheets. She had beads of sweat pouring down her forehead, which I wiped with a wet, cool cloth. She turned her eyes up toward me and smiled, which was then replaced by a deep, penetrating look of pain. Her eyes welled up with tears as she asked me what was happening to her. I asked her what she thought was happening. Estelle, with an astonishing clarity, said that she was dying, but that her daughter wanted her to fight. She said to me, "But I don't think I have any fight left in me."

She also talked of being scared of dying and facing something she knew nothing about. Was it going to be hard? How would her daughter handle it? She burst into tears as she told me of her deep love for her daughter and not wanting to leave her yet. There were no answers. I just held her and stroked her head as she cried. My own tears streamed down my cheeks as I felt her pain within me. After a few minutes, I heard her saying a prayer for her daughter. After she finished, I hugged her and suggested that I might speak to her daughter, and I encouraged Estelle to tell her daughter what she told me. She squeezed my hand, smiled, and went back to sleep. Later, talking to her daughter, I found out that the daughter felt the same emotions but was fearful to speak to her mother about dying. We both went to her mother's room and initiated a conversation. Once the subject of dying was brought out into the open, both mother and daughter talked, cried, and hugged. I left unobtrusively, knowing the connection had been made and that Estelle and her daughter would be all right. For me, the grace of that encounter was being open to the unplanned mystery of life and to intuition, or what I believe is the sacred within all of us. What if I had not listened to my inner voice and not taken the time to listen to Estelle? Estelle would die, her daughter would be sad, but I believe both were now healing. Healing is more than a physical cure or treatment. Healing is the restoration of wholeness and a sense of balance and meaning in one's life. Healing can occur at any time and often is unpredictable.

Compassion

In order to walk with someone in the midst of his or her suffering, one needs to be aware of that suffering. This means being aware of the suffering in our own lives. The more fully we understand suffering in all its forms, the deeper will be our ability to be compassionate. This requires an awareness of the brokenness and pain in our own lives. It is from that brokenness that we find the commonality with others. This is the basis of the human bond of connectedness that we establish with each other. Our own pain, fear, and woundedness allow us to trust another person.[5] Compassion is the foundation for the connection we form with another as two human beings. Desmond Tutu wrote, "My humanity is bound up with yours. For we can only be human together."[6]

As I helped Estelle and her daughter, my tears were for Estelle but also for myself. My mother is aging and struggling with illness. I know that one day she will die. The very thought of her death fills me with such a profound sense of anticipated loss and emptiness that I want to run from those thoughts and live in a fantasy in which she will continue forever. But by confronting that pain and fear inside me, I feel that I am better able to hold another's pain and suffering without running from it. In holding Estelle, I was also holding my mother, my father, Eric, and all my loved ones who suffer or who have died. By facing the pain and loss in my own life, I am able to experience another's pain and not run. I am able to love others from a place of healing within me, embracing the emotions without labeling them or avoiding them, and without being destroyed by them. That is what grace is for me; that is what the divine within me and within all of us is. That is the spiritual basis of the practice of medicine.

Compassion is also the foundation of all spiritual values. From it flows patience, perseverance, forgiveness, kindness, generosity, and tolerance. The fruits of being compassionate are joy, love, gratitude, peace, and meaning in life. We often run into ethical dilemmas in the clinical setting, but if there is genuine compassion for another, "ethical conduct is automatic."[7] In times when I have been rushed with patients, I found myself confused and unable to come to clarity about what should be done. But when approaching my patients with compassion and attention, I usually have been able to find the ethical and appropriate therapeutic recommendation or solution. Fundamental to this process is the partnership between the patient and me. That partnership is present in compassionate relationships, so that decisions are formed between two people wherein wishes and beliefs are respected and valued. If patients are to be treated as whole persons, they must be respected as whole persons—biological, psychological, social, and spiritual beings. It is critical that the patient's hopes, fears, dreams, anxieties, wishes, and values be considered before a course of treatment is recommended.[8]

When we are genuinely compassionate, or as the Dalai Lama, from the Buddhist tradition, writes, "When we begin to perfect our compassion,"[9] we have no self-interests or hidden agendas. The other person's appearance, behavior, or position does not affect our response to him or her. In the Greek, this type of love is called *agapē*, which is understood as unselfish love of one person for another. Stephen Post has written that the "essence of love is to affectively affirm as well as to unselfishly delight in the well-being of others, and to engage in acts of care and service on their behalf; unlimited love extends this love to all others without exception, in an enduring and constant way."[10] In the Christian tradition, it is the love of a Christian for other persons, thus corresponding to the love of God for humankind.[11]

When treating patients as whole beings and with compassion, medicine then becomes a spiritual practice. As Post writes:

> Widely considered the highest form of virtue, unlimited love is often deemed a Creative Presence underlying and integral to all of reality: participation in unlimited love constitutes the fullest experience of spirituality.[12]

Thus, in loving our patients, we are engaged in spiritual work, for compassion is the foundation of the spiritual care we give to patients and their loved ones. The basic motivation for care of another is derived from love of and benefit to another, rather than self-aggrandizement or benefit to oneself. The caregiver is dedicated to understanding what is causing the suffering of the other and then works with the patient in helping him or her overcome both the suffering and the causes of that suffering, if possible. The relationship between physician or other healthcare provider and patient becomes a healing partnership rather than a business relationship.

Healing as Partnership

Spiritual care, then, involves a partnership between two people. To understand spiritual care, it is helpful to define what spirituality is. One definition developed by a consensus group of medical school educators and clinicians with the Association of American Medical Colleges (AAMC) is:

> Spirituality is recognized as a factor that contributes to health in many persons. The concept of spirituality is found in all cultures and societies. It is expressed in an individual's search for ultimate meaning through participation in religion and/or belief in God, family, naturalism, rationalism, humanism and the arts. All of these factors can influence how patients and healthcare professionals perceive health and illness and how they interact with one another.[13]

This definition is important in that it defines spirituality as related to health, not just illness. The definition is intentionally broad. How people find meaning in their lives varies, and it is important to be open to all sources of meaning and purpose in a person's life. In this definition of spirituality, a critical element has to do not only with the patient's spirituality but also with spirituality as the substance that bonds the physician and patient, as well as the physician and other professional caregivers. It is from this spiritual base that the healing partnership forms. That partnership is the basis for how people behave in the relationship.

Timothy E. Quill (2001) defines the key elements of medical partnership as:[14]

- Sharing power and expertise
- Mutually influencing and understanding one another
- Clarifying commonness and difference
- Negotiating differences
- Ultimately patient centered

Underlying all these elements are the basic principles of respect, listening to another, and being fully and compassionately present to the other person. One can attempt to implement the elements described above, but, without the love and commitment to serve, the partnership will not exist. To be a true partner in a medical relationship, one needs to see oneself as the server of the patient. Most physicians go into medicine to serve patients. Most physicians want to have meaningful relationships with their patients. Many physicians find their own sense of meaning and purpose from serving others. But the training of physicians, as well as the current healthcare system's business focus, mitigates against a partnership model. Much of medical training is focused on curing and fixing problems. The approach is to diagnose correctly, find the appropriate therapeutic intervention, and carry it out with the aim of a cure. While this is an excellent goal, in many cases problems cannot be cured. In fact, most people deal with chronic, sometimes lifelong problems, be they stress or chronic illnesses such as diabetes, hypertension, cancer, or depression. There may not be a cure, but there is always an opportunity for healing. Even though a person may not receive curative therapy, he or she can still find meaning and purpose in life. This search for meaning and purpose is what spirituality is about.

Healing occurs in a person's spirit. In end-of-life care, the focus is mostly on healing, which is why, particularly in end-of-life care, spiritual care is so important. Therefore, the spiritual basis of our work as physicians and the spiritual aspects of the compassionate partnership are what enable the patient to heal and to find hope in the midst of despair. Healing—the restoration of wholeness, hope, and meaning—occurs in the framework of the physician-patient relationship. In that moment of healing, the physician and patient share a profound and deep connection in a process that is sacred, holy, and filled with mystery.

Emphasis on Service in Partnership

Dr. Rachel Naomi Remen writes:

> Helping, fixing and serving represent three different ways of seeing life. When you help, you see life as weak. When you fix, you see life as broken. When you serve, you see life as whole. Fixing and helping may be the work of the ego, and service the work of the soul.[15]

The emphasis in medical education should be on service. A partnership is composed of two people who work together for a purpose. In the medical partnership, the purpose is the identification of, and attempt to relieve, the suffering of another. The patient benefits because he or she receives quality compassionate care and an opportunity for cure (if possible) and healing at all stages of the illness. The physician or other caregiver has the opportunity to have a meaningful relationship with the patient, to find meaning from a life of service to another. The Dalai Lama (1998) writes of a "feeling of freshness rather than dullness" that occurs when one feels that connectedness with another.[16] The physician may have the opportunity of finding joy in his or her work because of the genuineness of his or her commitment to the well-being of the patient and love of that patient. In my own practice, I have learned so much about life and death from my patients. They are my true teachers, more so than the books I read. Sally Leighton (1996) writes the following after a difficult experience with a physician and her dying aunt: "The physician will do better to tune in carefully on what may be transpiring spiritually both in order to comfort the dying and to broaden his or her own understanding of life at its ending."[17]

My very first patient in medical school was a young woman named Sheila who had sickle-cell disease. Sheila had a twin sister with the same illness who had just died. I met Sheila in the emergency room as she was bargaining with me about the dose and type of her pain medication. It became very clear to me that pain medications were the focus of her life and that she was the one calling the shots. As a new medical student, I struggled with her to gain some control over the situation and to help her decrease the narcotic use and find some other ways of dealing with the pain. What I did not realize was that my focus was totally wrong. I did not listen to Sheila and to her pain. Over the next 2 years, I learned that she feared the same fate her sister had: pain, crisis, and then death, with little else in between. As a resident and then attending physician, I continued to care for her. We started talking about hobbies, parents, faith, and love. Sheila cried as she told me she had nothing in her life but her illness.

Over the next few years we worked together to find another focus for her life. She began to get more involved with her church and joined some social groups in which she made friends. She started having parties and having fun. As her focus in life shifted solely from her illness to other things, so did her focus on narcotic use. She was able to find a regimen that worked for her and allowed her to function. Few changes were made in dosage, and she remained relatively pain free. Her other sister had a young daughter with whom Sheila became close. It became Sheila's dream to take her niece to Disney World. By this time, Sheila was wheelchair bound. Her church group helped her find a group of young people with chronic illnesses with whom to go to Disney World. She took her niece, had a wonderful time, and brought back pictures to share with me. She told me she never imagined her life could be so full and rewarding.

Three years later, Sheila was severely anemic and had liver failure from the numerous transfusions she received. After many discussions, she decided to forgo more treatment and tests. She felt at peace with her life, with God, her family, and her relationships. She came regularly to my office; no tests were done—I did not even use my stethoscope. We just sat and talked about her life, her relationships, God, her mother, and her dying. We laughed and cried, sharing the highlights of her life and our work together. During her last office visit, as we shared our usual hug, she asked me if I would go to her funeral. I cried, held her, and told her I would be there. Three weeks later, I visited her at her home. She was very weak but comfortable. I thanked Sheila for being in my life and for the privilege of being able to care for her. She smiled, told me she was at peace, and then, with her impish grin, she said that she did not even need any pain medication, that she was finally healed. I kissed her on her forehead and she squeezed my hand as we said our final good-byes. The next day, her mother called me and told me Sheila had asked to be carried to her mother's bed. She died peacefully in her mother's arms. I went to Sheila's funeral. There, I joined her family in our expressions of joy and sadness. She is still with me, in my heart, to this day. Relationships do not die but continue to live on within us and in all we do. I believe that the relationship I shared with Sheila is as important, if not more important, than all the tests and technical handling of her illness. Out of that relationship blossomed the opportunity for healing. Interestingly, the healing, as is the partnership, is a shared healing.

Crisis in Medicine: Anti-Partnership

The medical system is in a crisis as we enter this new millennium. Medicine has gradually become a business, due to the high cost of healthcare, malpractice insurance, and decreasing government support of programs such as Medicare. As a result, physicians are seeing patients in rushed and inefficient environments. There is no value placed on the doctor-patient relationship. The value is rather on the revenue that is generated. This mitigates against a partnership model, which is so important for good patient care. There are studies that document the importance of the doctor-patient relationship.[18] Dr. Francis Peabody wrote in his 1927 medical classic, *The Care of The Patient*, "One of the essential qualities of the clinician is interest in humanity, for the secret care of the patient is in caring for the patient."[19] This relationship can have a positive impact on healthcare outcomes, compliance, and patient satisfaction.[20] Vaillot (1970) suggests that it is the relationship between the caregiver and the patient that sustains the presence of hope.[21] Helping dying patients find hope is central to their healing process and to their finding meaning in the midst of their suffering. It is critical that as we change our evolving healthcare system, we create one that is value- and relationship-centered. It is then that we will be able to provide the best medical and spiritual care possible.

Reverence for Mystery

Life presents us with mystery all the time. Rabbi Lawrence Kushner (1994) writes, "The first mystery is simply that there is a mystery. A mystery that can never be explained or understood. Only encountered from time to time."[22] The mystery that confronts us in situations of death and illness has to do with the lack of control that we ultimately have in our lives. Not all illnesses and life conditions are curable and fixable. One reason may be that we need more research in order that answers may be found. But if history has any lessons for us, even with technological advances, death and suffering cannot be avoided. In spite of all the advances of the last half-century, people still die, people still suffer. There are questions that we cannot answer. So often my dying patient will ask, "Why is this happening to me?" My residents or medical students usually try to answer with a biological response such as, "You have a genetic predisposition for this." But this question is not about answers. It is a plea for an opportunity to be heard about the deep pain and suffering that the patient is experiencing.

There simply are no answers to these types of questions. Part of spiritual care is recognizing when to simply sit in silence as the person grapples with his or her own quest for meaning. Honoring the mystery is sitting in silence, being present to another's as well as our own grief and sadness while surrounded by unanswerable questions. Life and death become more precious when we unlearn our need to fix and control and simply learn to be present to another, to ourselves, and to the mystery.

One of the greatest stressors around illness and dying, for both patient and caregivers, is probably created by the ambiguity regarding the patient's health, including the prognosis, the capacity of the family to provide support and care, and financial concerns.[23] There is a tremendous amount of uncertainty with any illness and in life in general. While science and medicine may have some answers to many of the physical aspects of disease and illness, there are so many aspects of being ill for which there are no answers. Some of the questions patients, professionals, and family caregivers ask are:

- Who am I in the midst of the stress of my or my loved one's illness?
- Why am I suffering, or why is he or she suffering?
- Why do I feel angry, sad, and afraid?
- What is the meaning and purpose of my life in the midst of this experience and in the midst of this stress?
- Why would God do this to me?
- Why is this happening?
- Why can't this illness be cured?
- How long can I or my loved one function like this?
- When will my loved one or I die, and how?
- Why can't I do and be everything to another person? Why can't I be who I used to be?
- How will I cope with my own or his or her death?

These questions of uncertainty, limitations, meaning, and purpose are essentially existential or spiritual questions. Burton (1998) writes, "Spirituality is the expression of self-in-relation, incorporating both material and non-material realities, and reflecting the tension between the possibilities and limitations of human existence in history."[24] Henry and Henry (1999) suggest that people need mystery. They write, "If there is no wonder there is no holy."[25] Uncertainty may trigger the spiritual questions that lead to an awareness of mystery. It is then that the struggle of the spiritual journey may lead to an honoring or acceptance of the mystery.

Part of the journey in living and dying is spiritual, and people may have spiritual experiences for which there are no answers. There are many claims of miraculous recoveries, a few of which I have witnessed in my professional life. At this time in medicine, however, there are no scientific explanations for these types of recoveries. Patients may talk about spiritual or mystical experiences that may manifest as visions, feeling God's or a deceased loved one's presence, altered states of consciousness, locutions, or sensory experiences (e.g., unusual smells, sights, and sounds). From the clinical standpoint, there is a debate as to the difference between spiritual experiences and psychopathology. Many patients close to death often talk of seeing loved ones or angels in the room. Some physicians will medicate patients if these experiences cause the patients distress or agitation. This assumes that spiritual experiences are comforting versus psychopathological, which could cause agitation. Theologians would argue that, in fact, not all spiritual experiences are comforting and that medicating people in the midst of a spiritual experience might be in conflict with the patient's beliefs and religious tradition.

There are no clear-cut answers to these questions. Spiritual or mystical experiences may be part of a person's life, but those experiences have nothing to do with how well people communicate, either with God or with the spiritual practices inherent in religions, such as prayer or virtue. Neurotheologians suggest that we may be "wired for God"[26] or that evolution has programmed the brain to find pleasure in transcending the self. St. Teresa of Avila and other mystics regarded spiritual or mystical experiences as special gifts of God, but not essential to spiritual growth.

Science can offer many answers, but not all of them. In the realm of the spiritual, it would be reductionistic to attempt to explain God's existence or spiritual grace in scientific terms. Thus, in the clinical setting it is important to recognize the limits of science and to relinquish the need for reductionistic explanatory models for spiritual beliefs and experiences. Much of what happens to our patients may have no explanations. Illness causes us to ask questions that are deeply spiritual and scientifically unanswerable: Who am I? Why am I suffering? What is the meaning of my illness and suffering? Illness, in and of itself, is a spiritual journey that may include emptiness, joy, despair, hope, and mystical experiences. As physicians and caregivers, our job is to support our patients as they go through this journey.

Dying is a process that no one can control. When physicians give an estimate of how long a person has to live, they are simply just that—estimates. I know of many patients who have outlived both their physicians' predictions and the physicians themselves. And I know of other patients who die far ahead of the predictions. We all know of the parent who lies on his or her deathbed, waiting for the child to come, and then dies within minutes of the child's arrival. The moment of death, either of a family, friend, or even a pet, is cloaked in the beauty of mystery and awe.

Dying is a process, and we are participants in that process, whether as the dying patient or the loved one or the caregiver. Whatever our role, we are simply companions to the dying on their journey. Spiritual care involves walking with another on this journey, not trying to fix or change it but simply being there, experiencing all that process has to offer. For the professional caregivers this may be hard, because of our need to fix and improve. For the family member or friend, it may be sad to see a limited journey of togetherness. The way to be a companion is not an easy way. But by loving the patient in an altruistic sense, there can be a trust that the process has a meaning and purpose that is out of any of our control, and that the meaning and purpose has inherent value in a spiritual sense.

Self Care of the Caregiver

The process of caring for another who is suffering, and of being compassionate, means opening oneself up to another's suffering. In order to do this, it is critical that one is first honest with oneself about his or her own experience with suffering, as well as an awareness of our own mortality. There are training programs for residents[27] that include experiential classes, which enable them to encounter their own issues about their mortality, their suffering, and grief. Once we face our own issues we can then recognize and help another with theirs. So in spiritual care, a prerequisite is to reflect on what suffering and loss you have encountered in your life and how you handled it; to recognize that you, too, will die, and what that means to you; and to ponder what values you have in your life that give you meaning.

In being compassionate, as previously described, you allow the person's suffering to touch you and affect you but not debilitate you. What allows you to do this is the intent with which you open yourself up to another's suffering. As a caregiver you love another out of the intent to serve and do something for the higher good of another person. The compassionate partnership with the patient results in a sense of connection and commitment to the good of another. The positive aspect of service to another overrides the negative experience of suffering. The spiritual nature of the work and the commitment that comes from that gives one the strength to be able to support another's pain. Many physicians talk of being called to the profession of medicine, as I very much feel in my own life. That calling is spiritual, and that gives me the drive to transcend the stresses of my work. For me, as a Catholic and a Carmelite, my medical practice is also my vocation, my spiritual practice. Many physicians and other healthcare providers find meaning in their work in the context of their spiritual beliefs and values. In the Jewish tradition, for example, it is written in the Talmud, "Who hath compassion for others receives compassion from Heaven."[28]

The pain and suffering my patients and their families face become part of me as I work with them. But if I had no place to put that pain, I would become immobilized and unable to function. I spend time at the end of the day reflecting on the day and on what my patients shared with me. Often I am deeply moved by what I experienced earlier. Sometimes I weep for my patients and for myself; sometimes I experience a profound joy. I am not afraid of crying as I rekindle the emotions I experienced with my patients and their families. Expressions of sadness and joy, however, must be followed by a letting go and acceptance of the impermanence of emotions and situations. In my belief system, I know that there is little I am in control of. I may be able to ease my patients' suffering to a degree or to help control physical symptoms and make good diagnostic and therapeutic decisions. But the ultimate existence of suffering and dying is out of my control. How patients handle their illness and their dying is their decision, not mine. I am an active partner in the process, but the ultimate experience belongs to the patient. So, at the end of the day, I thank God for giving me the skills, knowledge, and ability to serve others; I place my patients and their families in God's hands and ask for his help for the next day. The prayer that most helps me is the Serenity Prayer:

The Serenity Prayer

God grant me the Serenity to accept the things I cannot change;
the Courage to change the things I can; and
the Wisdom to know the difference.[29]

Another prerequisite for doing spiritual care is having a spiritual practice. For the religious physician or healthcare provider, it might be a practice in a tradition such as prayer or service attendance. For others, their practice might be meditation, yoga, rituals, relationship with others or the divine, or art and music. A spiritual practice can help one encounter the transcendent and realize a higher value or meaning in life and enable one to be truly compassionate to another. Most mystics, such as St. Teresa of Avila, see spiritual practices as "leading them beyond themselves to the practice of charity and love of neighbor."[30] In addition to medicine being my practice, I also meditate and spend quiet time by my altar in my room. On the altar I have placed symbols that help me focus on spiritual issues I am dealing with. My father, a very spiritual person, and I were always drawn to stones, and ever since I was a child, we collected stones on the beach. Then he would tell me a story that touched on a spiritual theme. He makes beautiful stone sculptures, which I use on my altar. They speak to me of the stories my father and I shared and the lessons learned from him, as well as my patients, about God, mystery, hope, living, and dying.

My relationships with my family and friends, my cats, and my colleagues are also critical to self-care. Talking with others about my experience (in a confidential manner, to protect the identities and details of my patients' lives) makes an enormous difference in how I handle my stress. Having someone offer a different point of view, an alternative explanatory model, or just a hug and a welcoming shoulder for tears make me aware of how connected we all are to each other. Often, one can feel so alone in the midst of professional stress. My loved ones remind me that I am not so different from the rest of the world and not so alone in my experience. An affectionate head butt from my cat Zoey makes me laugh and feel warm and loved. Max, my other cat, insists on my putting aside my work and playing with him, which reminds me of the spiritual power of play. The connection with my friends, family, and cats is a healing and supportive one.

It is essential that when we care for others, we also care for ourselves. So in addition to a spiritual practice, exercise, proper nutrition, and sleep are critical. It is also important to have a support system for caregivers. Working with the dying can be enriching, and that often gives meaning to our lives. But it can be draining as well. It is important to have people with whom you, as the caregiver, can share your feelings—grief as well as joy and awe.

For some people, caring for others who are suffering is too difficult. Some people avoid others' suffering. Part of the reason is that it is painful and may be too hard to handle. Another reason is that another person's wounds spark in us the recognition of our own wounds. It is just as critical to address the pains and suffering of the healer as that of the patient.[31] By facing our own suffering, insecurity, loss, and grief, we are more able to support our patients in their suffering and grief. In this process we are able to gain an insight into ourselves and into our inner spiritual lives and consequently open ourselves to the opportunity for our own healing. An awareness of our own pain, suffering, and loneliness helps us better understand the suffering of another. In the process of reaching out to another in need, we form a connection that heals the loneliness both people feel in the midst of their individual pain.

When you extend yourself so that you feel another's pain, you begin to feel a sense of responsibility to the other and a connection to that person. That level of responsibility may be too much for some people. This is why it is so critical to be honest with yourself about your ability to provide care to another. At different times in all of our lives, it may be harder to give of oneself, even for the most compassionate caregiver. It is important that we take the appropriate breaks and time away from work in order to be able to be more present and give more fully when we do work with patients who are seriously ill and dying.

Serving others has many magical moments of blessings and joy, as well as sadness. Life becomes ever more full and rich when we allow those moments into our lives, when we allow ourselves to connect with others. Out of these magical moments, healing becomes possible. In the end, it is the healing of not just our patients but of ourselves as well.

Spiritual care has many aspects, some more easily practiced than others. In its most esoteric form it is relational, immeasurable, and unique, often difficult to describe. I am frequently asked if one can teach these principles—aren't they just inherent to certain personality types? Yes, these principles can be taught and learned. There is no personality type that is a prerequisite for providing spiritual care. All of us are capable of serving and of giving to another. But there are certain skills that are necessary in order to talk with patients about spiritual issues, in order to be present to patients in a compassionate way, in order to develop a spiritual care plan, and in order to interact with others on the interdisciplinary healthcare team. In Chapter 15, we will look at some practical tools to use in our care of our patients.

4

Spiritual Stages of Dying

CHRISTINA M. PUCHALSKI

The spiritual journey can be challenging and difficult. From my patients, I have learned to be open to questions, struggles, and challenges and to continually deepen my relationship with God. In the very first visit I had with Louis, my patient, he shared his struggles with his faith. He wanted to find something deeper and more meaningful beyond "simply going to Mass." I referred him to a spiritual director who helped Louis look deeper into his relationship with God. Over the next ten years, in the midst of his struggles with cancer, Louis worked on his relationship with God—intensely, honestly, and with commitment. He faced doubt, anger, and uncertainty with grace and steadfastedness. While he was dying, he shared his trepidation about the unknown. In the midst of tears and sadness, he exclaimed that he was "chicken about this whole process . . . but I know God is there and I am not alone." Now I try not to run from questions or discomfort in my own spiritual life but face uncertainty and struggle with the grace I saw in Lou.

Christina M. Puchalski

Spirituality

Spirituality, as seen from the research, has the potential to impact health outcomes, particularly regarding the way patients cope with illness and their dying. It also has implications for how loved ones cope with the stress and grief of a loved one's dying and death. But spirituality is more than just a tool. People find meaning in their lives through their spirituality; they connect to others, to a transcendent, or to God/Divine through their spiritual lives; they experience the awe of a brilliant sunset through their spirituality; and, they come alive from listening to a Bach cantata or a Mozart symphony through their spiritual selves. Just as one's spirituality can affect the experience of people, so also can nature, music, art, and illness affect our spirituality.

This chapter will discuss some ways people understand spirituality, what the spiritual stages of dying are, the spiritual issues people face in chronic and serious illness, and, finally, practical ways of dealing with these issues.

St. John of the Cross (1542-1591) writes of spirituality as being in its essence relational.[1] It is the sixth sense we use to fully understand and love God or the transcendent, to love another person or animal, to respect and honor nature, and to perceive the meaning of art and music beyond their color and sound. God, or the transcendent, affects our spirituality if we are open to him or to the presence of the transcendent. People and animals, as spiritual beings, can help us recognize the holy and divine in our lives.

Illness or loss challenges us to ask questions about the essence of who we are, why we are alive, and why we eventually die.[2] A relatively stress-free and unchallenged life can make us complacent and comfortable in our present situations. There may be no reason to change or grow if all is smooth and uncomplicated. A diagnosis of cancer, diabetes, stroke, or any illness that affects our uncomplicated routine; the death of a loved one; a broken relationship; an act of terrorism or war—all of these can rip us from our cocoons and force us to grow and to take steps in directions we may not want to take. It can force us to look at our lives and ourselves in a brutally honest and self-revelatory way: Is this the person I want to be? What do I want to accomplish before I die? Is my work meaningful, or "just a job?" Are my relationships honest and loving? Where is God or the transcendent in my life? Am I living in a way congruent with my values? Am I able to love? Who am I at my deepest core? Why is this happening now in my life? These are inherently spiritual questions, and the triggering event may find us at a major crossroads in our lives. We can face the questions and struggle with the suffering to find answers for ourselves, or we can turn away from the discomfort and struggle to create another, familiar cocoon.

Spiritual Growth

The process of spiritual growth takes time, support from others (including professionals), guidance, and self-reflection. Some people turn to their family's religious or spiritual roots for answers. Others explore new directions of questioning and seeking. In the end, our greatest task is to face ourselves in stark nakedness, stripped of all the prejudices, patterns, dependencies on others, social status, job title, and expectations and goals we may have had. Ultimate self-reflection occurs in the solitariness of our being. Being alone is difficult for many. In fact, people may sit in solitude, but when given the option to connect to others, they do so to ease the experience of solitariness. Dying accelerates these challenges because of the realization that dying is a journey we ultimately face alone and one that we cannot run from. In dying, the comfort of presence from others, while helpful, does not help one avoid the inevitable: a confrontation of self in naked isolation.

Living and dying are ultimately spiritual beyond all else. Dying may be the ultimate spiritual challenge we face, because death is an unknown. While all of us have encountered uncertainty in everyday experiences—predicting outcomes of relationships, job interviews, and so forth—there are no easy answers or concrete solutions to the process of dying or of life after death. The mystery surrounding life and death can frighten us because certitude may be the lifeline to which we think we need to cling. Spiritual journeys can be shaped and challenged by the facing of uncertainty and mystery. Previous beliefs, such as the universality of God's power, the belief that prayer brings cures, that one's community can help overcome all suffering, or that science has all the answers, might not be of help in the face of inevitable death. Some of my patients cry out about the injustice of an all-powerful, good God allowing suffering, a distant, uncaring God not answering a prayer, or a deceptive medical treatment that held promises of a cure, yet failed. People may give up entirely on their beliefs or may be spurred to evaluate their beliefs on a deeper level.

People may integrate religious dogma and beliefs as less definable, spiritual beliefs. Emily Chandler distinguishes spiritual journeys from religious beliefs, in that spiritual journeys "involve us in the mystery of experiencing the holy, the mysterious."[3] Is it possible to have meaning and purpose, an implied knowledge of self, in the midst of mystery and unknowing? Reinhold Niebuhr, a twentieth-century philosopher, insisted that mystery and meaning are interwoven.[4] While we may not have the full meaning of mystery, mystery itself does not leave us without meaning. Meaning can be found in many places—in relationships, in God, in the illness itself, in service to others, and in love. But even these meanings are surrounded by mystery. As Niebuhr wrote:

> Thus wisdom about our destiny is dependent upon a humble recognition of the limits of our knowledge and our power. Our most reliable understanding is the fruit of "grace" in which faith completes our ignorance without pretending to possess its certainties as knowledge.[5]

As one who cares for the chronically ill and dying, I have shared parts of others' challenges and spiritual journeys and witnessed tremendous sadness as well as joy. It is almost as if the journey is like a rainbow. Occasionally, the beautiful spectrum of colors is visible in its perfect arches. Sometimes only parts of the colors are seen, and often it is completely obliterated by rain. But if you keep following the rainbow, having faith that it is there, you will come to a profound joy and understanding of the meaning of life. People who have struggled with suffering and have managed to find some meaning for themselves in the midst of that suffering may not always be joyous and blissful, but they are often at peace and content with their lives and with themselves. They see themselves, others, life, and the transcendence of God with clarity, honesty, and love.

Hope

Spirituality, in the face of isolation and suffering, as discussed in Chapter 1, offers people a language of hope. Hope, in the face of an initial serious diagnosis, a loss or devastation, is usually for a cure or a resolution of a difficult situation. But as illness becomes incurable or unresolvable, hope may give way to despair. Moving from the darkness of despair to the light of another kind of hope is often a painful task. People may isolate, lash out in anger, or become numb. Moving through these emotions to a different source of hope heals people on a spiritual level. Hence, incurable does not mean unhealable. This different source of hope leads to less tangible but perhaps more significant goals. For example, it may be the hope to find peace, finish important goals, reconcile with others or God, and, in the end, hope for a peaceful dying and death. Religions offer people an organized and common set of beliefs and ways to find, within their different traditions, this hope in the midst of despair. Christians look to the Lord for hope: "The toughest thing to do is to search for the Lord in faith and repeat Peter's words—'Lord, it is good for us to be here'—with the hope that the Lord will bring light into our darkness."[6] For the Hindu, acceptance of suffering and death is seen as just retribution for past karma, and the hope is in making spiritual progress through this experience of suffering.[7] Many religions speak of the hope that life extends beyond the grave. In Judaism, for example, continued survival through one's family is the hope of many patients who are dying.[8]

For the dying person, hope is integral to living with dying. The spiritual aspects of hope help the dying and chronically ill person make his or her life meaningful. As caregivers we engage in numerous discussions about outcomes, percentage likelihood of surviving 5 years with a particular cancer, and so on. Physicians often struggle with how to deliver these types of difficult news to a patient. "Mrs. Smith, you have a 20 percent chance of being alive in 2 years without chemotherapy and a 40 percent chance of being alive in 5 years with chemotherapy." Mrs. Smith then becomes filled with anxiety and despair as she faces the real message, which is that she will die from the illness. With only those words spoken, patients can feel empty and desperate, without any sense of hope. We need to temper the medical information with a message of hope. Often the conversations are so technical that hope gets washed away with statistics. By listening to our patients' emotional and spiritual responses to each bit of medical information, one can get clues as to how to convey more information in language that does not obliterate hope. One can convey hope without being dishonest about outcome.

The technical data that are often conveyed are based on population studies but do not take into account an individual's resources, such as beliefs, support systems, and will to live. Rhonda, one of my patients who lectured to my students, said that she was a "statistic of one" and that her outcome would not reflect the data but would reflect her beliefs, her relationships, and who she was. So, the conversation with Mrs. Smith might go as follows: "Mrs. Smith, your cancer has progressed, and it is quite serious. How do you feel about what I have said?" Then after listening and experiencing her emotions and spirit, the physician might recommend a particular chemotherapy and describe the statistics but add that there are many factors that statistics don't take into account; for example, Mrs. Smith's strong spiritual resources and the support of family and friends. Perhaps just the power of presence and caring can convey to Mrs. Smith that her physician will be there for her during this time and help her in the journey with her cancer. That presence and relationship can be the trigger to help Mrs. Smith tap into her own sense of hope.

We as caregivers can help our patients and loved ones find hope in the midst of pain, suffering, and despair. Doka challenges the caregiver when he suggests that we do the spiritual work through our spiritual selves: "A spiritual person inspires hope more by who he or she is than by what he or she does. To be effective, hope—no matter how transient—must be realistic."[9] Physicians often say that all technical information must be completely realistic, even if the data is devastating. But what is more realistic—statistics or the actual presence of the physician for the patient? I cannot write a prescription for my patients that can be filled and provide an instant hope for her or him. But by loving them and being a partner with them on their journey, I can help my patients find hope for themselves. Thus, in our caring for others, we may not be able to give that person hope, for hope is something each person must find for her or himself. But we can be catalysts for that person, not through what we do for them but by our interactions and who we are for our patients and loved ones. In essence, we can be beacons of hope by being present and by loving one another.

Stages of Dying

Elizabeth Kubler-Ross is a physician who, in the 1960s, began to look at the process of dying and how people cope with dying. Her work was based on interviews with dying patients. Based on these interviews, she developed the five stages of dying: denial, anger, bargaining, depression, and acceptance.[10] While these stages are often described as sequential, they are in fact dynamic stages that people can experience throughout their journey. Patients do not automatically become peaceful once acceptance is attained. There can be many moments of denial and anger, even after some acceptance has been experienced. Getting through these stages is an emotional and spiritual process.

Dowling Singh describes the psychospiritual stages of dying as a process of moving from chaos to surrender to eventual transcendence.[11] Chaos is the initial encounter with illness and the prospect of dying. Surrender is a moment of awareness when one opens to one's deeper being, and transcendence is seen as going deeper into spiritual integration. As with Kubler-Ross's stages, one moves between these phases in a dynamic and fluid way. We may, in all of our lives, move toward a spiritual integration, which in its fullest, clearest form may be experienced at or near death.

Contemplation: Glimpses of the Divine

Many of the great mystics write of glimpses of the Divine while in deep contemplation. Meister Eckhart notes that "the great need of man is that his soul be unified with God; for this, a knowledge of God and his relation to the world, a knowledge of the soul and the way which it must go, are necessary."[12] The encounter with God or the Divine in contemplation gives one deeper knowledge and understanding of who God or the Divine is. St. John of the Cross writes, "Contemplation, consequently, by which the intellect has a higher knowledge of God, is called Mystical Theology, meaning the secret wisdom of God."[13]

One can achieve contemplation through prayer and meditation. Meditation involves many stages, contemplation being the highest but not consistently attainable stage. St. Teresa of Avila, a sixteenth-century mystic, uses the word *meditation* as a category of prayer. Prayer is the door to relationship with the Divine. Therefore, meditation as prayer leads up to an experience of contemplation.[14] St. John of the Cross taught friars, nuns, and lay Carmelites to "seek in reading and you will find in meditation; knock in prayer and it will be opened to you in contemplation."[15] Prayer and meditation are the experiences of being in relationship with God or the Divine. At times, during prayer and meditation, one can experience union and oneness with God the Divine. For me, the experience of God also occurs in relationship with others. Thus, encounters with my patients become prayers as well. The relationship is that of the Divine in each of us connecting as one. Therein lies the basis for spirituality as the foundation of medicine.

St. Teresa of Avila explains the process of meditation and prayer through the use of the metaphor of dwelling places in a castle as the places where one's spiritual relationship with the Divine is recognized and developed. The first three places are achievable through the human effort of prayer, meditation, and reading. The last four deal with the mystical elements of one's spiritual life, which one can call contemplation. She writes that the "door to the castle is prayer and reflection."[16] Contemplation is an awareness of and union with God's or the Divine's presence, which at times overflows into all of one's senses. St.Teresa and St. John caution us, however, that these experiences may be fleeting and not lasting. Nor are they necessarily blissful experiences. Contemplation and even spiritual integration can occur in darkness as well. St. John of the Cross expresses this journey beautifully in his poem, "The Dark Night of the Soul."[17]

The Dark Night of the Soul

1. One dark night,
    fired with love's urgent longings
    —ah, the sheer grace!—
    I went out unseen,
    my house being now all stilled.

2. In darkness, and secure,
    by the secret ladder, disguised,
    —ah, the sheer grace!—
    in darkness and concealment,
    my house being now all stilled.

3. On that glad night,
    in secret, for no one saw me,
    nor did I look at anything,
    with no other light or guide
    than the one that burned in my heart.

4. This guided me
    more surely than the light of noon
    to where he was awaiting me
    —him I knew so well—
    there in a place where no one appeared.

5. O guiding night!
    O night more lovely than the dawn!
    O night that has united
    the Lover with his beloved,
    transforming the beloved in her Lover.

6. Upon my flowering breast
    which I kept wholly for him alone,
    there he lay sleeping,
    and I caressing him
    there in a breeze from the fanning cedars.

7. When the breeze blew from the turret,
   as I parted his hair,
   it wounded my neck
   with its gentle hand,
   suspending all my senses.

8. I abandoned and forgot myself,
   laying my face on my Beloved;
   all things ceased; I went out from myself,
   leaving my cares
   forgotten among the lilies.

This poem describes one's spiritual journey, which ultimately leads to the perfect union with God or the Divine through love, as it is attainable in this life. A key element of the spiritual journey and union with God is love. Love of God enables us to see God and connect with God. It is that experience of love of the Divine that may enable us to genuinely love others, especially in the midst of their suffering and pain. It is therefore recommended that to be an effective and compassionate caregiver one should be attentive not only to the spiritual journey of others but also to one's own spiritual journey and practice.

Transformation

Spiritual journeys are ones of transformation. They lead us from an old way of experiencing life and ourselves in relation to life and others to a new and more profound way of life. Similar to Kubler-Ross's phases of dying, a spiritual journey also involves elements of grief. Joseph Campbell refers to this journey as a threefold process:

1. Loss of structure (denial, anger, bargaining)
2. Chaos: into the woods (chaos, depression, resignation)
3. Restructuring (openness, readiness, reemergence)[18]

Loss of structure can refer to the questioning of previously held beliefs and values, which, in the face of dying, no longer seem tenable to the dying person. The resulting feeling of emptiness, which can be expressed as abandonment by God or others, may cause immense pain, chaos, and suffering—independent of the pain, chaos, and suffering caused by the illness itself. It is critically important to be able to sit with the pain in the midst of aloneness. Into that space of ultimate uncertainty may come a profound wisdom and an acceptance of the beauty of mystery. In that acceptance comes openness to the divine, the sacred, or the holy, which ultimately leads to transcendence.

Jeffrey's Spiritual Journey

One of my patients, Jeffrey, was 40 years old when he died of AIDS. I met Jeffrey about 8 years prior to his death. At that time he was an angry man, in denial of his illness and unwilling to open up to anyone to talk about his anger. Initially, I approached these issues gingerly, only to be met by icy glares. For the first year or two our conversations focused on his physical condition and whether he would agree to take medication and do the appropriate tests. He continued to be resistant to medical treatment. After some time Jeffrey began to trust me, as we discussed his relationships, his homosexuality, and the guilt he felt—that his lifestyle may have caused his illness. I saw a person filled with self-hatred and confusion about his life, his meaning and purpose in his life, and how he was viewed by others in his family and church. As sad as this made me feel and as compelled as I was to convince him he was a good person, I held back and let Jeffrey struggle with these issues until he could let go of the anger. Without words, I showed my love for him by being present to him, seeing him often and supporting him in whatever phase of his journey he was in. We eventually got into profound discussions about God. Jeffrey had a deep belief in God and a longing for God's love, but he also felt that God was not there for him and that because of the mistakes he made, God would not forgive him. He refused a chaplain visit or counseling.

On one visit, I did share a book a chaplain had given me, with nondenominational prayers and writings for people with AIDS. Over the next few years, that book formed the basis of our discussions about God, forgiveness, and self-worth. Each visit started out with a hug, a new box of tissues for tears, and a hug at the end. Jeffrey struggled profoundly with guilt, forgiveness, and meaninglessness. But as time progressed, so did Jeffrey's intimacy with God. Eventually he started the process of self-forgiveness. His conversations with God deepened. He emerged from his dark night of the soul periodically with lightness and self- acceptance.

The last time I saw Jeffrey before he died was during his final hospitalization for AIDS-related fever and dehydration. His mental status had been progressively declining for the previous weeks. As I walked into his room, Jeffrey was lying motionless with a childlike smile on his face. The light from the window was streaming in, and for a brief instant I thought he had died. I also was profoundly aware of how much at peace he appeared. He turned his head toward me and told me he felt "funny and different somehow." Our conversation for the next hour fluctuated between tears and laughter. At one point he sheepishly confessed to me that he was fondling himself while talking to me. Without judgment, I accepted his action as self-comfort as well as a sense of intimacy he felt he could share with me. For a fleeting second I felt that I was his mother, father, sister-in-law, brother, and church community all rolled into one. But unlike his experience from others in his past, I did not chastise him. Jeffrey wept as he recounted the self-hatred and loneliness he felt over the years. He told me that for many of those years, I was the only person who really loved him. He also said that at last he has seen in himself all the qualities I saw in him and shared with him for many years. He said that finally he realized that he never did anything wrong and that he was a worthwhile person whose life mattered. There was no more shame, no more guilt, and no more self-loathing. Most importantly, he said he felt God's presence in a way he never had before and knew "without a doubt, that God loves me as I am." Jeffrey deeply believed he would die soon and be reunited with his mother, who had died the year before. He shared his vision of his mother and God welcoming him into heaven with open arms. As Jeffrey thanked me and told me he loved me, I was overcome by a deep sense of the holy. What had happened that day was sacramental, and for me, the highest experience of contemplation. To this day, as I recount Jeffrey's story, tears fill my eyes—tears of gratitude for being given the opportunity to know someone so special, for being privileged to be Jeffrey's physician, and for the experience of communion with the holy within another person. Those are moments of genuine grace in my life.

Teaching about Patients' Spiritual Journeys

In teaching medical students, residents, physicians, and other healthcare providers about caring for the ill and dying, specifically with regard to spiritual issues faced by patients in their spiritual journeys, I found that one of the greatest barriers to teaching this material was what is often seen as the esoteric nature of the concept of spirituality: What is it? How do we recognize spiritual issues? What do we do about it? How do philosophical and theological principles translate to the practical? "It is too complicated," is what many of my students and colleagues suggest. Critics of our work suggest that the medical model is too reductionistic to apply to deeper and less medical aspects of peoples' lives, such as spirituality.[19] But medicine is both a science and an art. The science aspect does conform to a reductionistic model, such as evidence-based care. The art of medicine, though, does not. So within the discipline of medicine, there is a tradition of nonscience-based practice. Listening to patients'

stories, getting to know about patients' families and cultural background, and forming relationships are all out of the realm of strict scientific discourse. However, just
as important as it is to teach the scientific skills necessary to train good diagnosti-
cians and therapists, it is also important to teach the skills needed to practice artful
medicine as well. Therefore, I have developed some practical concepts and tools so
that physicians and other healthcare providers can more easily address spiritual issues of the dying. Some of these tools are described in Chapter 15. In this chapter, I
will present some of the spiritual issues patients face and a way to address the spiritual stages of the dying.

Spiritual Issues of the Dying

As people face their dying, there are some spiritual issues that come up that can
be recognized from their spiritual history or from talking with the dying person
about what they are going through emotionally and spiritually. Many of these are
amenable to clinical intervention. However, unlike treating physical pain with
medications, there are no quick or standardized solutions to the care of people's
spiritual issues. Most of the work in dealing with these issues is done by the patient
as part of his or her spiritual journey. The caregivers—professional, family, and
friends—can be present to their loved ones as companions in a supportive and compassionate role. Some of the spiritual issues faced by chronically ill and dying patients are listed in Table 4.1.

TABLE 4.1
Spiritual Issues

- Lack of meaning and purpose
- Hopelessness
- Despair
- Not being remembered
- Guilt/shame
- Anger at God/others
- Abandonment by God/others
- Feeling out of control
- Spiritual pain/suffering
- Mistrust
- Lack of forgiveness/reconciliation

In the following section I will describe patient cases from my own practice and some potential ways for caregivers to approach these issues.

"My Life Is Meaningless"

Dave is a 67-year-old successful businessman with Parkinson's disease who now has mild cognitive impairment and physical impairments that require him to get assistance with all his activities of daily living. He has been very active all his life. His meaning in life came from his work and accomplishments, but now he is unable to work, and he feels life has no meaning anymore.

How does he make sense of a world that does not seem to be intrinsically reasonable? Dave never faced these spiritual issues of meaning until he became seriously ill. His sense of meaning was in his work and relationships. Now he can no longer work, and he feels that since he is no longer successful in his own eyes, his friends and family no longer value him.

Intervention

The goal is to help Dave move beyond defining himself by what he did to a deeper and more intrinsic meaning and value of himself as a person. By reflective listening, one can first learn more about past sources of meaning in life and whether those sources still apply. One can ask questions such as:

- What have been important events in your life? What is important now?
- What is the most important thing you have ever done? What could be the most important thing you could do now?
- Have you loved and have you loved well? Do you still love?
- What has inspired you in your life? What inspires you now?
- What gave your life enthusiasm? What gives your life enthusiasm now?

If a patient is religious and/or expresses a belief in God:

- Ask what the person's relationship with God is like.
- Does that relationship with God or religious belief provide a sense of peace or meaning in life?

Most religions speak of an intrinsic value and meaning. Ask the patient what he or she thinks his or her beliefs indicate about that meaning and purpose. Sometimes people find meaning in their struggle, sometimes not. But as caregivers, we can support them in looking beyond the extrinsic and into an intrinsic sense of value in themselves. In addition to listening to these issues with the patient, the physician/ healthcare provider could consider referral to a cognitive therapist, chaplain, pastoral counselor, and spiritual director for more counseling and discussion.

Dave has been working with a psychiatrist and a priest on these issues, as well as talking with his family and me. While there have been no quick fixes, he has been able to create activities he can do that give him some sense of control. Over the years, being in control and being the person that others lean on have been critical to him. The challenge now has been to accept being dependent on others. Dave understands this as a stage of spiritual progress—out of dependence arises some lesson about life's meaning. Over the years, I have seen in him a gradual acceptance of who he is on a deep level, where accomplishments no longer hold the same importance. He seems more at peace but continues to struggle with these issues.

Hopelessness

Rhonda was a 52-year-old female with end-stage ovarian cancer. Seven and a half years after good outcomes with multiple surgeries and chemotherapy, she was faced with an advanced disease for which there was no longer any treatment. Her hope has always been for a cure. She now faces a deep sense of hopelessness; her hope is gone.

Hope can be expressed in many ways. It may initially be for a cure, but when that is no longer possible, people may still find hope in finding important projects, making peace with others, and having a peaceful death.

Intervention

The most important intervention is to sit and be present to Rhonda as she struggles with the grief and despair of her impending death. Sharing the sadness and offering a supportive hug often may be the best first step. Later in the visit, or more likely in another visit, one can then start talking about other sources of hope for Rhonda. Some ways to get at those other sources of hope are to:

- Help the patient create a dream list.
- Talk about the relationships in the person's life. Is there any conflict from relationships that might need to be resolved? Any relationships which are strong and supportive, to lean on at this time?
- Ask about the person's sources of hope. What have they been in past life experiences in times of stress?
- If the person is religious, what does her religion say about hope? Is that meaningful to her?

Referral to chaplains or pastoral counselors might be appropriate in order to work on these issues in greater depth. Practically, I often deal with these issues in multiple visits, sometimes in phone conversations, in addition to the office or home visits. For many patients the search for hope triggers so many issues that stir up emotions and further questions. No one person on the interdisciplinary team or within the family or friend community needs to be the sole person helping the patient. Referral to chaplains, pastoral counselors, and spiritual directors, as well as therapists and social workers, is critical to afford the patient the most help possible. Lay spiritual companions are excellent sources of support. These volunteers meet with patients regularly and talk with them about their spiritual issues.

Rhonda worked hard on her journey. She worked with a rabbi on the issue of "how Jewish people die." He told her that Jewish people die the way they live. In saying that, he helped her celebrate her life. She was able to appreciate the richness of her life, her accomplishments both in her work and her relationships, and the impact that she made on others in her life. Her hopelessness turned into hope for a meaningful time before she died. Her heart opened even more than it had been through all of her life. She could accept the love that surrounded her daily from her family and friends. The day before she died, her family and I sat around her bedside and sang, told jokes, reminisced, hugged, and cried. The room was filled with profound love, joyful energy, and connection. It was a hope-filled experience for everyone. The hope came from Rhonda, who inspired all of us to live life to the fullest and to love beyond limits.

Despair

Susan was a 46-year-old female with metastatic breast cancer. She was an attorney, married with two children, ages 13 and 15. Her goal had been to live to see both children graduate from high school and start college. In the last 2 months, she had a rapid decline. She wanted to try an experimental treatment at the National Institutes of Health but was too weak and debilitated to be transferred out of the hospital.

When confronted with the possibility of dying, she panicked and said she didn't know how to die. In particular, she felt as if her life was being cut too short and that God may not be there for her. She was full of despair and sadness and not sure of where to turn. As a Catholic, she attended church but couldn't turn to that now. She was afraid of sharing her feelings with her family because she thought they were unaware of her dying and therefore would be unable to handle it.

Intervention

In listening to the patient, you may hear some issues that arise (e.g., a punishing God versus a supportive God) or the patient may sort out her issues while talking about them. Susan related a spiritual experience in which, during prayer, she became aware of how conflicted she was about God's absolute power and ability to change things. Then Jesus appeared to her in her prayer and wrapped his arms around her. She had an insight that while God may not be all-powerful, he is ever present to her. That brought her comfort and eventually a way to come to terms with dying. She also talked about the deep experience of God's presence in some of her times of prayers, moments similar to St. Teresa of Avila's description of contemplation. During these times, she was able to experience a sense of wholeness and peace that gradually increased as she approached her death. These experiences were so important to her that she requested that her pain medications be adjusted so that she could be more alert during the times she meditated.

Susan found the following actions helpful:

- Prayer, meditation, or other spiritual practices
- Exploring issues of giving up versus letting go
- Inviting conversations with family members and clergy.

Susan did not feel she could approach her priest about the issues she was facing, but she was willing to talk with the hospital chaplain. The hospital chaplain was a rabbi and also a mother, so Susan was able to talk with her about many of the fears she had about dying and leaving her children. Susan discussed her feelings with me about dying and of giving up. Susan saw dying as giving up and felt that her children would not be proud of her but rather see her as a failure for giving up. We discussed the concept of dying as one of letting go rather than giving up. When she was able to see it as letting go, she was more able to see dying not as a failure but as a part of life. Meditation became part of her daily prayer practice. She received strength in being an example to others, especially her family, as to how to die with grace.

Her family was very much aware of her dying, but they were hesitant about discussing death with Susan for fear that she would find that discussion difficult. This led to strained and superficial discussions, where true feelings of sadness and grief were covered with social politeness. Both the chaplain and I met with the family and helped facilitate the discussion between Susan and her family. This enabled all parties to start having meaningful talks about Susan's illness and eventual dying. The children were able to express their feelings, and Susan was able to see that her family would survive her dying. After her death, Susan's husband told me that the last few weeks of Susan's life were the richest and deepest moments they had ever experienced. The intensity of his love and the children's love for Susan was so brilliant that he never imagined such a love was possible. In the end, the connection and unity the whole family felt was again a time of grace and acceptance of life, love, and mystery.

Not Being Remembered

Monica was a 32-year-old woman with ovarian cancer who was dying in hospice. She had three children, ages 8, 6, and 2. She became very depressed and, in spite of medication, was not being relieved of her symptoms. While talking to her, the hospice nurse and I elicited a spiritual history, in which Monica told us that as a Jew she believed that she would live on through her children. As she told us this, she broke down in tears, relating her fear that her 2 year old will never remember her, and thus part of her will always be dead.

Intervention

There are many ways clinicians can help people be remembered. Clinicians can elicit the patient's goals and dreams. Then, they can work with patients on ways those goals and dreams can be accomplished that are feasible for the patient, given his or her clinical status. It may be adjusting the patient's chemotherapy schedule in order to provide the opportunity to travel to an important reunion. Or it might be helping the patient reach an acceptance that certain goals and dreams might not be accomplished but that there are other ways the patient can be remembered. Referrals to chaplains, counselors, or spiritual directors can be helpful. Use of tools such as writing journals or legacies, videotaping, and recording can also be powerful ways that people can use to be remembered.

The hospice nurse and I recommended that Monica write a journal for her children. We helped her make a video of herself giving messages to her family. This gave Monica a sense of meaning for her last month of living and a way to be remembered. Her depression resolved itself almost immediately. Clearly, in this case, Monica was not suffering from a clinical depression but rather from grief about not being remembered in her children's life and not being able to participate in their lives anymore.

Guilt/Shame

Sharon is a 28-year-old female with HIV, newly diagnosed. She had an abortion after a rape as a teenager and has been "waiting for God's punishment, and this is it." She is Baptist and is active in her church.

Intervention

- Listen to the patient. Find out why she feels the way she does.
- Ask about her relationship with God. If God is a punitive God, she can't go to him, especially now that she is vulnerable. She needs help in dealing with the image of a punitive God.
- Ask about her religious beliefs. People may incorrectly interpret what their religion says about sin and/or punishment. A referral to a chaplain or inviting the minister to join the patient and you may be helpful.
- Be supportive and accepting of the patient.
- Give her time to work through these issues.
- Some people can talk themselves through issues such as this. Often, feeling so strongly about punishment comes from shame about something. As people talk about shame, they may come to another awareness of the event(s) that led to the shame. They may bring an adult perspective to it. They may be able to forgive themselves and move on.

Sharon spent a year talking with me regularly at office visits. Most of the office visit time was spent discussing these issues. She also spoke regularly with her minister and had a few visits with a chaplain. Over time, she was able to see God in a different way, as a forgiving and compassionate God. Eventually she forgave herself and was able to move on. Today she has remarried, finished college, and has a great job. Her children are doing well, and she is very content with who she is.

Anger at God or Others

Teresa was a 38-year-old female attorney with both ovarian and breast cancer. She was raised as a Catholic and prayed a lot, but when it became clear that she would not be cured, she turned away from God and her church community. She also felt distant from many others.

Anger at God or others is a normal expression of frustration and of not being in control of one's life, of not being able to determine the process of one's life or illness. The book of Job is an example of this, in which Job calls out to God in despair over the plight of his life. God does not change Job's circumstances right away but helps Job understand that God is the one ruling the universe. Eventually Job accepts his place in creation, and God ends his suffering.

Intervention

Talk with the patient and listen to her. Let her reveal her own feelings. Often these emotions are so deep that bringing them up and giving light to them help the patient confront her own feeling of helplessness. Don't contradict the person. Use reflective listening; after you hear the person describe an emotion or a situation, you might ask a question to elicit more information and to encourage the patient to develop other interpretations of the events. Chaplains have training in this process and are wonderful resources.

Teresa faced her dying with anger. At that time, I felt a need to make sure that everyone was at peace when they died. The image of friends surrounding the bedside, singing Gregorian chants, the patient with a glowing smile and a gentle, happy dying process were what I hoped people could attain, or at least a portion thereof. Teresa taught me that people die in their own genuine way, and if their path is one of anger and fighting, then that is their way of dying. Teresa never resolved her anger in any obvious way. She struggled with her issues, she yelled at a God she claimed no longer existed, and she pushed many of us away. But she let all of us in on her time when she was ready for interaction. I suspect that all of her anger was her way of coping with the tremendous pain and frustration her life situation caused her to feel. In her anger, Teresa was alive and filled with questions, emotions, and reactions. She was able to be clear about the injustice of life and her desire to have had a different life experience. She was not about "to go gentle into that good night," as Dylan Thomas wrote; she wanted to leave kicking, and that she did. In her anguished discourse with God, she touched a spiritual chord within herself that was deep and genuine. It was what I think of as contemplation in anger—fierce, intense, and very real. I have come to realize that Teresa's journey of anger was one of the most spiritual journeys I have ever witnessed.

Abandonment by God or Others

Jeffrey, my patient who died of AIDS (described earlier in this chapter), had a deep sense of abandonment by God. Dying is something one does alone. A sense of abandonment is often seen in patients. Jesus felt abandoned by God when he called out during his dying, "Why have you forsaken me?" Patients may feel abandoned by God or by other loved ones. This experience of abandonment may be the final purification of faith. One believes in total emptiness—having no proof, no feeling, yet one still believes. Abandonment is a spiritual experience, but abandonment can also have some roots in family life. A lot of issues may come up from childhood. People's response to a sense of abandonment may be either working through the despair and ending up with a deeper belief or faith or saying there is nothing but being at peace with that sense of nothingness.

Intervention

While no one can take away that profound sense of abandonment, we can offer comfort, presence, and support. As Jeffrey struggled with his illness, he felt abandoned by God and others for many years. My role, in part, was to be a loving presence for him when he felt no love, to be accepting of him when he could not accept himself, to see him for his true inner worth when he saw himself as worthless. Perhaps, when we are a loving presence to our patients, they will start to see in us what they cannot see in God and others. Eventually, Jeffrey started to see that others loved him as well— his mother, the rest of his family, his church, and God.

Feeling Out of Control

Dave, my patient with Parkinson's disease, described earlier, experienced the frustration of being out of control. When I asked him if he was in control before his illness, he said, "No, but I had the delusion I was in control. Those delusions are now gone."

Intervention

Being in control is very important for people, and it is critical that we enable people to regain as much control as possible and support them in finding peace with not being in control of the things they use to have control over. Religious and/or spiritual beliefs may help people find a sense of control, especially feeling that they are in God's care. Cornelius Bennhold, professor of physics at George Washington University, in his experience with illness, found healing in recognizing what he could control and what was out of his control (see Chapter 22 for more details). By turning the uncontrollable things—whether he would have a recurrence of his cancer or when he would die—over to God, he could focus his energies on the things he could control, like the type of chemotherapy he would use.

Dave has a supportive family who help him find ways to maintain control, even in the face of a progressive neurological decline. They encourage him to express choices whenever possible and to maintain as much independence over his environment as possible. His family members are ardent defenders of maintaining his dignity. Part of that involves treating him with respect and affording him the ability to have a choice whenever possible.

Spiritual Pain and/or Suffering

Paul was dying of pancreatic cancer. He was quiet; he seemed to be in pain but not able to identify the source of his pain. His family noted that he seemed down but not depressed—just hard to reach. Paul mentioned that he couldn't put his finger on what was hurting him, but he felt a deep internal pain.

Generalized spiritual pain is often hard to diagnose, since there may be no objective symptoms. Some people talk of deep, existential, or spiritual pain. It is often hard to diagnose, as there may be no objective symptoms. This type of pain may come from a sense of meaninglessness, hopelessness, despair, and an unmet need. Thus it is important to talk to the patient and elicit these potential sources of distress from the patient. But the pain may also come from a deep and profound spiritual crisis. St John of The Cross, a sixteenth-century mystic, writes of "The Dark Night of the Soul," where the pain is so intense that it may be unbearable. This type of spiritual distress may be the most profound step toward enlightenment. Some religions see this type of suffering as necessary for redemption. In fact, religious tenets may help a person frame this suffering in a concept such as redemption that helps him or her deal with it. It is important for the healthcare professional to honor spiritual journeys, however difficult they may appear. To medicate these experiences as if they are merely physical pain or experiences to be fixed or avoided may do the patient spiritual injustice. There are many aspects of dying that are unknown and indeed are mystery. Such deep experiences, I believe, are in the realm of mystery.

Intervention

- Listen to the patient. Patients can be helped by having people around them to support them through these journeys.
- Respect his or her beliefs and ask how the patient's beliefs can help relieve the suffering.
- Ask the patient when he or she felt like this before. What helped relieve the suffering? (e.g., prayer, music, nature, and art are all ways that might help people tap into whatever is the spiritual stirring within them.)
- Refer to therapists and/or chaplain.

Spiritual pain may represent an unmet need, so ask what is the source of pain—abandonment, despair, frustration, or lack of control. In Paul's case, it was a profound sense of abandonment. He recognized that people loved him and felt appreciative of all the love and presence. But he also felt that no one wanted to really hear about his pain. People changed topics when he started talking about his anger and the despair that he felt because he would die. He wanted to be heard and to be accepted as he was. He once said, "Why is everyone sugar-coating the fact that I will be dead in a few months." I shared this with family members, and some told me they just could not handle it. That is perfectly acceptable. We all need to be aware of our own needs and limitations. Several family members and friends were able to listen to his pain. In the end, each member of his community of support helped him in whatever way he or she could. Paul's needs were met as well, and his spiritual distress was lessened. Paul had a philosophy that we are all on earth for the greater good of all people, so his actions reflected that belief of doing good for others. Paul found meaning in a redemptive quality of suffering. He saw his suffering as an offering for the pain and suffering of others in the world.

Mistrust

Samuel was a 75-year-old man who was dying from lung cancer. Samuel's father had abandoned him when he was a child. He grew up in poverty and in difficult circumstances. He was raised as a Christian, and while very regular in his religious practice, he always had a difficult time with the concept of relationship with God. As Samuel faced his dying, he experienced difficulty in trusting others and God. This manifested as poor compliance with treatment recommendations, minimal conversations with his healthcare professionals, and a sense of loneliness and isolation.

Intervention

Trusting others and God can be difficult for anyone. Family dynamics and past experiences can affect how willing one is to trust others. People's relationships with God often mirror their relationships with people in their lives, particularly parents. Being able to trust one's healthcare professionals is important. The therapeutic relationship, in order to be effective, has to be rooted in trust. For people who believe in God, trust that one's welfare is in God's hands or that one will be with God after death is fundamental to many religious beliefs. Thus one's relationship with God also needs to be rooted in trust within those belief systems.

One can help a patient move from mistrust to trust by exploring issues from the past that may be affecting the patient's current ability to trust. Referral to therapists, pastoral counselors, and chaplains can be helpful in this process. But, in addition, healthcare professionals can, by their interaction with patients, provide a living example of a consistent, healthy relationship in which patients can place their trust. In effect, the healthcare professionals can help patients heal their past hurts by giving the patients the opportunity to experience unconditional love and acceptance from another. This may be one of the most healing aspects of the therapeutic relationship.

Samuel came irregularly to my office over the years that I treated him. Rather than chastise him for missed appointments or noncompliance with treatment plans, I welcomed him and showed my delight in his being there for the appointment. I invited him to share whatever he was comfortable sharing. I ignored his attempts to push me away with his occasional sarcastic comment. Over time, he gradually began to trust me. Eventually, he accepted my recommendation to see a pastoral counselor. In the sessions with her, Samuel was able to let go of past hurts and start trusting others in his life. He was able to see that his image of God mirrored that of the experience he had had with his father. Healing the relationship with his father enabled him to fully experience a trusting relationship with God.

Lack of Forgiveness and/or Reconciliation

Mike was a 60-year-old man dying from pancreatic cancer. He was being treated in an inpatient hospice unit. He was in severe pain, yelling out in agony frequently. Even though medications were available that would treat his pain, Mike refused them. He told the medical staff that he was "no good" and did not deserve to be pain free.

Intervention

The need to be forgiven or to reconcile can be so powerful that it can affect one's sense of worth and value. Having an opportunity to explore these issues, and then seek forgiveness from and reconciliation with another or with God, can be a powerful step toward inner peace, acceptance, and healing.

Many complicated emotions can arise in the exploration of these issues. In some cases, a wrongdoing can be so severe that anger, either from the patient who was wronged or the loved one the patient wronged, may be justifiable. Some people also hold a deep belief, rooted within personal or religious values, that there are some deeds that may never be forgiven. It is critical that patients be referred to therapists, pastoral counselors, or chaplains who can support the patient and/or family as these issues are explored. Specific forgiveness interventions can be used to help the patient or family reconcile, if that is appropriate.

Mike worked with the hospice chaplain, who helped him to acknowledge wrongdoings from his past. Through talking with the chaplain, Mike was able to ask his wife and God for forgiveness. Eventually, Mike and his wife were able to reconcile and share an intimate deepening of their relationship. Mike was able to accept pain medication, and he died peacefully with his loved ones at his bedside.

Spiritual Stages

How do patients move through the stages of dying in a spiritual way? By looking at the questions that serious illness triggers and attempting to find answers to these questions for themselves. Most of these questions have no specific answers, but they often lead to other questions that patients can answer for themselves. For example, "Why is this happening to me?" may lead to a life review and a new insight that helps the person understand themselves, or the Divine, in a new way. "Who am I?" may be the impetus for a deeper search into self, with a resultant deeper meaning of self. Reconciliation and forgiveness may be the key elements in achieving inner peace and intimacy with God and others. Finally, a hope for living on, either eternally or through others or one's accomplishments, may be the initial confrontation with one's mortality. These stages can be described in the form of an acronym: LIFE. This acronym summarizes some of the key steps that may occur for people in their spiritual journeys.

LIFE (for the spirit)©

L   Life Review
I   Identity
F   Forgiveness/reconciliation
E   Eternity

L. Life Review

The awareness that our lives are limited, while true for all of us and acutely real for the terminally ill person or for one who is faced with a life-threatening illness, can prompt many of the spiritual questions and issues addressed in this chapter. A *life review* includes an analysis of one's past, in which people reflect on their past relationships, accomplishments, and dreams, both lost and gained. People may revisit their life and evaluate the meaning of their life, past and present. Many issues can come up for people during this time, such as failed or problematic relationships, perceived career failures, and unaccomplished dreams and regrets. It might involve acknowledgment of wrongdoing and the need for forgiveness and reconciliation. People may become depressed or anxious during this time. Some experience guilt and anger. Some people are able to forgive; others hold a grudge and may even isolate from people, especially loved ones.

It is critical to address all dimensions of care. Depression may need to be treated with counseling and/or medication. A forgiveness intervention may be appropriate. Spiritual issues need to be identified and worked with, either by a chaplain or other healthcare providers. Ideally, people should be given all the resources needed to address these issues and achieve some resolution of their issues.

As people review their lives, they may reframe past experiences in a different way in order to give a new and more significant meaning to their lives.[20] Past hurts or failures may be understood as stepping stones for successes that occurred later in life. Broken relationships might be seen as openings to newer and perhaps more intimate experiences. But, as with Kubler-Ross's stages, the process of life review is dynamic. It is not as if one day someone awakens with an optimistic insight and is happy until death. People may waver between joyful insight and deep moments of despair. This journey can provoke deep spiritual suffering and needs to be supported. In the end, the life review can lead to a sense of integration and peace.

I. Identity

Identity refers to the questions people begin to ask—about who they are and what gives their life meaning. As described in many of the patient stories, many people do find a renewed and deeper sense of who they are. Often it is more congruous with their inner self than any definition they had in their earlier lives. The reflection that ensues, after the realization that one may die or is dying, affords one the opportunity to go deeper, to pause and reflect and discover a new self. People may develop a sense of deeper self-worth and learn to accept love and caring from others. Relationships, ideas, and titles that used to hold meaning for a person may no longer do that. Friends may be surprised that their loved one is a "new person." The patients themselves may realize a new peace and inner calm. This process, however, can be tumultuous and painful. As a butterfly struggles to emerge from its cocoon, so do we, as we let go of old beliefs and perceptions. All of the stages discussed by Joseph Campbell—loss of structure, chaos, and restructuring—occur during this time.[21] Again, support from trained spiritual care providers, as well as healthcare providers and family and friends, can help people as they go through this struggle. But ultimately the journey is one that is done alone, as the person reaches in to touch him- or herself and the Divine.

F. Forgiveness

Forgiveness plays an important role in each of our lives, on a personal as well as a relational and societal level. On a personal level, forgiveness of self can help us achieve an inner peace as well as peace with others and with God. Wrongdoing against others and ourselves can result in guilt and resentment. This can then lead to self-recrimination and self-loathing. It also can create a distance or disconnect from self and others. Resentment can give way to hate and intolerance. As a result, forgiveness is the first stage of self-love and acceptance. It is also the basic building block of loving relationships with others.

There have been many studies looking at the role of forgiveness in relation to health. Forgiveness can impact health outcomes. Unforgiving persons may have increased anxiety and depression, whereas the act of forgiveness can result in less anxiety and depression, increased coping with stress, and increased closeness to God and others.[22] There have been numerous studies looking at forgiveness interventions.[23] These interventions involve counseling and exercises that are used to help people move from anger and resentment toward forgiveness. In many of these studies it was shown that people who are able to forgive are better able to find peace and to have improved relationships. One can postulate that anger with

God can similarly cause distress and that a forgiveness of God may be an appropriate intervention.

From my own clinical experience, I frequently encounter in my patients themes of self-loathing arising from guilt about a perceived or actual wrongdoing. For example, patients come to understand their illness as a punishment from God. This perception may hinder their ability to heal or to seek appropriate treatment. Self-loathing can result from an inability to forgive one's self or from hatred and resentment of others.

Religions offer people ways to forgive or at least to understand wrongdoing. In the Christian tradition, for example, forgiveness can occur when we deepen the virtues of faith, love, and hope in our lives. With faith and love, hope is the normally expected fruit of prayer, especially contemplative prayer. One adjunct of healing, then, is prayer. Hope, then, gives birth to change. Without hope, there is no possibility of changing, and there is no future without hope. The inability to forgive blocks hope, and that is why it sets the stage for depression. St. John of the Cross wrote, "Attachment to a hurt arising from a past event blocks the inflow of hope into our lives."[24] So, without forgiving, we cannot feel God's presence. Harboring resentment and hatred for self or others even while praying blocks one to the openness that comes from prayer and from relating to God or the divine. This creates a barrier between the person and God, between two people, and between the person and the self. Forgiveness is the act of being restored to a good relationship with God or others, and self-forgiveness brings wholeness back to these relationships and ultimately to ourselves. Forgiveness of self brings wholeness and integrity to self.[25]

E. Eternity

Finally, *eternity* refers to the variety of beliefs people may have about what happens after one dies. A patient of mine, who died of natural causes at age 97, believed that once one died that was the end of one's life. She said, "One dies when it is time to open up a space for a new person on earth." She believed that all of us are privileged to be on earth and should do the most to contribute to others and to society. She said that we will live on in the memories of others and in our good deeds. So, for her, the connections she made with others in her life, a review of her life works, and knowledge that she made a difference were vital to her ability to let go. Other patients of mine have a variety of beliefs about life after death, such as being with God, the Divine, or a higher power. Others find comfort in the belief that they will be reunited with loved ones. Still others speak of a new role for themselves, becoming guides or angels for their loved ones left on earth. When I was a medical student, during my pediatrics rotation, I cared for a 7-year-old girl who was dying of osteosarcoma, a cancer of the bone. Her mother and the staff were reluctant to discuss dying with her. One night, as I was drawing her blood, she asked me if I ever knew anyone that died. I told her of Eric, my fiancé, who died of cancer several years earlier. She broke out into a joyous song, "Eric and Christina, sitting in a tree, k-i-s-s-i-n-g." After a long pause, she looked deeply into my eyes and said, "And that tree is in heaven and when I get there I will tell him 'hi' from you." She then turned to her mother and said, "Don't worry, mommy, I am not afraid and I will always be with you. . . . I will be your angel."

For people who do not believe in a life after death, there are other significant belief systems that help people feel that they will be remembered. For some, it is living on through one's family or accomplishments. During this time of reflecting on the next stage or on the end of one's life, people may start to bring closure to personal and community relationships. Some may begin to give special gifts to loved ones as a way of saying good-bye.

Lessons Learned

Each of the stories I have shared with you in this chapter are from people who taught me the principles discussed here. Is your spiritual journey going to be like theirs? Probably not. Your journey will fill the pages of your life; it will be uniquely yours and will help you define who you are. The knowledge I have gained from other colleagues, from philosophers, from friends, and from my patients is a guide to help you in the journey you face, either as the person who is ill or the person taking care of the ill and dying. The journey can be challenging and joyful as well. There are people around you who can help you if you are open to the possibilities of love. By taking the time to listen to and to be aware of not only your body but also your spirit, you give yourself the opportunity to become whole and to heal.

5

The Spiritual Issues Faced by Children and Adolescents at the End of Life

PATRICIA FOSARELLI

A Personal Story

As a pediatric intern, I was once responsible for a unit full of elementary school children, because my resident was tending a crisis in the emergency room. Around 2:00 AM I was called to restart an IV line for a 6-year-old girl who needed her medication in the middle of the night. She had very few veins left as a result of all the medicines she had been receiving to save her life. To make matters worse, like many interns, my skill at starting IV lines was rudimentary. The more I stuck her, the more she cried. The more she cried, the more I missed—on and on. Finally, I decided to give her and my nerves a break. Through her tears, she looked at me hard. "Does God want you to hurt me?" she demanded. Startled, I didn't know how to answer her. If I said "yes," what would that do to her sense of God? If I said "no," she might say something like, "Then why do you keep hurting me?" Finally, I stammered something about God wanting me to help her and, at this point, that meant giving her an IV so she could get her medicine. She shook her head, "I don't think God wants anyone to hurt other people."

Even though that episode happened 27 years ago, I remember it as if it were yesterday. At a time when I was an agnostic, this child brought me face to face with speaking about God in the midst of pain and suffering—something, up to that point, that I had avoided. It was probably the first step in the journey that led me to become a physician-theologian.

Patricia Fosarelli

Introduction

That infants, children, and teenagers become ill and die is repugnant to most adults. In the natural order of things, young people are not supposed to die before their elders. Their bodies are supposed to be much healthier than those of older people; their immune systems are meant to be more resistant to the ills that befall older persons. In addition, they have so much to live for, so much life ahead of them.

But infants, children, and teens do die. Each death is a tragedy, a sorrow over what might have been. Each death is a profound loss, not only for an individual family but also for society as a whole. Societies cannot flourish if their youngest members die, for their deaths rob older members of their hope. And when much suffering precedes a child's death, a sense of anger, frustration, and despair may overtake those attending that child.

In most Western industrialized societies, after the immediate neonatal period, the death of an infant or child is uncommon. Yet, in most countries of the world, the death of infants and children is a commonplace event. Conditions such as infectious diseases and malnutrition, entities that rarely cause death in richer countries, routinely take the lives of the youngest and weakest members of poorer countries. The parents and siblings of dying children in poorer countries grieve them as much as do parents and siblings in wealthier countries. Even in our own country, there are certain urban and rural areas in which the mortality rates are far higher than in other urban or rural areas or in more affluent suburban communities. Societal problems—such as poverty, lack of prenatal care, substance abuse, and violence—cause countless deaths of our nation's young. The parents and siblings of those who have died in these areas mourn their losses as much as do parents and siblings in healthier (and wealthier) communities.

Regardless of where people live, the death of a young person prompts many questions: Why? Could it have been avoided? Did something or someone contribute to the death? Will it happen again? When the people experiencing the loss of a young person believe in God, other questions may surface: Why did God take my child? Did I do something wrong? Am I being punished? Was he or she being punished? If God didn't cause my child to die, why did God permit it? Is God testing me? Is God angry at me? Does God love me?

These questions are all natural human questions when faced with some of the most traumatic events one can face. Children, too, ask their own set of questions, very much like those of adults but geared to their age-appropriate way of thinking and understanding. Their level of development affects how they will interpret any situation, which, in turn, influences what they will most need from caring adults in their lives.

This chapter begins by reviewing the usual stages of cognitive, emotional, and spiritual development experienced by children and teens as they mature. An understanding of these stages is necessary to understand, in turn, the most common spiritual issues faced by dying children. A review of common reactions of parents and siblings will also be included for each age group. The chapter will conclude with some general suggestions as to what is most needed by dying children and teens (and their families).

Stages of Normal Development in Childhood and Adolescence: Piaget, Erikson, and Fowler

Piaget: How Children Learn

Jean Piaget, the great Swiss psychologist, was interested in how infants and children learn. By observing his own children as they grew, he developed his theory of development. There are four stages, progressing from infancy to adolescence. Piaget called the stage in infancy *sensorimotor*. Infants and young children normally learn about their world by exploring it through their senses—looking, smelling, listening, touching, and tasting. In fact, many parents are concerned that their young infant places everything in her or his mouth . . . even things which are clearly nonedible! By the end of the first year, infants develop the ability to walk or otherwise move about, and they can then go after what they want, rather than waiting for the object to come to them.

Piaget's second stage, the *preoperational*, applies to preschoolers. Once children can talk and express themselves, they eagerly do so. Adults find that preschoolers have very fanciful ways of discussing their world and why they think things happen. To make sense of their world, preschoolers use a logic all their own, which is not logical in the adult sense of the word. Preschoolers are convinced that their ideas are right and that anything is possible, from tooth fairies to Easter bunnies.

In the elementary school years, children must learn many skills (such as math, reading, writing, and categorizing) if they are to succeed in school and in life. Piaget called this stage *concrete operations*. Children learn by doing, by working with *concrete* objects. For example, to learn to count, children use their fingers; to add or subtract, children must first have actual objects in front of them, to which they add (or subtract) other objects. They learn about science and nature through projects or walking outdoors and handling objects of interest.

Piaget called the final stage of development *formal operations*. Teenagers do not need concrete objects in front of them in order to count, do math, spell, and so on.

Furthermore, they can imagine themselves in situations or places in which they have never been. They can imagine what it might be like to be another person. They can imagine a future, even one which is very different from their present.

Erikson: Forming Relationships

Erik Erikson, considered to be the father of psychosocial development, was interested in how human beings form relationships throughout the human life span. Erikson believed that each age had a developmental process to master; if one failed to master that process, future progress in development would be affected. For the purposes of this chapter, only Erikson's stages of infancy, childhood, and adolescence will be discussed.

Erikson's first stage is called *trust vs. mistrust*. Young infants can do nothing for themselves; others must meet all of their needs. If these needs are met in a timely, compassionate fashion, they will learn to trust people, objects, and their world. If the needs are ignored or ridiculed, or if they are abused, they will learn not to trust, and might, instead, learn to fear.

The next stage, *autonomy vs. shame and doubt*, reflects the fact that toddlers and young preschoolers are learning to do many things on their own, such as feeding, dressing, and toileting themselves. Insofar as they are successful, they become increasingly autonomous; if they fail (as they will, at least in the beginning) and if they are ridiculed, reprimanded, or punished, they will experience shame and doubt their abilities. If a child's treatment is particularly harsh, it might be particularly hard for her or him to try to do anything on her or his own.

Erikson called the third stage *initiative vs. guilt*. Preschoolers have an increasing desire to do things on their own, especially to help others. If this initiative results in a job well done or praise, they will continue to take initiatives. If their attempts to take initiative result in failure or in more work for others, they will experience guilt. Just as in the previous stage, if they are treated harshly for their failures, they are less likely to take future initiatives.

The stage of elementary school-age children is known as *industry vs. inferiority*. Children in school must work hard to succeed. They must learn many new skills, such as counting, naming, spelling, writing, and so on. Because they want to succeed and to please, they will work hard. If their hard work results in success or praise, they experience their reward. If all their hard work does not bring the results that they want, they will experience a sense of failure or inferiority. All children naturally experience lack of success in some area of their lives. But if they can succeed in other areas that are important to them, then they will generally be able to weather a few failures. This is especially true if loving adults support them when they fail, encourage them to try again, and act as their advocates or cheerleaders regardless of the outcome. When children are not supported or are ridiculed or punished for their failures, they are more likely to experience themselves as inferior or as failures.

Erikson called the stage of adolescence *identity vs. role diffusion*. The task of adolescence is to separate from parents—to forge an identity separate from that of one's family. Thus, the adolescent tries a variety of roles (friends, activities, etc.) to determine her or his identity—who she or he really is in her or his own right. Such behavior might seem unfocused to many adults. In their concern, loving parents usually place certain limits on role changes that entail anything illegal or immoral. Yet, in the end, for better or for worse, most teens end up with values and goals much like those of their parents. If a teen has been lovingly supported by parents throughout childhood, it is highly unlikely that she or he will do things that are completely contrary to her or his upbringing.

Fowler: Forming Faith

James Fowler, an ordained minister and psychologist, was interested in how faith developed across the life span. To develop his theory, he interviewed many people of different ages. In addition, he seriously considered the work that Piaget and Erikson had done before him and based some of his work on their theories. Although "faith development" is not synonymous with "spirituality," they are closely related, especially if the word "faith" has a more inclusive meaning than simply a collection of denominational beliefs. As such, it can serve as a proxy measure of spirituality in childhood. In childhood, thinking of spirituality as "finding meaning in life" would be foreign, since abstract concepts like that are not understood until the preteen years (if then). Children need more than the abstract (as we have seen in the theories presented earlier). That does *not* mean that children have only concrete ideas about God; far from it. But thinking about God as a person or as something they have experienced helps young children not only to understand others but also to express themselves.

Fowler thought about infancy as a time of *undifferentiated faith*. Like Erikson, he believed that an infant learns to have faith (or to trust) by being treated well. Furthermore, if an infant learns to have faith in those whom she or he can see, then she or he can learn to have faith in a God whom she or he cannot see. This is especially true if parents speak lovingly of God and have special rituals that are associated only with God, such as folding one's hands or closing one's eyes in prayer. On the other hand, if parents are inconsistent in their treatment of their child or if they speak of God sloppily, irreverently, or in negative terms, even an infant can pick up negativity (or confusion) about God.

Fowler's stage of faith development in the preschooler years is called *intuitive-projective*. As Erikson noted, young children have very different ways of looking at the world. Sometimes their ideas are fanciful, and sometimes they are quite insightful or intuitive. However, because of their limited experience, they also tend to project— that is, place onto a new situation, place, thing, or person attributes of a previously encountered similar situation, place, thing, or person. In terms of God, young children can have amazing insights into God. But they also project onto God both the positive and negative attributes of important people in their lives, especially their parents and authority figures. For example, if such individuals are loving, preschoolers will say that God is loving; if such individuals are angry, preschoolers will say that God is angry.

According to Fowler, the stage of faith development in elementary school children is called *mythic-literal*. Piaget noted that children of this age are very concrete in the way they learn. Fowler agreed that they *are* very literal. Fowler also noted that children of this age love myths and especially Bible stories that describe larger-than-life persons who conquer evil with goodness. In terms of God, children of this age love to hear stories in which God is doing mighty things, and they take these stories literally. They also think of God as a friend and have the same expectations of their friend God that they would have of other friends. For this age group, the Golden Rule says it all. Hence, if they do something for God, God should do something for them.

Fowler called the faith stage in early adolescence *synthetic-conventional*. Conventional is the norm, the usual. Coming out of their literal period, this aspect of the young adolescent stage is somewhat expected. But the other aspect of this stage says something very different. In a synthetic stage, young people are trying to put together the different experiences, opinions, and insights they encounter. For perhaps the first time, they are able to come into contact with others who might hold very different beliefs than they do. This is true not only for persons whose faith traditions are different from that of the young person but also for those who are of their same faith tradition but whose beliefs are very different. Following from their previous literal stage of surety, such differences can be a bit of a shock. Essentially, in this stage, a young person is wondering what beliefs his or her faith tradition holds (and why) and why others don't hold these beliefs.

In the stage of older adolescence and young adulthood, *individuative-reflective*, a young person struggles with what she or he believes and seeks to discover in which tradition those beliefs might fit. This period is "individuative" insofar as she or he must do the work alone; it is "reflective" in that much interior work must be done to sort it all out. This stage may take many years, even decades, to complete, and some people never completely emerge from this stage—even though they live many years.

How does serious illness affect these normal stages of cognitive, relational, and faith development throughout childhood and adolescence?

Spiritual Issues Faced by Dying Children and Their Families

Common Issues across Age

Regardless of age, two fears usually present in those who are dying are the fear of pain and the fear of abandonment. Both of these can cause untold suffering, if not physically, then certainly emotionally.

Relentless pain is all-consuming; one can think of nothing else. A dying child of any age might become frantic in response to both the intensity of the pain and its duration. Modern pediatric practice has a number of potent pain-relieving medications that can assist in making most children more comfortable; naturally, some medications might be more appropriate for certain children than others, because of age, the ability of a child's body to handle the medication internally, interactions with other medications being received, and so on. Potent pain relievers might make a child drowsier than usual, or even somnolent. Parents should be aware of the side effects of the particular medication that their child is receiving, but parents should not withhold such medications from their dying child because of any fears of developing an addiction or because of bias against pain relievers as a whole, especially if their child is in severe, constant, or intensifying pain. Parents and members of the medical team can assure children and teens that they will do their best to keep them as comfortable as possible.

Most children like the company of others, especially those they know the best. Ill children want—*and need*—company even more than their healthier counterparts. Many dying children share a fear common to most dying adults: that they will die alone; that their parents, siblings, friends, and even doctors and nurses will abandon them in the most frightening time of their lives. Parents and members of the medical team should allay this fear by assuring children (and teens) that they will do their best to prevent this. *Every* effort should be made to reassure a dying child, of any age, that she or he will not be abandoned; arrangements may have to be made to have someone present as needed, even around the clock. Parents should *not* have to feel personally responsible to be present at every moment, for they will need a break if they are to remain available emotionally for their child.

Infants and Toddlers

The Dying Children Themselves. As Erikson and Fowler noted, infants and toddlers need to be treated well if they are to develop trust and faith. When infants and toddlers are dying, their usual daily routines are completely disrupted. They might not be able to eat what they want or to engage in their favorite activities. This is especially true if they must be restrained so that an IV does not become dislodged. If an IV line becomes dislodged and a child needs intravenous medication, attempts must be made to reinsert the line; this might be quite painful. As Piaget noted, children of this age learn through exploring through their sense organs and by moving about. If a child is restrained, she or he cannot move about, bring objects to her or his mouth, or even touch treasured people or objects. Parents might not be able to hold their child in familiar ways, which frustrates both child and parents. These young children might cry inconsolably when their parents are out of their sight.

Furthermore, serious illness brings discomfort or even frank pain. Because these children are too young to speak and have limited receptive language, adults cannot know exactly why they are crying.

Although infants and toddlers may experience spiritual crises, it would be nearly impossible to know for certain, since their expressive language is so limited. We can only know from their cries and their behavior that they are distressed.

Parents. Parents (and other loving relatives or significant adults in the child's life) are themselves frustrated because they cannot relieve their child's distress and pain, nor can they adequately explain to the child what is occurring or why certain activities must be prohibited. These parents may feel helpless, hopeless, angry, and guilty, especially if they believe (rightly or wrongly) that they played a role in their child's illness or condition. Unfortunately, even the youngest of children can detect these negative feelings and may become even more irritable. Thus, a vicious cycle might be set up as negative emotions feed on themselves. Parents may express their frustration and anger at the medical and nursing staff, visitors, or pastoral care staff. They might cry uncontrollably or "hold it in" in an attempt to be strong for an ill child or other family members.

If parents believe in God and if they pray, they might wonder why God has not answered their prayer or whether God is angry at them or is punishing them for some real or imagined transgression. If they are angry at God, they might express this anger at a pastoral care provider or representative of their church. Alternatively, they might lose their faith in God altogether ("If there is a God, how could he let babies suffer?"). Parents who do not believe in God might use the illness of an infant or toddler as proof that God could not exist.

Siblings. Siblings are also affected by the illness of a younger sibling. They frequently resent that their parents must spend more time with the ill child or must spend time away from the home at the hospital, clinic, doctor's office, and so on. They may be jealous of all the attention that the ill sibling is receiving, not only from their parents but also from other significant adults in their lives. If they resented or were jealous of a sibling before his or her illness, they may have said things or wished bad things for him or her at that time that scare them now that he or she is ill. For example, an older sister wished that her baby brother would "just go away" when he first arrived, and now he is far away in a hospital. Or an older brother hit his younger sister and wished she was dead several months earlier, because she played with his toys; now, she is dying from leukemia. In both of these examples, the siblings are likely to be filled both with guilt and fear.

If they pray to God, but their ill sibling does not get better, they might wonder if they are being punished or if God is mad at them or doesn't love them. These feelings are especially likely to be present if they hear significant adults in their lives express similar feelings. Finally, children may blame themselves for their sibling's illness, even when it makes absolutely no sense for them to do so. Again, this is especially true if they have heard their parents or other significant adults express guilt. Siblings might also be afraid that they are going to be the next to die or, alternatively, that they weren't good enough or that God didn't love them enough to call them to heaven. Either way, older siblings suffer when their sister or brother is dying.

PASTORAL APPROACHES

Because babies and infants have such a limited ability to verbally communicate, words are not the best means of communication. Gentle expressions and a calm tone of voice are far more reassuring than are words. Siblings can be reassured that God loves us all and cares a great deal for each person. This is true even when we don't know why certain things happen. Parents can also be reassured that God is not punishing them or has ceased loving them. Compassionate listening, as they speak about their fears, questions, and sorrows, might be the greatest gift any parent can receive from visitors. Before asking members of their congregation to visit, parents should always be asked if this would be helpful.

When parents don't believe in God, one can give them the gift of compassionate presence, without judging their belief system. Interestingly, when adversity comes, many children (and a few adults) who have never thought much about God will begin to pray or ask questions about God. These individuals should be supported.

Preschoolers

The Dying Children Themselves. Like younger children, ill preschoolers are frustrated because they cannot do or eat whatever they want. Because they are in the normal developmental stages of seeking autonomy and taking initiative, serious illness halts those processes, as it is likely that their parents will *not* permit ill children to do things on their own. Children at this stage might regress to behaviors typical of them when they were much younger, such as soiling themselves, thumb-sucking, or temper tantrums, especially when their requests are denied or their attempts at doing things themselves are frustrated. They might throw themselves down, scream, kick, throw objects, hit, or bite. Although some of this behavior is understandable, children must not be permitted to physically hurt others. Much of the preschooler's anger and frustration is directed at his or her parents (who are the safest) and medical or nursing professionals (who are the ones causing at least some of the pain). Ill preschoolers may cry inconsolably, rejecting all efforts to bring them comfort. This behavior is especially present when parents or other loved ones attempt to leave the room. This, too, is understandable, because all they want is to feel better, go home, and escape all the painful procedures and pain-causing adults in their lives.

Unlike younger children, preschoolers *are* old enough to speak and receive explanations. That, however, doesn't mean that they will listen to them or that they will not have their own explanations for what is going on. In this Piagetian stage, when children have a logic all their own, they frequently have their own explanations for why they are sick or why people are hurting them; it is common for them to feel that the more pain they experience, the "badder" they must be or have been in the past.

In terms of Fowler's stage, such children might project onto God all the meanness that they perceive in the people hurting them (albeit for their own good, which they cannot understand). They might be angry at God for not making them well or fear God, whom they believe is punishing them. They might refuse to pray. On the other hand, some dying preschoolers come closer to God and like to pray. Some have visions of God, angels, or loved ones who have gone before, who reassure them that everything will be OK. Even in their pain, some children radiate a sense of joy. Such children bring comfort to all with whom they come into contact. Why certain children are at peace while others are in turmoil is not understood, although the reactions of loved ones certainly plays a role.

Parents. Parents of preschoolers have much the same feelings as do parents of younger children. However, there are two important differences. First, parents can talk with a preschooler and can explain what is going on and why certain procedures are needed. This gives the parent a greater sense of competence.

Second, parents can listen to what a preschooler has to say, which wasn't possible when she or he was younger and could not yet speak. This is a mixed blessing, since the verbal preschooler might say things that the parent doesn't want to hear, like "I hate you, Mommy! Why won't you take me home?" "Daddy, why don't you make the doctors stop hurting me?" The ability to communicate back and forth means that parents have to carefully watch what they say, so that they neither lie nor tell the truth too bluntly. Preschoolers tend to have endless questions, which may wear their parents out and down.

Parents who believe in God might wonder why God doesn't answer their prayers or wonder if they are being punished for some real or imagined offense. They might question God's love, concern, and even existence, while at the same time needing God more than ever. They might be angry at God and everyone and everything that reminds them of God. They might resent those whose children are healthy and accuse God of playing favorites. Parents who don't believe in God might use the illness of a young child as proof that God does not exist.

Siblings. The reactions of older siblings have been described in the previous section on infants. Infant and toddler siblings of an ill preschooler will be able to detect that something is wrong, but they won't know what it is. Because of their limited ability of verbal expression, they express themselves behaviorally. They might respond to the stress by becoming more demanding, fussy, or clingy. They might not want to let their parents out of their sight. Their own routines of sleep, activity, and diet may be affected, placing even more demands on their exhausted parents.

PASTORAL APPROACHES

Ill preschoolers should be treated as intelligent beings. There is no need to talk to them as if they are still infants. Although one might use simple language in conversations with them, such conversations *should* occur. Questions should be answered as honestly as possible; simple, direct questions merit simple, direct answers. Responses to siblings should be appropriate for their developmental level, but the message that God loves us all and cares a great deal for each person should be given. This is true even though we don't know why certain things happen. Sometimes, children just want someone to listen to them. Because young children love to draw, if they are able, they might be encouraged to draw what they're feeling or "draw a prayer" for God, if they believe in God. When adversity comes, even many children who have never thought much about God will begin to pray or ask questions about God; they should be supported.

Parents can also be reassured that God is not punishing them or has ceased loving them. Parents need someone with whom they can talk freely. Not everyone qualifies for that service. Therefore, before asking clergy or members of their congregation to visit, parents should always be asked if this would be helpful. Some parents will welcome such visits, and some will not. When parents don't believe in God, one can give them the gift of compassionate presence, without judging their belief system. This is not the time to convert them or "set them straight." Such attitudes might be what led to their alienation from church or God in the first place. Compassionate listening as parents speak about their fears, questions, and sorrows might be the greatest gift they can receive.

Elementary School-Age Children

The Dying Children Themselves. Elementary school-age children have a daily routine outside their homes in terms of school and friendships. Unlike younger children, their friends are very important to them, and their lives center around the rhythm of a school day. Thus, when ill, they still miss school and the activities there; some dying children try to attend school up to the last days of their lives. Ill children also miss their friends and are especially hurt if their friends do not visit or maintain some kind of contact (e.g., phone calls, letters, and e-mails). Like younger children, they might react to departures of their loved ones in marked ways (e.g., anger, frustration, and weepiness)

Like younger children, they may react poorly to pain or to taking medications and may act out in aggressive ways, regress to behaviors more typical of younger children, or cry inconsolably. However, unlike younger children, they understand the permanence of death and can more readily accept logical explanations for illnesses. Naturally, this ability evolves over time, and many younger elementary school children may still have a bit of magical thinking going on as to why they are ill. Dying children may believe that they are so ill because they ate the wrong foods, went to a wrong place, or disobeyed a parent. Furthermore, the sicker they are or the more pain they are in, the more likely they are to think that they *really* did something very wrong: a kind of cause and effect.

Children of this age are in the Piagetian stage of concrete operations; hence, they are usually very interested in the details of their illnesses. They may be very eager to see medical instruments, X-rays, vials of blood, and so forth, and they may like to hear about the gory details of procedures and surgeries . . . or even death itself.

Because this age group focuses on industry, they really believe if they work hard enough (e.g., eat the right foods, say the right things, and do the right activities), they can make their illness go away permanently. Hence, they are very disappointed when this does not come to pass. In fact, they feel cheated if they believe that they have kept their end of the bargain (e.g., taking all their medicine without complaining) and they are not rewarded with good health or just the privilege of going home, eating what they want, or going where they choose.

This dovetails with their understanding of God. God is a friend, and friends keep their promises and do things for each other. So, if God is a friend, God *should* help them. If the ill child prays for a cure and doesn't get one, he or she feels cheated, because he or she kept his or her promise (by praying each day), but God didn't keep his promise by helping out when most needed. The elementary school-age child is completely comfortable with an all-powerful God and an all-loving God; if God is both of these, then God *is* able to produce a miracle and cause an immediate cure. If God doesn't produce a cure, the child might believe that God is unfair, angry, punitive (for some real or imagined transgression), or doesn't love him or her. He or she might be angry at God and any person, place, or thing that is associated with God in his or her mind. If a child should ask, "Why doesn't God make me all better?" a good response might be, "I don't know; I wish that would happen, too. What do you think?" Such an interchange gives one the opportunity to see if the child has any erroneous ideas.

Alternatively, some dying children come to a real peace about their imminent death and even have visions of God, angels, or loved ones who have gone before them, telling them everything will be OK. This might even be true of children who have never before expressed a belief or interest in God. In their dying process, they grow closer to God and pray a lot. They may even bring a sense of peace to their parents, siblings, and other significant persons in their lives.

Parents. The reactions of parents described in the previous stages (anger, fear, frustration, helplessness, and hopelessness) may be present. A major difference between parents of dying elementary school children and those of dying younger children is that the former can have some very deep, significant conversations with their children, whom they have come to know over years. Both parents *and* children mourn the fact that they may not grow into adulthood, unlike the previous stages, in which the parents did the mourning but the children could not, because they were either preverbal or didn't understand the concept of "future." For example, the parent of a dying, bright fifth grader mourns the fact that the child's dream of becoming a doctor will never come true. Parents also mourn when their children are not visited or contacted by their friends; they feel deeply their children's sense of abandonment.

As described previously, questions of why doesn't God answer their prayers and grant a miracle cure may be present. Parental anger or disappointment with God can be stated or unstated. Elementary school children (and their siblings) can easily pick up on these sentiments, even if they are not stated.

Siblings. Reactions of both siblings older and younger than the seriously ill or dying child have been discussed previously. This stage is a little different, because the healthy and the ill siblings might be each other's best friends. Hence, the healthy sibling will keenly feel the weight of the sibling's illness and might experience a sense of helplessness, anxiety, fear, or anger when thinking about losing his or her best friend. He or she might wonder why his sibling is ill and not him. On the other hand, if there was a fair amount of friction between the two siblings before the illness, the healthy sibling might feel guilt about his or her health (while the ill sibling feels resentment over his or her illness).

He or she might also blame his parents for not taking better care of the ill sibling, so that he or she would not have become ill in the first place, or he or she might blame him- or herself for not being a better sibling; such reactions are not necessarily logical or reality based. Although siblings might be jealous of all the attention that the ill sibling gets (and even develop some symptoms of their own to attract their parents' attention), they are generally very concerned about their ill sibling and are willing to help in any way they can.

Children who believe in God may include praying in their coping mechanisms. Even some children who don't believe in God might "try" prayer to see if it will help; they might "bargain" with God, saying, "If you make him better, I'll always believe in you from now on." Naturally, the nonbelieving ill child might say the same thing. Children may pray a great deal for their ill sibling and will enlist their friends and teachers to do so as well. Their belief in God or in the power of prayer may well be shaken if the desired result does not occur; this may lead to anger at God, with a subsequent refusal to pray, attend church, or be involved in other religious activities. The death of a sibling may affect their faith for many years to come. This is especially true if the relationship with the ill sibling was a troubled one even before the illness occurred.

PASTORAL APPROACHES

Every child needs to be taken seriously, along with their fears, hopes, beliefs, and questions. If one doesn't know the answer to a question, it is perfectly acceptable to say, "I don't know; what do you think?" or "I don't know; whom should we ask to get the best answer?" Children need to know that adults are in solidarity with them, even when they don't have the answers. Sometimes, all children really need is the nonjudgmental presence of a caring adult. Children and their siblings should be reassured that God loves them, even though we don't always understand why God lets certain things happen. If they feel well enough, children might want to use art to expresses what's going on inside them. When adversity comes, even many children who have never thought much about God will begin to pray or ask questions about God; they should be supported.

As has been stated earlier, parents can be reassured also that God is not punishing them or has ceased loving them. Before asking members of their congregation to visit, parents should always be asked if this would be helpful, in terms of who is doing the visiting. When parents don't believe in God, one can give them the gift of presence, without judging their belief system. This is not the time to convert them, for such previous attempts might be what led to their alienation from church or God in the first place. Compassionate listening as parents speak about their fears, questions, and sorrows is what is most needed and appreciated.

Preteens and Adolescents

The Dying Young People Themselves. Of all the age groups discussed, dying adolescents have the greatest potential for emotional and spiritual suffering because they, unlike younger children, have a much deeper appreciation of what they are losing. Because they are in the stage of formal operations, they can place themselves in another situation or imagine a future very different from their present. They suffer because they know what they could once do (and what their friends can still do) but what they can no longer do and maybe never will do again. Similarly, they realize that they probably will not have a future like their friends will have, and they might not have a future at all. They also suffer because, in their age of wanting increased separation from their parents and families, they must depend increasingly on their parents for care, even performing the skills that they had once done for themselves, like toileting, bathing themselves, or feeding themselves. Although they love and need their parents, they may resent their increasing dependence on them, and so, they may lash out at them. They may both want and not want their parents around—*at the same time.*

At a time when friends are of the greatest importance, these adolescents may feel abandoned by friends who do not visit or make contact (usually because they do not know what to say or do). Frequently, they feel angry, cheated, helpless, and hopeless. They mourn the loss of their physical attractiveness and vitality, and although they want friends to visit, they may be too ashamed of their appearance to encourage those visits. Some may consider suicide, because the pain is too much, the future is too uncertain, or they don't want to suffer anymore; others may engage in risk-taking behavior to assure themselves that they are still alive and OK.

These children may experience a troubled relationship with God. They may ask God, "Why me? Why was I born if I was just meant to die before I got to do anything, to make my contribution to the world?" Of course, there is no adequate answer for such questions, but simply allowing the teen to express his or her sorrow and frustration, without judgment, is essential. These young people may question God's love, concern, abilities, or even existence. They may feel abandoned by God and may be angry at God and those people and things that represent God to them. Alternatively, their experience may draw them closer to God and to others. Like younger children, they may have visions of God, angels, or loved ones who have gone before them, assuring them that everything will be all right. Such young people experience a sense of relief and peace, and they positively affect all those with whom they come into contact. These experiences can even occur with teens who have never before expressed a belief in God or any interest in God.

Parents. Common parental reactions have been discussed at length in the previous stages. The difference for parents of teens is that they may consider their children to be friends as well as offspring. Thus, they are losing a young friend, one with whom they may have shared hobbies, activities, or increasingly mature conversations. Parents' struggles with God as to why their child must die is ever present. For some, this can alienate them from God and people, places, and things associated with God; for others, it draws them even closer to God.

Siblings. Common sibling reactions have been discussed at length in the previous stages. An important added reaction is that the dying sibling might be the oldest child, the one to whom the younger siblings look up. In such a case, they face the devastation of losing their role model, and they worry what might become of them when they reach that age. If the seriously ill or dying adolescent is the baby of the family, the older siblings might feel that they are losing a part of themselves, since they were there for the ill sibling's entire life and even cared for her or him when she or he was a baby.

For siblings who believe in God, their struggles with God as to why their sibling must die are ever present. For some, this can alienate them from God; for others, it draws them even closer to God. These older siblings might take their lead from their parents' reactions, or, alternatively, because of their own life experiences, they might have vastly different reactions from those of their parents. As with other age groups, even children and teens who have never expressed an interest in God before the illness may begin to speak about God or even to pray. This should be encouraged.

PASTORAL APPROACHES

Preteens or adolescents should be encouraged to express themselves and ask their questions; they *need* to feel free to do this without judgment or ridicule. Even if one cannot answer the question, it is acceptable to say, "I don't know; what do you think?" These young people want to know that they are not alone in their struggles. Sometimes, just being present is really all the teen (or even the siblings) really needs. Give that gift. Reassure all concerned that God does love them and that the illness is not punishment. Even though we do not understand why God lets certain things happen, we can be confident that God does love us and will give us the strength to endure. If the young person is up to it, encourage her or him to create art work to express her or his feelings, or to write down thoughts, with the assurance that they will be kept private.

For suggestions on working with parents, see Pastoral Approaches in the previous two sections.

Some General Guidelines for What to Do and What Not to Do

What to Do

1. Illness affects all members of a family, not just the obviously ill member. Take that into account in working with ill and dying children; their parents and siblings need concern, too.
2. Before visiting, find out how the ill child or teen looks or is feeling, so that you will be prepared when you enter his or her room.
3. Treat each ill child in an age-appropriate, respectful manner. Use the information in this chapter as a guide.
4. When visiting an ill or dying child, always greet him or her first, even if there are adults in the room.
5. If the child or teen you are visiting doesn't want to talk or doesn't want you to visit, respect his or her wishes.
6. Never lie to an ill or dying child or teen. If you don't know the answer to a question, say so and offer to try to find out the answer. Better yet, ask the child or teen what he or she thinks the answer is.
7. Permit the ill or dying child or teen to ask questions or to express his or her feelings without judgment. Physical injury or verbal abuse, however, is not acceptable . . . no matter how angry or frustrated the ill child or teen is.
8. Before praying, ask the child or teen if this would be OK. If prayer is welcomed, ask if she or he wishes to choose the prayer or lead it; many young people do.
9. Make no promises to an ill or dying child or teen that you cannot *personally* keep. He or she is experiencing enough disappointment in life already.
10. Above all, support the ill child or teen in the way that she or he most wants; this is true for the family as well. This means that you may have to ask what is most needed. Never make assumptions based on what *you*

would want. And finally, remember that it is not your job to cheer up ill children, teens, or the adults in their lives. Your job is to be there, to listen, and to do whatever is most needed that you are able to provide.

What Not to Do

1. Don't visit without checking first to see if it is OK.
2. Don't overestimate or underestimate a child's or teen's development.
3. Don't ignore a child or teen in order to speak to the adults present.
4. Don't make judgments about how a child or teen feels or about what he or she says.
5. Don't make judgments about the parents' care of their child or teen, or the medical care that is being given.
6. Don't take sides in disagreements between family members.
7. Don't offer unsolicited advice. Even when your advice *is* solicited, offer it sparingly. You might not have all the information to provide the best advice in a given situation.
8. Do not pray with the child or teen unless he or she says that it's OK to do so. Never insist on prayer or visits by clergy or chaplains for either the ill child or teen or for family members.
9. Don't reprimand ill children, teens, or their parents, who wonder why God permits illness or who doubt God's existence.
10. Don't forget the needs of the parents or the siblings. If you can't meet those needs, don't try. Suggest someone who can or, if you don't know who can meet those needs, try to assist them in finding out.

These are only general guidelines. For an in-depth discussion of working with ill and dying children, by age, and their families, see Fosarelli, P. (2000). *Whatever You Do for the Least of These: Ministering to Ill and Dying Children and Their Families.* Liguori, MO: Liguori Publications. For a more detailed discussion about praying with children, see Fosarelli, P. (2003). *Praying with Our Children.* San Jose, CA: Resource Publications.

6

The Healthcare Professional as Person

The Spirituality of Providing Care at the End of Life

DANIEL P. SULMASY

*A patient of mine was dying of breast cancer, and I performed a thera-
peutic thoracentesis to help with her dyspnea. I accidentally sheared
the tip of the catheter off within her thoracic cavity, and I was devastated by my error. After talking it over with a senior colleague, I approached the woman and her family and explained what had happened. I was sweating. My heart felt as if it had crowded out my lungs
and had taken over my entire chest. And then she said, "That's OK,
dear. You know better than I do that I'm dying anyway. It doesn't hurt
or anything. Don't worry about me. You just take care of yourself."*

*To receive that sort of forgiveness from a dying patient is a lesson
for living.*

Daniel P. Sulmasy

In the last century and a half, the health professions have enjoyed untold successes.
They can now offer help and even cure diseases that for the first 24 centuries of
Western medical practice could not even be imagined as treatable. They prevent in-
fections with vaccines and prevent tooth decay with fluoride. They supply hormones,
such as thyroxine and insulin, when patients cannot make their own. Antibiotics are
only a bit more than 50 years old. Healthcare professionals open people's hearts, fix
their valves and arteries, close them up, and not only do they survive, but these treatments now actually extend their lives and relieve their symptoms. They put people
inside huge magnets, bombard them with radio waves, and explore the inner work-
ings of their brains. They administer people drugs when their bodies are riddled with

cancer, and sometimes the cancers go away. Hippocrates couldn't have imagined this as being possible. Healthcare professionals now consider it routine.

Physicians and other healthcare professionals have put great faith in their own technological prowess. They have begun to harbor the belief that there is no healthcare problem that they can't solve. If they just do enough science, use enough machines, throw enough money at "It" (whatever "It" is), they can solve it. Cures for cancer, AIDS, and cerebrovascular disease are all just around the corner. They're just a scan or two, an enzyme or two, or a nucleotide or two away.

Health professionals are now fascinated with the dials, the machines, the switches, the injections, and the pills. They pull the levers. They have a pill for everything. Want to lose weight? Take a pill. Want to quit smoking? Take a pill. Want to feel happy? Take a pill. Stop going bald? Take a pill. Have children? Take a pill. Not have children? Take a pill. Live forever . . . ?

Patients want answers, and physicians write prescriptions. But what has become of the human person in the midst of all this? That question is too rarely asked. It has become almost trite to lament that the patient is no longer a person. The patient has become, for many physicians, merely a pretext in which to display their power.

All talk to the contrary is now dismissed as silly, anachronistic, idealistic tomfoolery. Patients are consumers—amorphous blobs of undifferentiated medical preferences. Physicians are the providers. They provide the power—the means of satisfying consumer demand. There is nothing very personal to all this. It's about supply and demand for gadgets and pills. And physicians have learned to make quite a good living behaving in this fashion.

So, physicians, nurses, and other healthcare professionals should be deliriously happy. But despite all the good news, despite the fact that they're capable of doing so much more for their patients than any of their predecessors, healthcare professionals are among the most dissatisfied of all professional groups in America today.[1]

Technology has begun to bite back. The burdens of iatrogenic illness grow daily. Most "buffalo humps" and "moon faces" are caused by physicians, not by pituitary tumors. More and more, patients feel imprisoned by the very technology that was supposed to set them free. The intensive care unit, the paradigmatic symbol of technological prowess, the place where physicians control the horizontal and physicians control the vertical, has become for many persons the symbol of the very worst fate that could befall them. Patients feel increasingly alienated from their healthcare professionals. They feel depersonalized and dehumanized, as if they were extraordinarily complex biological machines at the mercy of mechanics and engineers.

Increasingly, also, healthcare professionals themselves are becoming alienated from their patients and their work—viewed as mere expertise and technology. Looking through a fiberoptic scope and inspecting human colons a dozen times a day can become as boring as inspecting chickens in a poultry processing plant. Both are just applied science—the practical use of highly specialized knowledge.

Physicians are becoming increasingly cynical and bitter. Patients are often seen as burdens. It is easier to look at their X-rays than to talk to them. I know some internists who make their rounds at 6 AM, in part to avoid meeting their patients' families. Whenever anything goes wrong, physicians are quick to blame patients. In turn, patients blame their physicians. And patients also bring lawsuits.

Physicians have been knocked off their pedestals. Their expertise has been popularly interpreted as thinly disguised greed. Now physicians are only regarded as heroes on television. In real life, physicians are greeted with suspicion. People blame physicians for taking up 14 percent of the GNP. The response of insurers and the government has been to throw the lives of healthcare professionals into utter chaos, in an effort to control healthcare inflation.

In the setting of caring for those at the end of life, all of these problems are amplified many times over. Death beats its wings and fans the flames that engulf the dispirited world of doctors and nurses. The reality of death intensifies bureaucrats' complaints about healthcare expenditures in the last 6 months of life. The reality of death confuses patients, who view themselves as consumers, and death as an option they do not choose for themselves. The reality of death contradicts medicine's belief in its own omnipotence.

Many forces have converged to bring us to where we are in healthcare today. I believe healthcare professionals are nearing a point of desperation, caught in the crosscurrents of all these conflicting forces. Morale among healthcare professionals is low. But at the deepest depths of this maelstrom, despite the fact that its substrate is social, economic, and political, I believe the most fundamental element of this crisis is spiritual. The spiritual element of this crisis is especially acute in the context of end-of-life care. But from the smoldering ashes of Death, that obvious and ominous presence that sits right in the middle of the healthcare field, spiritual stirrings have begun to rise.

Clinicians know in their hearts that there is a better way to do health care. The gnawing feeling in doctors' and nurses' bellies when they return from work each night, in frustration with the system and with themselves, is not caused by *Helicobacter pylori*. The only source of satisfaction for their hunger is spiritual.

Spirituality

But if I am to convince any reader that the malaise among healthcare professionals is spiritual in nature, I ought to define spirituality. Many people equate the term "spirituality" with "religion." However, even though they are conceptually related, these words are not synonymous.[2]

In one sense, spirituality is the broader term. One's spirituality may be defined simply as the characteristics and qualities of one's relationship with the transcendent.

Everyone may thus be said to have a spirituality. One may call the transcendent "God." One may also live in relationship with the transcendent and refuse to personalize it or call the transcendent "God." Even if one explicitly rejects the existence of the transcendent, one still has a relationship with the transcendent, at least by way of rejecting it.

And so, even an atheist has a spirituality, because an atheist must search for personal meaning and value in light of his or her rejection of the possibility of a transcendent source of personal meaning and value. Many atheists consider themselves spiritual persons.

By contrast, a religion is a specific set of beliefs about the transcendent, usually in association with a particular language used to describe spiritual experiences, a community sharing key beliefs, as well as certain practices, texts, rituals, and teachings. Not everyone has a religion.

So, while in one sense spirituality is very broad, in another sense it is more specific than religion. Within every religion there will be groups of people who share the key beliefs of the religion and remain part of the community of believers, yet have slightly different ways of praying and other slightly different ways of living out their relationships with the transcendent. Ultimately, since every human personality is unique, every human relationship with the transcendent is also unique. Spirituality is therefore ultimately personal. Only persons can apprehend, question, and live lives that engage the transcendent.

What does any of this have to do with the practice of medicine? Abraham Heschel, the twentieth-century Jewish philosopher and theologian, once said in an address to the American Medical Association (AMA), "To heal a person, one must first be a person."[3] If they are committed to healing patients as whole persons, Heschel suggests that physicians, nurses, and other clinicians must understand not only what disease and injury do to their patients' bodies but what disease and injury do to them as embodied spiritual persons grappling with transcendent questions.

In the midst of all that is being written and said these days about spirituality and healthcare, it is therefore surprising that so little has been said about the spiritual lives of healthcare professionals. As Heschel reminds us, if physicians and nurses are to heal patients as whole persons, they themselves must seriously engage the transcendent questions that only persons can ask. If they are to be true healers, they must rediscover what it means for healthcare to be a spiritual practice.[4]

Illness, Death, and Healing as Spiritual Events

Illness is a spiritual event. Illness grasps people by the soul and by the body and disturbs them both. Illness ineluctably raises troubling questions of a transcendent nature—questions about meaning, value, and relationship. These are spiritual questions. How clinicians answer these questions for themselves will affect the way they help their patients struggle with these questions.

Illness is always a disturbance in relationships.[5] But illness disturbs more than relationships inside the human organism. It disrupts families and workplaces. It shatters preexisting patterns of coping. It raises questions about one's relationship with the transcendent.

Healing is often characterized as a "making whole." But I think it is more instructive to understand that healing, in its most basic sense, means the restoration of right relationships. What genuinely holistic health care means, then, is a system of health care that attends to all of the disturbed relationships of the ill person as a whole, restoring those that can be restored, even if the person is not thereby completely restored to perfect wholeness. A holistic approach to healing means that the correction of the physiological disturbances and the restoration of the *milieu interior* is only the beginning of the task. Holistic healing requires attention to the psychological, social, and spiritual disturbances as well.

The wholeness of persons includes the finitude that is part of human nature, and the relationship of all persons to this essential fact about themselves. Health professionals who are genuinely dedicated to healing patients as whole persons will facilitate their patients' grappling with these questions, especially at the end of life, when ultimate finitude is most obvious.

Aequanimitas

Clinicians often underestimate the healing power of their own relationships with their patients. Rachel Naomi Remen tells the story of a patient who kept asking for more chemotherapy, even as his cancer became so advanced that even he was certain that further treatment would not be effective.[6] He had just grown so to appreciate his relationship with his oncologist that he feared their relationship would end if the chemotherapy stopped. He feared the loss of his relationship with his oncologist more than he feared the loss of his hair.

A clinical attitude of cold, scientific detachment from patients breeds a spirit of alienation and deadens the spirit in healthcare. Sometimes physicians appeal, mistakenly, to Oslerian "Aequanimitas" to justify this attitude. But William Osler didn't quite mean this by the title of his famous speech. If one reads his speech carefully, one notes that he does recommend keeping calm in the face of adversity for the sake of the patient. And much of that is good. Patients do not want their physicians and nurses to turn into gelatin whenever they disclose bad news. Nor do they want physicians and nurses who are so flustered by circumstances in the hospital that they forget why they're working there—to serve the patients. But Osler was not prescribing a cold, aloof, detached, totally scientific attitude. What he actually wrote was,

> Cultivate, then, gentlemen (sic), such a judicious measure of obtuseness as
> will enable you to meet the exigencies of practice with firmness and courage,
> without, at the same time, hardening "the human heart by which we live."[7]

Today, Osler would understand that he would not be talking exclusively to gentle-
men. But his sentiments are essentially correct. The equanimity he urged physicians
and nurses to cultivate had more to do with the adequacy of their *attachment* to patients than with their *detachment.* He goes on to write:

> Curious, odd compounds are these fellow-creatures, at whose mercy you
> will be; full of fads and eccentricities, of whims and fancies; but the more
> closely we study their little foibles of one sort and another in the inner
> life which we see, the more surely is the conviction borne in upon us of
> the likeness of their weakness to our own. The similarity would be intol-
> erable, if a happy egotism did not often render us forgetful of it. Hence
> the need of an ever-tender charity towards these fellow creatures. . . .[8]

Osler's idea of equanimity was more about avoiding the temptation to blame the
patient than it was about maintaining one's distance from one's patients or preserv-
ing an icy coolness. This is interesting to reflect upon, because today there is an epi-
demic of blaming the patient. One hears frequent, sneering remarks from healthcare
professionals about "self-abusing patients." House officers complain that "Mrs. Jones
died on me last night," as if Mrs. Jones thereby somehow had been disrespectful to the
house officer. Many proposals for healthcare reform have included plans to tax ciga-
rette smokers differentially because they are consuming valuable healthcare resources
through their "sins." Osler's point was that the more closely we clinicians study our
patients, the more striking becomes "the likeness of their weakness to our own."

Recognition of one's own foibles is a necessary ingredient in becoming a good
clinician. The first stage in the process of becoming a good healer is recognizing that
one is wounded and in need of healing oneself.

Osler also meant a bit more by "Aequanimitas" than putting up with the foibles
of patients. He also reminds healthcare professionals that:

> It is sad to think that, for some of you, there is in store disappointment,
> perhaps failure. You cannot hope, of course, to escape from the cares and
> anxieties incident to the professional life. Stand up bravely, even against
> the worst.[9]

Healthcare professionals are often far too convinced of their own perfection and of
their own invulnerability. Doubtless, the system of training that physicians undergo

helps to foster thoughts of invulnerability. But these thoughts are delusional. The inevitability of the death of each patient ought to prove this. And delusional healthcare professionals are dangers to patients and dangers to themselves. Unless healthcare professionals are convinced of their own fallibility and vulnerability, they will either make serious mistakes, or begin to take out their angers and frustrations upon patients, or both. The virtue of "Aequanimitas" can only be cultivated by healers who know their own wounded nature.

It is easy to understand how this delusion of perfection and invulnerability develops. Americans, in general, lead very privileged lives. This is especially true of physicians. Donald Nicholl has observed, however, how bad this can be.[10] He notes the curious paradox that perhaps the worst thing that could happen to anyone would be to have perfect health, never to have failed in any endeavor and to have had all personal plans fulfilled, to be financially secure, to be warmly loved, and never to have suffered. Under such conditions, observes Nicholl, every one of us would become a monster. In fact, it is not precisely true of anyone. But the closer one's life comes to such conditions, the greater the danger of becoming a monster. And I'm sure that most healthcare professionals have known colleagues for whom this danger has become more reality than fiction.

Beatitudes

These are troubled and uncertain times for healthcare professionals. But it may be instructive to note that Jesus of Nazareth lived in troubled and uncertain times as well. To be a Jew living in Palestine under Roman occupation 2,000 years ago was to live in a time of uncertainty, doubt, suffering, change, and social upheaval. It was to people who lived in such circumstances that Jesus said, "Blessed are the poor in spirit; the sorrowing; the meek; those who hunger and thirst for righteousness; the merciful; the clean of heart; the peacemakers; and those persecuted for the sake of righteousness" (Mt 5:3-10).

I am told that the formulation, "blessed are you when . . ." is more literally translated as "you are in the right place when." In the face of the present turmoil in healthcare and the tremendous pressures of caring for patients at the end of life, this formulation may be a real source of spiritual insight. "You are in the right place" when all your patients die and no one else wants to have your job. "You are in the right place" when desperate family members demand cures you cannot provide. "You are in the right place" when the HMO utilization review official says the company will no longer pay for the care of your patient with intensive palliative care needs because "nothing is being done" for the patient. Paradoxical? Yes. Spirituality is full of paradoxes. What would happen if you were not there? Or fled to some other place? What other place would be the "the right place?" Where else would blessings lie? The "right place" is the place of blessing.

This spirit of the beatitudes must, of course, be tempered by realism and humility. Any healthcare professional who begins to think that he or she can do it all is not "in the right place." This is the greatest temptation for those who really do care—to think that it all falls on their shoulders. But the sheer mass of the world's sickness is far bigger than any physician or nurse. There is no such thing as Superman or Superwoman. The sociological crucibles from which the modern plagues emerge are quite beyond the reach of healthcare per se: injection drug use and AIDS in the inner city, and cocaine, alcohol, and inflammatory bowel disease on Wall Street. No individual can possibly fix all these problems. But like Dr. Rieux in Camus' *The Plague*, physicians and nurses have a choice. They can either flee or stay at their stations and do whatever they can do. No more can be asked of them. No less will be required of them. And in this experience, perhaps, they will come to the insight of Fr. Paneloux, who tells Dr. Rieux that through the experience of living through the city's plague, he has finally discovered the meaning of grace.[11]

Grace comes in the midst of the stuff of life. It comes in our struggles and in our triumphs, in our daily attention to what is ours to do in the midst of our hopeless inadequacy. Understanding what grace means is a lifetime's work. It is on his deathbed that the curé in *The Diary of a Country Priest* comes to the recognition, "Grace is everywhere."[12]

But while grace saves even those who are naive enough to think that there is nothing from which they need to be saved, we also know of those who find clinical life all too burdensome. Some are racked by cynical bitterness even before they come to the healing professions, driven by pride, greed, or parental expectations that don't fit their talents and personalities. Others try to *be* Superman or Superwoman and burn out. Healthcare professionals need to be attentive to signs of burnout in themselves and in their colleagues. And they need to be quick to intervene before it is too late. In this regard it is interesting that there appears to be an inverse relationship between burnout and religiosity among staff treating patients with cancer.[13]

I do not wish to imply, however, that these themes are relevant only for those healthcare professionals who are burned out. Even that majority who are managing to cope with the stresses of their work still need to acknowledge their wounds and look for healing and strength for themselves. All physicians, nurses, psychologists, social workers, and chaplains make mistakes. All fail. All have feelings of guilt that need to be dealt with. Almost all physicians have been or will be sued and will know the pain, doubt, and isolation that this brings. Healthcare professionals need to acknowledge these feelings of failure, inadequacy, guilt, and of being overwhelmed by the sheer mass of patients' needs. To suppress these feelings invites the danger of becoming unfeeling. Many need to unburden themselves. Some may even need counseling.

The holiness of the beatitudes is not about being perfect. It is about the courage to acknowledge imperfection. It is about the courage to act in the face of imperfection. It is about the courage to be less than superhuman and yet more than the irredeemable, dismal, rational maximizer of self-interest that some philosophers and some economists say represents the reality of all that human beings can ever be.

Recently, for instance, I had been told by a case manager that a 90-year-old woman with dementia who had been living independently was now ready for discharge, 12 hours after having been transfused (yet again) for another cryptogenic GI bleed. The house staff agreed. As often happens, when I entered the room as the attending physician, the picture was different from the description at the morning report. The patient was actively hallucinating. I went out to the nurse's station to stop the patient's hospital discharge, and when I returned to finish my exam, she was standing at the side of the bed urinating on the floor and not very steady. I held her up. The urine began to pool around my shoes. Tragically, she had enough insight into her predicament to say, "I'm so embarrassed, so embarrassed." I muttered, "That's OK. Don't worry. These things happen." The nurses came, and we eased her back into bed. I washed my hands and my shoes.

Later that night I reflected on that moment. Moments like this happen often in practice. I had walked into it. I had no anticipation of what would happen as I entered that patient's room, as I really can have little anticipation of what will happen when I enter any patient's room. At that moment I had felt helpless and impotent— trapped in an awkward and unpleasant situation. But I was given, in that moment, the grace to decide to treat this woman with respect—to recognize her value and her deepest dignity precisely when her value and her dignity were most in doubt. I was given the grace to reach out to her, for a moment, in a healing relationship—a relationship as imperfect and as partial as all of the frail humanity that physicians and nurses share with their patients. And later that night I was given the grace of reflection that helped me to understand that this moment had been filled with profound meaning. I came to realize that I had been in the right place that morning. I wept as I thought about her and about that moment. I am afraid that I am often ungrateful for the gift that I am given of having such moments in my life. The Divine comes to us, I am convinced, disguised as our professional lives.

To be a wounded healer is to be a physician or nurse who is present and receptive to the moments of grace that come one's way when one least expects it. It is to be holy, not by virtue of any saccharine practices or hypocritical pretensions of perfection. But holy by virtue of honesty. Holy by virtue of courage. Here. Now. In the stuff of it.

Barriers

Multiple barriers presently stand in the way of this "repersonalization" of medical practice as a spiritual enterprise. The present economic reconstruction of medicine is surely one of these barriers. The culture's massive denial of death is another.

The spirituality of medical practice must therefore begin with a frank acknowledgment of how much physicians are suffering today. Many physicians now long to be able to give the spiritual questions of practice their due. But too many find their efforts thwarted by demands to shorten the time spent with patients, fill out more forms, refer patients to specialists they have never met, and treat them with formulary-approved drugs they have never used before.

Yet no amount of economic transformation can alter the fundamental meaning and value of healthcare, nor can it ever eradicate the interpersonal nature of the healing relationship that begins when one person feels ill, and another, highly skilled and socially authorized, asks, "How can I help you?" The spirituality of medical practice at the dawn of the twenty-first century in America therefore demands great virtue—courage, hope, perseverance, and creative fidelity.

It is certainly not easy to be a healthcare professional today. But when all is said and done, physicians and nurses still touch patients in remarkable ways. The spiritual meaning of medicine will outlast all mergers, all managed care organizations, all Medicare and Medicaid cutbacks, all bogus accusations of fraud and abuse, all malpractice suits, all direct-to-consumer advertising for drugs, and all manner of profiteering at the expense of patients. If spirituality is real, it is real for times of trial as well as times of triumph. Money can't buy spirituality. And money can't make it go away.

How?

How might one cultivate a spiritual sensibility in medical practice that will be credible in the twenty-first century?

Personal Religious Practices

First, if one takes one's own religion seriously, one should begin to deepen one's spiritual life within that religion. Religion makes it easier to grapple with spiritual questions. One has a community of faith and support. One has a ready-made language with which to describe one's spiritual struggles and joys. One has practices and texts that can be starting points for a deeper exploration of one's own spiritual life.

Patients, particularly those at the end of life, struggle with all the big questions. What is the meaning of my illness? Why must I suffer? Is there anything about me that is valuable now that I am no longer "productive?" Is there anything of value about me that will endure beyond the moment of my death? What is broken in my relationships that I somehow feel called to fix, now that my body is broken? Can my doctor possibly understand what I am going through?

A physician or nurse or psychologist who has begun to explore these questions in his or her own life will be better prepared to help patients struggle with these questions. If one has a religion or some set of spiritual beliefs, practices, and traditions, that is a good place to start. Genuine religions don't give pat answers to questions that are so fundamental to the human condition. Physicians who have taken these questions seriously will not trivialize or dismiss the questions of their patients, or dispense spiritual bromides to those who struggle with the mysteries of being human in the face of illness and death.

Funerals

An inevitable question that arises for those who care for dying patients is whether to attend patients' funerals. I have done so on a few occasions.

The most memorable funeral I attended was for a woman with whom I had shared very frank religious conversations over the course of her terminal illness.[14] Her name was Wilda. She was a devout Episcopalian. I learned from her family the day after her death that she had specifically requested that I read the prayers of petition during her funeral.

Wilda had severe coronary artery disease. She had discovered that I was a Franciscan friar shortly after her left main coronary artery bypass operation. Several days after the operation, which had been highly risky and was at least initially successful, she told me that she had known that it would be OK. The night before the operation, she said, she had a dream that a man in a long brown robe and a hood had stood at the foot of her bed and whispered to her that it would be OK. And she knew it would.

Like many things in the spiritual life, this could have been a coincidence. However, if one believes that God is never absent from human experience, one's interpretation of the miraculous depends more on the way in which God's presence is made manifest than it does upon God's presence or absence. I do not believe that God was any more or less present to this patient than to any other patient. But my interpretation of her experience, and her interpretation of her own experience, and her willingness to share that experience with me, constituted the miraculous in that event. In any case, I was, of course, flabbergasted and had to share with her the fact that I was a friar. "It was St. Francis," she replied. "I knew it. I just knew it."

Two months later her bypass graft clotted and she was declared inoperable, and she began to experience a long series of small heart attacks. In that final year of her life, I was privileged to watch a woman of enormous faith and goodness face her death with the fullness of human dignity. We talked often about God, family, life, and death. She had not asked for suffering. She had not asked to become so dependent upon her family. But she did not flee from suffering when faced with the choice of either to love or to avoid love and the suffering love entails. She did not flee from suffering when faced with the choice of either to embrace life or to annihilate life and the suffering life entails.

Wilda's family rallied around her. When we decided that hospitalization no longer served any purpose, we decided together to treat her subsequent presumed myocardial infarcts with nitroglycerin and morphine at home. Her daughter and the hospice nurse probably treated three more small heart attacks at home in the last 3 months, until her long Lent came to an end at last. She died on Easter Sunday morning.

If I had not been asked, I guess I probably would not have attended her funeral. But that would have been a mistake. I needed to be there. And in her own way I guess she knew that. I needed to be there to mourn the loss not just of a patient, but of a spiritual friend—a holy woman who inspires me to this very day.

I don't really know whose funerals to attend or with whom to pray. I have no secret formula to offer other healthcare professionals. Perhaps I have attended too few funerals and prayed with too few patients. I know also that I have neither the time nor the stamina to attend the funerals of all my patients who die. But I do know that on certain occasions it is absolutely the right thing to do. It can be an enormous spiritual experience and a source of inspiration, even on those dark days when I am harassed by Utilization Review nurses and the 800 number of the patient's insurance company.

Personal Spiritual Practices

The second general way one might begin to cultivate one's own spirituality as a healthcare professional would be to begin to develop specific, personal spiritual practices in relationship to medicine. Given the way I have defined spirituality, this can be done even if one is not explicitly religious, but all the more so if one is religious. In neither case will this be easy.

Many healthcare professionals will complain, "I don't have the time." And it is also probably not a wise idea to have one's neurosurgeon floating away into a mystic rapture when she has her thumb in the left hemisphere of one's cerebellum. But there are ways. Steve McPhee, at the University of California at San Francisco, for instance, says that he takes just 10 seconds before he sees each patient. He takes 10 seconds to quiet himself, reflect, and to draw a few deep breaths. Ten seconds to re-mind himself that he is about to enter deeply into the presence of another person. Or, one may prayerfully remember one's patients at the end of the day. If one had the ex-perience, one can recover the meaning through such prayerful remembrance, even if it rushed by too fast to notice as it was happening.

This is how it happens for me. I find myself incapable of processing the spiritual moments as they are happening. The press and flow of clinical life is too intense for me to become conscious of its spiritual meaning while it is happening. But that meaning is there. I recover that meaning in prayerful reflection. It is through that re-flection that I come to understand what my dying patients have taught me about life and its meaning, value, and nexus of relationships. It is through that reflection that I come to understand how a family I might have met the day before had made their dying loved one's room into a sacred space—one wherein I should enter only after having removed my shoes. A space where what really matters has become clear; a space where the extraneous has been stripped away; a space where the fire of love burns pure in perpetual brightness.

One finds such spiritual spaces through reflection. The precise method one uses to get there is not important. Perhaps one might even consider keeping a spiri-tual journal of one's practice as a disciplined way to reflect and to cultivate spiritual sensitivity. The spiritual happens. Spirituality requires effort. Effort will be required to cull from one's practice its personal and transcendent dimensions. Or else one will have had the experience but missed its meaning.

Collegial Discussions

Third, one can find fellow physicians, nurses, and other healthcare professionals with whom to engage these sorts of questions. One has to start somewhere.

In some institutions, this has taken the form of evening discussion groups, get-ting together monthly to read a chapter from a book, or discussing scriptural pas-sages in relationship to healthcare among those who share a common religious text. This can be an excellent opportunity to bring disciplines together, uniting physicians, nurses, psychologists, chaplains, social workers, and even volunteers in significant sharing. At the St. Vincent's Hospital Manhattan, for instance, we have invited out-side speakers from a variety of faiths to discuss themes such as "Forgiveness and the Care of the Patient" or "Hope and the Care of the Patient," followed by case discus-sions, all attended by a variety of healthcare professionals.[15] The Intensive Care Unit at the Boston Children's Hospital holds a monthly "Death Rounds"—an interdiscipli-nary meeting to share feelings, hopes, beliefs, difficulties, and prayers around one particular patient who died that month.

What is the meaning of medicine, nursing, psychology, chaplaincy, or social work? What is the value of these practices? What does it mean to care for the dying? What does it mean for one's patient to die? What does hope really mean? What are right and good healing relationships about?

These are spiritual questions. They arise ineluctably for believers and nonbelievers—for all healthcare professionals who take both being a practitioner and being a person very seriously. These are not questions that are often discussed in the doctor's dining room, but silence can constitute its own conspiracy. We can learn from our patients and from each other. How do we deal with our fallibility? With death (our own as well as that of our patients)? Can we move beyond complaining about the pressures we now face? Can we see our work as service? Do we ever pray for our patients? Or pray about ourselves as healers? Have we ever experienced the transcendent in our work? Can such peak experiences sustain us? Is there any meaning or hope for us? Without talking about these issues, we might begin to doubt the fundamental soundness of our own spiritual struggles.

To heal a person, one must first be a person. The healing professions will never recover from their spiritual malaise until they realize this. I have the hope and the faith to believe that it is not too late.

7

On Sacred Ground—The Role of Chaplains in the Care of the Dying

A Partnership between the Religious Community and the Healthcare Community

THE REVEREND STEPHEN MANN

In my years as a healthcare chaplain, I have always felt that interacting with individuals during the most vulnerable (and arguably the most intimate) moments of their lives, as they face their own mortality, is a supreme privilege—an invitation to walk with them through the sacred ground of their own souls.

Rev. Stephen Mann

High Tech and Out of Touch

The senior resident on call for the Intensive Care Unit stood at the bedside of his patient along with about a dozen family members holding vigil in the room with him. He watched the patient's cardiac monitor flatline and then turned to the family and said, "I'm sorry . . . he's gone" and then quietly left the room. The family was dumbstruck as they watched the retreating back of the doctor and then turned to look at their loved one lying in bed, whose chest continued to rise and fall with each puff of air supplied through the bedside ventilator. Several family members grasped the patient's wrists and remarked on the pulse they still felt coursing through his arteries and the odd blip which still appeared on the heart monitor . . . actions of the left ventricular assist device, which had been surgically implanted earlier in the patient's stay. Others commented that his skin was still warm and dry, thanks to the warm-air blanket that had been in place for days to help maintain the patient's normal body temperature. "How can he be dead?" they murmured among themselves, "when he is still breathing, has a pulse, and is warm?"

The chaplain who had been holding vigil with the family excused himself and went in search of the young physician and found him at a computer workstation entering the time-of-death note into the patient's electronic record. "Excuse me, doctor, but would you please turn off the equipment in Bed 10?" said the chaplain politely. "The family is having some difficulty accepting Mr. Parker's death with all the artificial life support equipment still running." The resident looked puzzled. "Hhmmm, I don't know. I probably need an attending physician to authorize that," he said uncomfortably. "If you've already declared the patient dead, turning off the machines is hardly a complicated matter . . . and it would go a long way to help the family begin to grieve his passing," replied the chaplain. The resident sighed resignedly and returned to the patient's room.

"I'm just going to disconnect all these machines so you can all have some quiet time in here," he said to the assembled family, and proceeded to do just that. As soon as everything was turned off, a chorus of sobs and wails from the grieving family members filled the cubicle. The resident gave the chaplain a look that seemed to say, "See what you made me do?" and then left again quickly to finish up his paperwork, clearly distressed at the display of emotion by the family.

The Newest Flower in God's Garden

The family had been camped out in the Pediatric Intensive Care Unit for days since 7-year-old Shanelle had been brought in with severe burns covering almost 85% of her small body. Several score of family members, neighbors, and friends had been coming in regularly to offer support to Shanelle's parents during her struggle for life. The family's pastor, Rev. Wilson, a respected minister in a large urban congregation, had been in the hospital a number of times, and when another member of his congregation had called to say that Shanelle was not expected to live out the day, he went immediately to lend spiritual support to Shanelle's parents, who were longtime members of his congregation.

With Shanelle's parents, grandparents, and an aunt and uncle seated around the table in the unit's conference room, along with Rev. Wilson and the Pediatric Chaplain, the Pediatric Intensivist compassionately informed everyone that despite all his best efforts, Shanelle had regretfully died. Expressing his own sorrow as the parents wept, tears streaming down his own face, the physician simply hugged both parents and waited patiently until Shanelle's father asked if they could go be with her for awhile, to which the doctor nodded his assent wordlessly and led everyone back to the little girl's bedside.

At the bedside, the patient's father said, "OK, preacher, I guess it's time for a prayer," indicating Rev. Wilson. Their congregational minister then prayed an eloquent and pious prayer affirming the sovereignty and majesty of God and God's loving care for all God's children. After concluding the prayer, the long-time pastor turned to the grieving parents and repeated a phrase he had apparently used to great effect during many a funeral service in the past. "God has just added Shanelle as another flower in the heavenly garden," he said softly, and was completely unprepared for the reaction he received from Shanelle's father, who grabbed the startled preacher by his lapels and shouted into his face. "Why did God have to take my baby girl? He's got lots of children, and I just had Shanelle. It's just not fair!"

Finding Joy in Strange Places

The physicians, nurses, and chaplain in the neurocritical care unit had worked together with a number of family members whose loved one was heading down the path to brain death. They knew many families had difficulty understanding how the concept of brain death was different from coma, and that brain death, as far as medicine and law were concerned, meant that their loved one was just as dead as if his or her heart had stopped. Only their heart hadn't stopped yet. And the fact that federal and state law dictated that the family members of the dying patient had to be offered the option of organ donation only confused the issue even more for some. The healthcare team was prepared for emotional turmoil such situations occasioned upon families— the shock, the anger, and the grief—but they were somewhat surprised by the laughter.

The patient was an older African American woman who had suffered a number of severe strokes that were rapidly depleting her brain of needed blood and functioning. This was a woman who had a number of children and grandchildren, but who had moved into a lesbian relationship late in life, occasioning a considerable amount of controversy among the extended family. But following the family conference, when everyone had been told about her grim prognosis and the certainty of brain death, within a few hours everyone had acknowledged the inevitable and had gathered around the patient's beside until the final diagnosis could be rendered. And there, seated or standing around the patient's bedside, were the woman's longtime lover, a couple of daughters and a friend, each sharing a humorous memory or story about their dying loved one, accompanied by gales of laughter.

The woman had apparently been quite a character, very independent in her thinking and full of life and delightful mischief. She had lived a long and satisfying life and had kept lines of communication open between herself and family members who were uncomfortable with her chosen lifestyle (and had indeed been able to find some reconciliation with many of them over the years). She had experienced a whole host of debilitating medical conditions in recent years and knew she would probably be dying soon and had had a variety of conversations with many loved ones about her wishes when the inevitable came. The patient had been prepared, the family had been prepared, and they had cried their tears, and they knew that more tears would need to be shed later, but for the moment laughter seemed more important to share.

When the family was told about the confirmation of brain death, the woman's partner volunteered the idea of the patient being an organ donor, to the unanimous agreement of other family members. They all seemed to agree that the patient would like the idea that part of her would live on, bringing life to someone else even in her passing. And after the family left the hospital, the physician asked the hospital chaplain how all the laughter had gotten started in the patient's room. Somewhat chagrined, the hospital chaplain had to admit that it was probably his fault. "I just told them that she had been unconscious the whole time I had been on the unit and that I really didn't get a chance to know her. I just asked them to tell me about her, to tell me what she was like before she became so sick. Apparently, she was a very funny person," he shrugged with a smile, remembering all the stories her loved ones had shared with him.

The Importance of Religious, Spiritual, and Cultural Awareness in Care for the Dying

Although in practice these three terms—religious, spiritual, and cultural—sometimes get muddled together as if they were synonyms for one another—Irish Catholic, secular Jew, African American Muslim—it is instructive to tease apart the differences between the terms. The term *cultural* usually implies that set of beliefs, values, and practices arising out of the primarily secular community with which a particular individual identifies. Despite hugely different religious and political differences that may exist between Irish Catholics, Irish Protestants, and even Irish Jews, there is still a set of beliefs, values, and practices that are uniquely Irish and quite distinct from, say, English or American Catholics, Protestants, or Jews. In actual practice there may be a significant amount of overlap between one's cultural and religious practices, especially if an individual's culture borrows heavily from a dominant religious worldview, such as from Islam in the Middle East, Buddhism in the Orient, and Protestant Christianity in the United States, but for the purpose of highlighting the distinctions, the cultural perspective will be considered as the secular component of an individual's identity within their community.

The innate differences in the terms *religious* and *spiritual* are perhaps less obvious, and in fact the terms are generally used interchangeably, although there are striking differences in their meanings. Religion, from the Latin *religare* (to bind again) and related to the medical term *ligate* (to bind, suture), captures the essence of the nature of religions—to tie down, to codify and institutionalize a very particular set of beliefs, practices, and attitudes. One's religion is not simply Christian, Jewish, or Muslim. One is Roman Catholic or Southern Baptist, Orthodox or Reconstructionist, Sufi or Sunni. The nature of religion is to define a particular orthodoxy and to establish norms for a particular community of faith. Religion circumscribes how the community of its faithful members believes and behaves, what it does not believe and what it proscribes. It is important to remember, however, that even when an individual self-identifies with a particular religious tradition, he or she may not be strictly orthodox in his or her belief across the whole religious landscape of the tradition, or even if he or she claims such orthodoxy of belief, necessarily be consistent in his or her practice of those beliefs. Being Roman Catholic does not mean that every individual agrees with every doctrine coming out of the Vatican, nor does being Jewish mean that one follows all the dietary rules of *kashrut,* nor does the fact that one is Muslim mean that he or she necessarily refrains from the intake of alcohol.

The heart of spirituality, as with religion, is the quest for meaning in human existence, the purpose of individual and collective human endeavor, especially in the presence of suffering and death. But whereas religion seeks to circumscribe corporate boundaries within which such answers may be found, spirituality locates those answers within the individual. Spirituality, from the Latin *spiritus* (breath, wind), carries connotations that are almost the exact opposite of religion. Whereas religion defines community, spirituality defines the individual; religion binds and spirituality blows free. Religion establishes norms while spirituality takes on an idiosyncratic individuality. This is not to say that religion is bad and spirituality is good, or vice versa. There is a necessary dialectic nature between religion and spirituality, each needing the other as a correction against the excesses of rigid formalism on the one hand or solipsistic arrogance on the other. Individual spiritual practices (prayer, meditation, and rituals) may arise out of one's religious tradition or may be incorporated from other religious expressions, secular or cultural practices, or from familial practices—or perhaps may even be something entirely idiosyncratic to a particular individual. Spiritual practices and beliefs can even be completely divorced from any religious connotations whatsoever, as in a musician who finds meaning and solace through music, or a painter through art, or a gardener through the natural delight of growing things.

Each of these elements—cultural, religious, and spiritual—may play a role in providing solace and meaning for patients who are dying, their family members and loved ones, as well as for the various caregivers also involved in the dying patient's final days. In Western society, death is an event that occurs increasingly within a healthcare context: hospitals, long-term care facilities, nursing homes, hospice—even home hospice involves a variety of healthcare professionals helping to maintain the patient's care in his or her own home environment—and within the healthcare context, it is often the healthcare chaplain who is tasked with the primary responsibility of identifying the patient's religious, spiritual, and cultural needs and resources, but it is incumbent upon everyone involved in the patient's care to be aware of the cultural, religious, and spiritual elements that help the patient and their loved ones cope with the stresses of dealing with human mortality, up close and personal.

Sorting through All the Providers of Spiritual Care

Medical research, spurred in part by growing patient demand for the inclusion of spirituality and other complementary health services, plus numerous articles in the popular American media over the past 10 to 15 years, has highlighted a growing interest in religious and spiritual dimensions. This interest is seen not only in patients, who arguably have always utilized religious and spiritual practices as an important adjunct to clinical medicine in coping with disease, disability, and the inevitability of death, but also in clinicians and scientists intent on discovering what effect, if any, spiritual practices have had in promoting health, reducing the likelihood or severity of illness, or on the outcomes of patient populations with specific disease processes. The standards asserted by the Joint Commission on Accreditation of Healthcare Organizations (JCAHO) are now beginning to recognize the importance of religious, spiritual, and cultural awareness in the total care of patients and have begun to recognize the role of the healthcare chaplain in addressing the religious and spiritual needs of patients in healthcare settings. In addition, federal guidelines on the provision of spiritual care in hospice have been in place for many years. All this popular attention in an era of greater toleration of more traditional and less scientific approaches to disease management has created a plethora of allied health professionals who claim provenance over the inclusion of spiritual practices in their overall care of patients—from physicians, nurses, and social workers to physical therapists, massage therapists, and acupuncturists. Some practitioners assert, from one end of the religious and spiritual spectrum, that their practice is "Biblically based and Christ-centered" (to capitalize on the market among conservative, evangelical, and Protestant Christians), or "spiritual care completely free of religious bias" from another end of the spectrum, to cater to a significant percentage of Americans who may claim belief in God but remain disaffected from mainline religious denominations. Ironically, the clinically trained professional healthcare chaplain, whose primary professional role is to provide spiritual care to persons in the healthcare environment, is often overlooked as a resource for providing an individualized spiritual care plan appropriate both to the patient's clinical course and the patient's religious and spiritual history and perspective. Although the importance of spirituality is beginning to be recognized in almost all contexts in the healthcare arena, it has long been a standard of care most notably among dying patients, whether from acute trauma or from some other terminal disease process.

As a foundation, this chapter has asserted the importance of an awareness, on the part of all healthcare professionals, of the spiritual needs and resources of patients in the management of end-of-life care for patients and their loved ones but will attempt to parse out the appropriate roles for a variety of spiritual caregivers from allied health professionals and hospital chaplains, to congregational clergy and denominational lay visitors. It will also attempt to lay out some goals of spiritual care not only for the dying patient but also for his or her family members and loved ones, as well as spiritual care for other professional or lay caregivers involved in the care of the dying patient.

The Healthcare Chaplain's Training and Role in Spiritual Care

A professionally certified healthcare chaplain must meet a number of educational and training requirements. The person in such a position is usually ordained, licensed, or otherwise formally recognized as a religious professional in a particular faith community and endorsed by that community for religious work beyond the local congregation in a specialized healthcare ministry. The chaplain must have earned at least a bachelor's degree, plus an additional 3 years of graduate theological education (often a master's level degree, such as a Master of Divinity, Master of Sacred Theology, Master of Arts in Hebrew Letters, etc.), and have engaged in at least 1,600 supervised hours of clinical pastoral education. Such professionals meeting these minimum standards can be certified by a variety of professional organizations in North America, including the Canadian Association of Pastoral Practice and Education, the Association of Professional Chaplains (APC), the National Association of Catholic Chaplains, and the National Association of Jewish Chaplains.

The hallmarks of the supervised clinical pastoral education training experience include the integration of theology and the behavioral sciences and the ability to correctly assess and provide appropriate spiritual care in an interfaith and pluralistic context. The competencies required for certification as a professional chaplain typically include the following, among others (excerpted from the APC):

- The ability to understand and articulate relevant aspects of one's history and personality and the manner in which these are reflected in one's behavior and relationships;
- The ability to provide leadership in pastoral care within an institution and a community with diverse faith and cultural traditions;
- The ability to integrate the insights of theology and the behavioral sciences into pastoral care assessments and practice;
- The ability to describe one's model of spiritual assessment, plans of care, and demonstrable outcomes;
- The ability to develop a comprehensive program of services appropriate to the setting of one's ministry;
- The ability to discern and involve oneself with ethical issues relevant to the setting in which one's ministry is practiced;
- The ability to conceptualize and communicate theologically the meaning of the crises experienced by persons in the setting in which one ministers;
- Participation in programs of continuing education and peer review.

In hospitals and other healthcare settings, the primary role of the professional chaplain is often to identify patients' religious and spiritual needs and resources, while carefully respecting each individual's religious or spiritual orientation. Then the chaplain offers spiritual care and support consonant with the patient's beliefs and practices or makes appropriate referrals to the patient's own religious community when appropriate, taking care not to infringe upon a patient's religious rights through proselytizing or otherwise violating a patient's religious or spiritual beliefs, rituals, customs, or practices.

With this specialized training and orientation, certified healthcare chaplains make it their mission to assess and understand the religious and spiritual language and worldview of the patients they encounter and to provide spiritual care and support appropriate to the patient's clinical and spiritual context, including emotional and spiritual support for patients who may view themselves as agnostic or atheist. The healthcare chaplain is also often a full-fledged member of the patient's healthcare team, working side by side with physicians, nurses, social workers, psychologists, and other allied healthcare professionals, and is involved in the total care of the patient, offering insights to the rest of the team members in providing care appropriate to the patient's cultural, religious, and spiritual background. Then, when appropriate, the healthcare chaplain's professional connection to the religious community also allows him or her to either provide or facilitate sacramental ministries, liturgies, rituals, customs, or practices requested by their patients, and/or to provide some liaison and education between the patient's congregational clergy and/or the patient's religious community and the healthcare environment around such practices.

Why the Need for a Certified Healthcare Chaplain?

There is a perception among some, both in the healthcare environment and among community clergy, that a healthcare chaplain is superfluous in addressing the spiritual and religious needs of patients. If a particular patient is religious, then having his or her own congregational clergy address his or her religious needs while hospitalized should be sufficient and perhaps even optimal; and if a patient is not religious, then there is no need for the services of a religious professional at all. Such arguments are simplistic and wrong-headed for a variety of reasons. In the first place, whether particular individuals have viewed themselves as religious or spiritual in the past, being hospitalized with a serious, potentially life-threatening illness, more often than not, will prompt an existential crisis. And whether a patient searches for meaning in such a moment through religious or philosophical means or cultural practices, the certified healthcare chaplain is trained to assist the patient using those religious, spiritual, and cultural modalities that are inherent in that individual's worldview.

Second, when the patient is a member of a local religious community, it does not necessarily follow that he or she would wish to have their own congregational clergy attend to all his or her religious or spiritual needs. For example, a Roman Catholic woman dying of cervical cancer may wish to receive the sacrament of the sick from her parish priest but may not wish to discuss what impact an abortion she had undergone as a young woman may have had medically and spiritually in her current terminal condition with that same priest, whereas she might be completely comfortable talking with a healthcare chaplain provided by the hospital. The healthcare chaplain would be able to alert the rest of the healthcare team about the patient's concern, enabling the medical facts to be explained and spiritual concerns to be addressed.

Third, even in those instances when a particular patient wishes his or her own congregational clergyperson to meet all of his or her religious and spiritual needs, that clergyperson may not be available or personally able to do so. While congregational clergy have many constraints upon their time and availability, a healthcare chaplain is frequently available to patient emergencies 24 hours a day, 7 days per week, 365 days per year, including religious holidays. It may also be true that the patient's congregational clergy may be equally traumatized by their congregant's impending death if they have had a longstanding and close relationship with the patient, and may be in equal need of spiritual support, in which case the healthcare chaplain is also prepared to assist community clergy in any way that may be desired. In this same vein, the healthcare chaplain is also available as a spiritual resource to all of the healthcare team, helping them all, individually and collectively, in dealing with the natural grief reactions experienced by all caregivers of the dying.

The Congregational/Community Clergy's Role in Spiritual Care

While all certified healthcare chaplains must meet the requirements for ordination and/or endorsement within their own religious community, and although most congregational clergy do not necessarily have the extensive clinical training that certified chaplains have in addition to those denominational requirements, many denominations either require or encourage at least some clinical pastoral education, and other clergy may have natural gifts in caring for the emotional and spiritual dimensions of their congregations. Whatever the individual community clergy's training, gifts, or skills, a patient's request for religious support from his or her own clergy, or a member of his or her own religious community should be respected to the extent that such resources are available, and if healthcare chaplains are part of the care team, they can assist in marshalling those resources for the patient.

   While the congregational or community clergy may not have the same degree of familiarity or comfort in the medical environment, they often have a prior relationship with the patient or at the least serve as a reminder to the patient that they are part of a wider religious community, both of which often serve as a source of consolation and support to the patient. The patient's priest, pastor, rabbi, or imam provides a reminder of the presence of divine concern for the dying individual in the language, religious symbols, and rituals that are a part of the patient's self-identified religious community and often the well-wishes of other members of his or her congregation. In addition, the community clergy may be able to marshal supplementary resources from within the congregation to some perceived needs (e.g., additional volunteer caregivers, meal preparation, and transportation assistance) that may lie outside the bounds of medical care but may provide respite or assistance to the patient or his or her family. Bringing forward such religious and congregational resources are the foundational elements that community clergy always bring in ministering with the dying patient.

While all clergy do not receive training in behavioral sciences nor take advantage of clinical pastoral education, some clergy have natural gifts and talents in responding to the emotional and spiritual concerns of patients—but these skills cannot be taken for granted. Religious leaders may or may not have had coursework in theodicy (the study of God's goodness and omnipotence in light of the existence of evil and human suffering), but even an academic study of suffering does not prepare clergy for dealing with the crises of faith experienced by patients acutely involved in the healthcare environment. Barring natural gifts and formal training, otherwise qualified clergy may find themselves ill prepared to deal with the existential, emotional, religious, and spiritual emergencies that may arise in the context of a dying patient. Such clergy, when confronted with the unfamiliarity of the acute fear, grief, or spiritual doubt that can accompany a dying patient, may find themselves resorting to the quoting of scriptural passages, reciting platitudes or clichés, or drawing upon prayers, liturgies, or homilies that may not be entirely appropriate to the context (e.g., prayers for healing, funeral homilies).

The Congregational or Religious Community Layperson's Role in Spiritual Care

The role of a religious layperson in caring for the dying can be even more variable than that of congregational clergy, from those who have had no formal training whatsoever to those who have had some foundational training (e.g., through Stephen Ministry, a nondenominational Christian training program for lay visiting, which includes an introduction to active listening techniques) to the extensive training involved in the Roman Catholic or Episcopal deaconate, which require several years of formal study. Whatever formal training, or lack thereof, the religious lay visitor can still play a significant role in the care of the dying. On the most basic level the religious layperson can be a sympathetic presence and a reminder of the patient's connection to the broader community and the divine. Such an individual may also be the one more directly responsible for marshalling the congregational resources mentioned previously or be the individual who is able to offer such services directly (e.g., food preparation, and transportation). For example, in the Orthodox Jewish community there is frequently a group of volunteers known as the Bikur Cholim who provide Jewish patients (usually of any Jewish tradition, and not just those who are Orthodox) with Hebrew prayer books, refrigerators for keeping kosher homemade food, as well as Sabbath candles, challah, and grape juice for observing the Sabbath, all of which can bring comfort and a touch of the familiar into an alien and frightening environment.

The Role of the Healthcare Worker in Spiritual Care

Even while advocating for the certified healthcare chaplain as the gold standard for the provision of spiritual care for the dying patient, there are two aspects of spiritual care that should be part of the healthcare worker's role in caring for the dying. First is an awareness of, and respect for, the cultural, religious, and spiritual concerns and resources that patients bring to bear or require to help them cope with the reality of their impending death. This should be accompanied with a willingness to allow the patient or his or her loved ones to incorporate those beliefs, values, behaviors, and practices into the total care of the patient. Second is the ability of the healthcare worker to be a comforting, nonanxious presence while caring for the patient. Although these two aspects of spiritual care seem simple, they nonetheless can be a considerable challenge for physicians and nurses, especially if the patient is in an intensive care unit of an acute hospital.

The intensive care environment of a typical hospital is replete with a plethora of sophisticated high-tech equipment (e.g., cardiac monitors, ventilators, and left-ventricular assist devices), a variety of tubes and lines regulating the input and output of bodily fluids (e.g., intravenous lines, central lines, nasal-gastric tubes, and urinary catheters) and a mind-numbing array of pharmaceutical wonder drugs, all of which require a considerable amount of human monitoring and active intervention. There are just so many things that need to be done that the average nurse or doctor in such an environment rarely has the time to just stand still for the few moments it may take to be a compassionate and nonanxious presence and just listen to the fears and anxieties of the dying patient and his or her loved ones or to suggest that any cultural, religious, or spiritual resources they may find comforting could be incorporated into the care plan of the dying patient.

In addition to the time crunch experienced by healthcare professionals in dealing with acutely ill patients, there is also a motivational challenge. Doctors and nurses faced with caring for multiple acutely ill patients often find themselves drawing away from the dying patient to attend to those who may still have a chance for survival. Some of this pull may have an ethical basis in terms of triage or the allocation of scare resources, but there can be psychological reasons for such shifts in focus as well. Healthcare workers choose their profession in order to help people recover from illness and injury, and caring for a dying patient can be especially stressful for a professional who has exhausted all of his or her means for preventing the patient's death. Doctors or nurses may feel professionally inadequate, or responsible for the patient's imminent death, or may think that the patient or his or her loved ones may blame him or her, even if the care was exemplary, or he or she just may be uncomfortable around the dying patient.

Ironically, this drift away from the dying patient to others on the unit may actually precipitate the patient's or family members' feelings of abandonment. When there is nothing that can be done, it can often mean quite a lot to patients or their loved ones to have their nurse or doctor just be there, standing quietly at the bedside during clergy- or family-led prayer—which very effectively signals to the family, even without words, "I have done all I can do professionally, but I can still stand with you, person to person, with human compassion."

As modern medical science has advanced, along with a mechanistic view of disease and injury that offers a technological or pharmaceutical fix for every symptom, an awareness of the cultural, religious, and spiritual dimensions of life can be an effective corrective for such a reductionistic assessment of human pain and suffering. As an example, one family member of an African-American patient was given to loud vocal and physical expressions of her grief over her loved one's death, and the healthcare team wanted to transport her to the hospital's emergency room and have her medicated. The healthcare team's plan would have removed a loudly demonstrative person, who may have been disturbing other patients, family members, or staff, but would not have assisted the woman in working through her natural grief reactions. As an alternative, the healthcare chaplain suggested finding an empty room in a remote corner of the unit where the door could be closed and the woman could give full vent to her grief in an appropriate venue, attended by other extended family members and her pastor.

Awareness of the Sacredness of Death

Since all the armamentarium of modern medicine is arrayed against death in the effort to indefinitely delay the inevitable end of every human life, it is important to note that not all individuals view death with the same professional vehemence as the dedicated healthcare worker or the fear of dying we suppose of every patient facing his or her own death. For some of the elderly, for some who have struggled long with severe and chronic illnesses of whatever age, or for those whose religious faith points to some spiritual realm beyond the veil of death, dying may be seen as an opportunity for the end of struggle and pain or for divine and eternal rest in the presence of God and their loved ones who have died before them. Every dying patient and every family situation will manifest through an unpredictable maelstrom of emotions: fear, anger, grief, peace, joy, love, relief, silence, or laughter. Indeed, the full spectrum of human emotion is possible during the last months, days, and even hours of the dying patient's life. The experience can be traumatic, sudden, and tragic, but it can also be full, meaningful, poignant, and touching. The ultimate goal of spiritual care with dying patients and their loved ones is to allow the patients and those closest to them to share the full richness of that experience in such a way that allows everyone to come to terms with their loss and grief in a way that promotes a healthy expression of emotions and enables each individual to begin to find some helpful meaning out of the experience.

Despite the work of many who have added valuable insights into the emotional and spiritual efforts of the dying, every death is as unique as the life of the individual prior to the moment when it ceases. There is no single way that one can categorize the process of a dying patient, or the reactions of his or her family and friends, and reduce it to a simple algorithm and shepherd everyone through the appropriate steps. There is no one ideal for a "good death." Human life is less predictable than our theories of human behavior of the dying or grief-stricken might suggest. But one thing everyone involved in the care of the dying *can* do is to treat each interaction with the patient and his or her loved ones as a sacred event. In religious terms, the essence of the concept of *sacredness* is to set something apart from common usage for special and holy use. And without necessarily intending the religious connotations of that word, treating every interaction with the dying patient and his or her loved ones as something sacred, special, unique, and acutely intimate, if not exactly private, acknowledges that all of the dying person's caregivers are interlopers, voyeurs if you will, into perhaps one of the most profound moments of human experience. There are very few moments in life that present with such an emotionally charged atmosphere, radiating issues full of existential, spiritual, religious, cultural, and relational concerns. And to be included within that circle, at whatever level and for however long, is an awesome privilege and should be treated with all attendant respect. To walk with people upon such a journey is to tread on sacred ground.

PART II

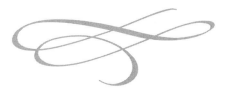

Theological and Religious Perspectives

8

A Buddhist Approach to End-of-Life Care

LOBSANG RAPGAY

Being with a dying patient, totally and completely, brief as it may be, helps us to be in the presence of death and dying in a deeply personal way, which has the potential of activating in us its constant presence. In being informed this way, we may value our daily experiences, both pleasant and otherwise, in a different way.

Lobsang Rapgay

For Tibetan Buddhists, life and death are seen as part of an ongoing cycle propelled by the power of karma—the law of cause and effect. The goal of each practitioner, therefore, is to untie the knot that binds him or her to cyclic existence. This chapter seeks to present the Tibetan Buddhist perspective that offers a rationale, experiential richness, and understanding in the area of death and dying.[1] This chapter will discuss the underlying principles of Tibetan Buddhism, which serves as the basis upon which death and dying practices are founded. It will also discuss the different practices during the various phases of death—the initial signs of death, the actual death phase, and finally the aftermath of death—and explore how many of these practices may be incorporated into present-day end-of-life care.

Buddhist teachings begin early, often at birth, in the life of a Tibetan Buddhist. The child is taught how to be compassionate toward all life by recognizing that every being is impermanent and subject to death. Such early training makes the child sensitive to how birth, sickness, old age, and death constantly play out in their environment, whether it is their pet becoming sick, the insect that is crushed, or the dying elderly neighbor.[2] Often stories and parables are used to reinforce the message. Many of the stories are centered around the Buddha's own life. One of the most powerful stories often told is about a day when Buddha entered a village as he and his disciples traveled from town to town, never staying at any one too long. A middle-aged woman came wailing up to the Buddha, crying out about the death of her only child.

She prostrated at the feet of the Buddha, pulling her hair apart, and in total grief said, "You are the Buddha, the Awakened One, you can do anything if you so desired, please save my child, bring her back." The Buddha listened silently as the woman wept. Finally, feeling deep compassion for her, he said, "Go to every doorstep in the village and see if you can find one family where death has not occurred, and when you do, come back with a mustard seed, and I will bring your child back to life." With great expectation and hope, the woman wiped her tears away and ran toward the first home. As she knocked at each door, she heard the endless sadness and misery of deaths that had occurred: of a father, a mother, a child, some sudden and unexpected, some after protracted illnesses. As she knocked at the last few doors, her hopes begin to diminish, and as she felt the heavy sadness of her pain return, she also became aware that there is no one who is free of death. Finally, with a heavy heart she returned to the Buddha, and as she reported that she had not found any family in the whole village who was free from death, the Buddha blessed her and patiently explained to her that death is an extension of life and that by accepting it can we find relief from our fears about it.

Practices and Beliefs about Death and Dying

When the novice observes that life and death are extensions of each other, just like the woman finally did in the story, he or she is then introduced to the formal practice of the nine cycles of death meditation. The intention is not to engage in a macabre preoccupation with death, but rather to develop a deeper recognition of death's eventuality and the need to acknowledge its presence in order to help us appreciate and live our lives more meaningfully. The practitioner begins by entering into a contemplative state of mind, to explore the three principal premises that govern death and dying. He or she meditates on the first premise in order to develop increasing awareness of the certainty of death, by looking for supporting evidence about the certainty of death as well as looking for evidence to the contrary. Once the practitioner finds evidence of the certainty of death, he or she meditates on this understanding for extended periods of time in order to integrate the realization into a conviction.[3]

Buddhists believe that insight alone does not lead to integration and that acquiring conviction about an understanding is critical for change. The technique of total concentration on the insight is the means by which conviction is achieved. Extended concentration on the insight for days and weeks results in a direct experience of the insight—described as being at one with the experience of that which is being observed and studied. Being convinced about death's certainty, the practitioner now contemplates its implications for him or her.

The above process of analysis and concentration is applied to the second and third premises, which are that the time of death is uncertain and only spiritual practice matters. A similar process described for the first premise is carried out, with the aim of acquiring convictions about these two subsequent premises. These convictions are then translated into daily living, by learning to accept death as it happens around him or her and by providing support to dying people as well as to those grieving for the loss of a loved one.

As the novice becomes more attuned to the play of impermanence, not only in death but virtually all human experiences, he or she is now introduced to an advanced training of death and dying practices known as the eight dissolution practice.[4] The purpose of this practice is to rehearse for death, a process conducted during meditation sessions. The practice is primarily designed for advanced practitioners, to help them activate a psychophysiological practice that involves control and regulation of autonomic sensory-motor activities as well as subtle mental and neurological activities during actual death, in order to minimize and eliminate all the negative processes of death. As a first step, the practitioner learns to identify both the gross and subtle psychophysiological processes involved during death. The training involves understanding how energies in the body sustain mental activities, becoming familiar with the physiology of the channels in which they flow. He or she then learns how a variety of factors can result in the cessation of these energies, resulting in the collapse of consciousness that signals the beginning of the death process. Such awareness of the functioning of the body during death is designed to help the practitioner to regulate these activities in order to facilitate the death process, which is conducive to spiritual practice.[5]

The Death Process

According to the Buddhist explanation of the psychophysiological process of death, the sequential dissolution of the energies that sustain the four elements—earth, water, fire, and air—results in final death.[6] Each of the elements of energy is associated with general and specific psychological and physiological functions, so that when the initial stages of death begin, these general and specific functions begin to deteriorate. During the first stages of death, the energies that sustain the earth element begin to gradually dissolve. The structures of the body that are primarily formed by the earth element—such as the bones, muscles, and so forth—begin to degenerate. The limbs become weak, the body loses weight and luster. The body feels as if it is sinking. The corresponding sensory organ of sight undergoes change. The eyes become weak and cloudy, with occasional hallucinations, and the dying person has difficulty closing or opening them. When the earth energy and the earth structures collapse, the water energy and its structure take over the lost functions. This cycle of elemental dissolution is repeated, and finally, after the elemental energies are dis-

solved, at the fifth cycle, the gross consciousness that deals with conceptual thinking begins to dissolve, while more subtle states of consciousness of white light, free
of gross conceptual processes, appear. This subtle consciousness eventually dissolves into a total state of vacuity and darkness, resulting in the person becoming
unconscious. In time, the dark vacuity dissolves into a clear state of emptiness. This
is the state known as clear light. Actual death, according to Buddhists, occurs at this
eighth cycle, not at the fourth cycle when clinical death occurs. It is believed that a
person may abide in the state of clear light for up to 3 days. Final death is determined
when there is discharge from the orifices. Understanding the psychophysiology of
death is critical to dying well, according to Tibetan Buddhism. By rehearsing during
life, dying becomes more familiar, easier to monitor, and therefore, contains the uncertainty of the changes that take place, as well as facilitates the appropriate cogni-
tion, affect, and spiritual behavior during each of the psychophysiological changes.[7]

As a staff psychologist at UCLA, I was consulted by the psychiatry department
to talk to a Hispanic family whose adult son was in a coma, dying from a major liver
disease. For weeks the family conducted a 24-hour vigil by his bedside. However,
they did not know what to do and say when they were with him and dreaded their
helpless feelings of watching him struggle and suffer. I explained to them that their
son was dying, and that changes in the breathing pattern and coloration of the skin
and lips are a part of the process. I also explained that there is a gradual dissolution
of sensory, cognitive, and motor functions, and that other parts of the body then com-
pensate for these losses. And though their loved one was in a coma and appeared not
to know or hear them, it is possible that if they held his hand from time to time, and
rubbed it in the more sensitive areas while they gently whispered to him, that he
might sense and hear them in his own way. The family began to do so and reported
how comfortable they now felt being with him through the long nights, knowing
that when he labored and suffered they could comfort and communicate with him.

Caring for the Dying

In order to provide care to a dying person, one has to first determine how conscious
the person is and whether the person believes in Buddhist principles and practices.
This differentiation helps to determine whether the individual is capable of conducting his or her own dying process. If the individual is unconscious, someone else may
help the person through the process. Furthermore, if the individual has any religious
belief, he or she is encouraged to utilize it, while those who do not have such beliefs
are simply asked to think positively about things they have done in their lives.[8]

Central to the dying process is the individual's personal spiritual teacher, who
plays a very important part in facilitating the initial phase of dying. He is often the

one who may let the person or family members know the time to begin the dying process and educate them on what to do. He teaches them the importance of dying peacefully and calmly and the importance of acceptance of death and how to work through their fears and concerns. The Lama also recommends specific prayers and rituals that may help the individual through this process, both symbolically as well as emotionally. One of the first instructions that the Lama may recommend is for the dying person to begin resolving family and material issues and conflicts, such as dividing up the family assets among the children, resolving individual disputes, and finding closure.[9]

Once the family concerns and disputes are addressed by the dying person, the Lama will then help the person and his or her family to begin the practices related to the dying process. The Lama will be consulted repeatedly throughout the entire process. When the final dissolution signs and symptoms begin, the Lama may recommend cessation of all medical treatment, since medical procedures during the dying process are seen as unnatural and, more importantly, a potential hindrance to the dissolution process. The Lama then instructs the family to set up a very quiet, spiritual environment in the home and to restrict the dying person to any exposure of major stress. The dying person, in turn, depending on his or her level of spiritual practice, is encouraged to engage in his or her personal practices within the context of the dissolution process and practice. At the same time, special prayers and rituals to facilitate dying are conducted by invited monks.[10]

Post-Death Practices

Once clinical death occurs, the appropriate rituals are conducted, and the body is preserved for a few days—averaging 3 days—to ensure final death. The cremation is conducted, and the ashes are mixed with clay to form the statutes of the deceased's personal deities. These statues are then distributed among close family members and friends, as well as placed in Buddhist holy cities all over.[11]

What Can We Learn?

What can we learn from these practices? The first is the need to prepare a dying person emotionally, physically, and spiritually for the process of dying. The second is the recognition and need to help the dying person first resolve his or her worldly conflicts and concerns before he or she can begin the dying process. Third, the dying person is educated about the various phases that he or she is likely to experience, based on the trajectory of the illness and the likely signs and symptoms that may occur at each phase, which helps the dying person differentiate between illness-related signs and symptoms and those associated with the natural dying process. Fourth, the spiritual minister and the family should be actively involved in the process. While the family's wishes are important to honor, the interest of the dying individual should be paramount. Consequently, if the family seeks to overlook important issues or concerns of the dying patient, the role of the minister and therapists is to help the family work through their fears and resistance to do what the dying individual seeks. Fifth, the goal—particularly when the dying person consents—is to facilitate the natural flow of dying, even at the cost of terminating medical care. Sixth, involve the dying person in planning his or her memorial.

What are some of the actual techniques we can use from the Buddhist tradition? Initially, listening to the individual and helping him or her to facilitate his or her thinking and expressing his or her feelings, based on his or her cues, are important steps. Confronting the patient or encouraging him or her to talk about his or her true feelings should be avoided. The task here is to facilitate the expression and completion of thoughts that the patient on his or her own has initiated. As an example, one can encourage the patient to complete a thought and identify the accompanying feeling. If feasible, appropriate sentence completion tasks may be proposed to the patient. When the patient begins to express feelings and thoughts more freely about his or her impending death, then explore if the patient acknowledges his or her impending death. If acknowledged, it is helpful to facilitate some challenges he or she may face. The challenges would include symptoms such as pain, dyspnea, functionality, and disability issues. One way to help the person process his or her issues around these issues is to mirror his or her subconscious thoughts verbally (after getting permission to do so). Another indirect, effective technique is to encourage the person to talk about how he or she feels regarding similar situations depicted in visuals such as photographs or movies, for example. In the Tibetan tradition, the wall painting depicting the cycle of existence, the 12 stages of the Buddha's life, and the personal deity of the person are placed in the room of the dying person to experience and reflect upon.[12]

Another important task for the dying person is to learn how to gradually manage and reduce noise and extreme stimulation, such as bright light. What is equally important is to plan a day-to-day schedule, by learning to pace medical treatment and care with rest, prayer, and TV. If the person is receptive and could benefit, it is also important to educate him or her about the potential physiological, psychological, and emotional changes that may occur over the course of his or her dying. The patient should be told about the processes and accompanying experiences and how best to deal with these phases. Often, breathing techniques can be used to facilitate rapport and connection with the other, by getting the permission of the patient to breathe like the patient and then asking the patient to also breathe with you.[13] Also, gazing into his or her eyes and their doing the same may be a wonderful way to communicate to each other. Touching, as well as whispering in the dying person's ear, is a another way to communicate, particularly when the patient is not fully conscious. It is equally important to let the patient know that he or she might have certain perceptions and explain to him or her that it may be normal when the dying process ensues to have such perceptions. I remember a professor who was dying from bone cancer who refused to be fed and would not respond or talk to anyone in the hospital. His young wife dreaded being with her husband and stayed outside his room. He was in constant agony from pain and could not lie down. I held his hand and began to place my warm hands on his pain area and very soon he began to relax. He gestured for the writing pad and for the first time communicated by writing down the words, "Why can't I love anyone?" I told him that he felt so alienated from others, and they from him. And because he chose not to communicate to others, they in turn gave up on him, and in the process failed to communicate to him by means other than words, such as by touch. Two days later he died.

Tibetan Buddhism shows us that death becomes more manageable when we see it as a natural process in our development, so that we can identify appropriate tasks to address when we are dying.[14] It is both an individual as well as a family process of letting go.

9

Spirituality in End-of-Life Care from a Catholic Perspective

Reflections of a Hospital Chaplain

MARY LOU O'GORMAN

David was 86, married, the father of 8 children and grandfather of 20. Upon learning of his terminal diagnosis, he wept for a few moments and then, with an infectious grin, said to those who surrounded him: "It's been a great fight." As the afternoon wore on, he quoted poetry and a treasured verse from Sanskrit and even sang a familiar song. His actions calmed and comforted those around him, assuring them that he and they would be OK.

Like so many other men and women, David taught me that the human spirit has an awesome capacity to confront adversity and death itself. Courageous men and women are able to draw strength from personal, social, religious, as well as other resources in order to write the final chapters of their lives and to die with integrity and authenticity.

Mary Lou O'Gorman

Narratives

James

James was 75, married and the father of three children. After suffering with lung disease for 6 years, he was informed by his physician that his disease was now "end stage." Since his retirement, James and his wife Margaret crisscrossed the United States to visit their children and seven grandchildren. On one such trip to Chicago, James' health rapidly deteriorated. His son drove him back home to be closer to his own physician. On arrival, James was so short of breath that his son drove him straight to the hospital, where he was admitted. He was immediately placed on a ventilator and remained on this machine for 3 days. Later on the day of his admission, he was anointed with oil by the priest. James, a lifelong Catholic, seemed to draw sustenance from this sacrament, the Anointing of the Sick. While on the ventilator, his sedation was light enough to allow him to communicate by nodding and mouthing words, and he made it clear to his family that he was eager to be off of the ventilator. Upon being successfully weaned from the ventilator, James made the decision with his physician and his family not to be reintubated. His family gathered and remained with him as he slipped into a coma. Later that day, Margaret requested a priest be contacted to give her husband last rites. When informed that death was imminent, that no priest was available, and that the patient had already received the sacrament that she referred to as last rites, the chaplain invited the family to join in saying the Catholic Church's prayers for the commendation of the dying. The chaplain shared the prayer book with Margaret. When they began the Litany of the Saints, a component of that ritual, Margaret began to lead her children and grandchildren in reciting its words. Suddenly, all in the room sensed Margaret's commitment to assume leadership in the family, a role previously delegated to James, as evidenced by her interactions with her husband and children throughout James' hospitalization. Margaret's manner and the words of that sacramental ritual seemed to contribute to a sense of peace for all.

Joan

In a single visit with her doctor, Joan was informed she had ovarian cancer, was not a candidate for chemotherapy, and had only months to live. She was 63, married and the mother of five children. The news was devastating for her and her family. Nevertheless, after a brief period of feeling almost overwhelmed by grief and loss, she rallied to make plans for her living and for her dying. Joan continued in her support group for people with cardiac disease and exercised three times weekly with other members of that group. The group worried about her and struggled with the probability of her death because of her pivotal role in their group. She also maintained her position as a leader in Alcoholics Anonymous (AA) and seemed to see that work as her mission in the waning weeks of her life. Joan attended Mass weekly at her Catholic parish and received the sacrament of the Anointing of the Sick from her pastor. She celebrated her 64th birthday with her husband and a large group of friends but discouraged her children from coming to that event. Instead, she invited each of them to come separately with their families for a visit, so that she could have "special time" with each family. She relished those gatherings and the opportunity to let her children and grandchildren know how much she loved them. Joan spoke openly of her death, executed a will, and planned her funeral with her husband and parish priest. With a broad smile she reminded her family, friends, and members of her support group, church, and AA that life is "a terminal condition." She assured her caregivers that she was grieving and that she and her husband wept together "often." At her request, Joan died at home with only her husband at her side.

John

John had suffered from heart disease since the age of seven, when he contracted rheumatic fever. In his thirties he underwent successful heart valve surgery. By his early forties he could no longer work and began to draw disability insurance. At the age of 45, John was hospitalized for an unrelated surgery. His physician asked him to consider the possibility of a heart transplant. Initially, he refused. His wife and three daughters, ages 18 to 25, begged him to reconsider, assuring him of their love and their need for him. John acquiesced. He waited in the hospital for 6 months before he received his new heart. Eucharistic ministers brought him Holy Communion daily. This sacrament was a source of strength for John. The chaplains and Eucharistic ministers, along with his own pastor, became a significant part of John's support system during that long wait. During those months John spoke frequently of his belief that his suffering was redemptive, a way of participating in Christ's suffering on the cross. Nonetheless, John struggled with the question of "why" this was happening to him. He repeatedly asked his caregivers—his physician, nurses, social worker, and chaplain—why they thought "bad things happen to good people." The meaning and purpose of this illness seemed to elude him, and he prayed about this question daily. Nevertheless, a belief in God's care for him seemed to grow through the long months of his illness. Shortly after receiving his new heart, John developed complications, and a month after the transplant he died, surrounded by his family.

Introduction

As a hospital chaplain for 20 years, I have accompanied many people, such as James, Joan, and John, to the threshold, to that sacred transition from this life to another. It is a privilege to witness the courageous and often awesome responses to dying and to death itself. As the previous three narratives reveal, each person's approach to dying is as unique as the approach to living, despite a shared Catholic faith. This is true of all people, regardless of faith tradition, churched or unchurched. Ministry to people facing the end of life requires attention to that person's spirituality—that is, to the essence of his or her life, to that person's story. Caregivers consider the individual's sense of meaning, purpose, hopes, goals and values, significant relationships, religious and cultural beliefs. The care given is never prescriptive; rather, it is evocative and attentive to the "wholistic" needs of the individual.

Contemporary literature devotes considerable thought to the potential for a death that is "good." One description of the good death includes the following: attention to the pain and suffering of all involved; the honoring of patient's and family's wishes; and a quality of death "consistent with clinical, cultural and ethical standards."[1] Additionally, the formation of artful, committed relationships is also fundamental to dying well. I have observed the transformational power of those relationships to encourage healing and to embody the presence of the Holy, even in the midst of the "valley of the shadow of death" (Psalm 23:4).

This chapter will discuss the spiritual needs, both universal and particular, of people facing the end of life, as well as the needs of family members and/or loved ones. The introductory narratives, as well as additional vignettes illustrating spiritual needs, are the reflections of a Catholic hospital chaplain and are acquired from ministry to people of many faiths. The beliefs and principles of the Catholic Church in regard to life and death and the sacraments and rituals specific to the Catholic Church will be identified. Specific ministry to Catholic people at the end of life will be described. Also, this chapter will delineate the obligations and relationships essential for professional or lay caregivers, regardless of specialty, who are engaged in this specialized ministry of care.

Spirituality

All people are spiritual. David Elkins defines spirituality as "humanity's single unifying dimension." It is "a way of being and experiencing that comes about through awareness of a transcendent dimension. Spirituality is characterized by certain identifiable values in regard to self, others, nature, life and whatever one considers to be the Ultimate. . . . [It is] that which gives one purpose, meaning and hope and provides a vital connection."[2] Spirituality encompasses relationships with art, science, music, or literature. A person's spirituality is dynamic and evolves through a lifetime. It is broader than religion. All are spiritual, while not everyone is religious. Religion is a way of expressing personal spirituality, demonstrated through a particular discipline or system of beliefs, rituals, practices, or sense of service.[3]

Attention to spirituality focuses on the fabric—the essence or "stuff" of a life. As a chaplain, I believe that spiritual care engages and blesses the significant relationships of a person's life. These include relationships with an Ultimate (many call "God") and with others and the self. Spiritual care at the end of life provides an opportunity to reflect on grief and sorrow, successes and failures, hopes and fears.

The framework for understanding a person's relevant spiritual needs and making treatment decisions is constructed from the individual's goals, values, and wishes. Additionally, cultural norms and formal religious beliefs contribute to the spiritual care plan.[4]

As a chaplain, I have discovered that one practices spiritual care while engaging in behaviors as diverse as honoring commitments to patients, comforting families, and supporting one's colleagues. Spiritual care is the responsibility of all caregivers and must not be delegated to the designated spiritual care provider, the chaplain or community clergy.

Spiritual care is always person centered, and its goals are the complex processes of integration and peace-making. When the nature of an illness precludes an individual from participating in planning and decision making, that person's surrogates may provide the only entrée to the person's story. "Family" may include one or more of the following: a spouse, significant other, children, friends, coworkers, or neighbors. Family is whomever the patient designates as family. In this chapter, "family" is used to describe those who provide support to the individual, regardless of relationship.

Spiritual Integration

Patient

In the face of life-threatening illness, the individual is faced with the challenge of integration. The goal of this process is to assimilate what is taking place and to organize the events that are occurring into a pattern congruent with the whole of one's life. This includes honoring significant relationships and commitments, exploring questions of meaning and purpose, engaging in relevant rituals, and making plans that flow from one's values and wishes. Integration also involves the difficult work of grieving and mourning the multiple losses associated with the ending of a life, a task neither time bound nor prescriptive. This process of integration may occur in hours or may require a lifetime. Integration is a spiritual process, providing healing, closure, and promoting a sense of dignity.[5]

I often marvel at the resilience of the human spirit. Daily, I witness the capacity of people to confront seemingly overwhelming experiences of adversity. Despite the implicit threats, they courageously engage in this integrative process: redefining purpose, ascribing meaning to the experience, and discovering a more viable hope for the future. In this section, I will discuss some aspects of spiritual integration for patients and their families.

The process of spiritual integration may begin with a diagnosis, deterioration of health, or on one's deathbed. One may begin to confront mortality when faced with a catastrophic illness, the exacerbation of a chronic illness, and/or when asked to make treatment plans or decisions about the desired level of end-of-life care. For Joan, described in the initial narratives, the knowledge that she now had cancer, in addition to advanced cardiac disease, propelled her to face death openly and to make decisions about how to spend the time remaining. Because of her cardiac disease, Joan had been keenly aware of her mortality. This new diagnosis convinced her that she could not waste time if she wished to accomplish her goals. For James this realization contributed to his decision to travel in order to spend as much time as possible with his family, who were scattered around the United States. For Joan and James, hope shifted from hope for a long life to hope for significant moments with their families. Joan also recognized that she could still provide a valuable service to others through her work with AA.

Many people find storytelling to be an essential component of integration. Reviewing one's life and reconsidering successes and failures provide opportunities to celebrate accomplishments as well as to acknowledge regrets. During John's 6-month hospitalization, his caregivers learned about those vital aspects of his life. It seemed to be therapeutic for John to share his story. He also discussed his more significant relationships and the meaning of each of those relationships. He reminisced about his associations with his family of origin, friends, former coworkers, his wife and children. This life review enabled John to see this illness in the context of a lifelong struggle with illness, to grieve past, present and future losses, and to begin to experience some acceptance of death.

Some people experience a sense of fulfillment in leaving something of themselves behind. One person wrote his memoir and died just after writing the last chapter. A man who had been a gospel singer recorded the songs for his funeral. A young mother made a video for her children to view when they grew older. During Joan's final visits with her children and grandchildren, she gave each a letter, sharing her gratitude for, and noteworthy memories of, her relationships with each of them.

Addressing unfinished business and mending broken relationships are aspects of spiritual integration. Joan found fulfillment in executing her will and making arrangements for her funeral. Life-threatening illness may contribute to a desire to make amends or to reconcile with a loved one. For one man with newly diagnosed lung cancer, his stated mission upon being discharged from the hospital was to reconcile with his son from whom he had been estranged for 12 years. Dr. Ira Byock summarizes reconciliation and farewell with what he calls the five last things: "Forgive me," "I forgive you," "Thank you," "I love you," and "Good-bye."[6]

Advance-care planning and treatment decisions are major components of spiritual integration. Most people make those choices based on desired quality of life, lifelong values and beliefs, and goals and hopes for time remaining. For James, discussions about reintubation led to his conviction that to be back on the ventilator would be intolerable. He was adamant in his communication with his physician and his family that he did not wish to spend his last hours or days on a ventilator. He did request medications for comfort so that he would not struggle for breath. Another person focused on dying at home. She apprised her family and caregivers of this desire and initiated contact with the local hospice herself.

Attention to suffering and pain, in all forms, is necessary for the individual to engage in integrative tasks. Symptom management requires an assessment of the individual's desired level of function and goals in regard to pain management. For example, one dyspneic patient may wish just enough sedation to be alert and maintain the capacity to communicate. For another, any shortness of breath may be intolerable and burdensome, thus requiring enough sedation to feel no pain. In my experience, commitment to symptom relief by caregivers may allow the individual to forgo unwanted aggressive treatment, such as mechanical ventilation, and make treatment decisions more consistent with lifelong values and goals.

Suffering is attributable to threats to personhood, to experiences that cause psychological or social disruption of the self and that place one's very existence in jeopardy. "Suffering is experienced by people, not merely by bodies."[7] I believe that suffering is essentially spiritual distress. Caregivers often hear this distress in the question, "Why me?" asked persistently by John. I believe that suffering is attributable to any one or more of the following factors: (1) experience of alienation, isolation, abandonment, and pain; (2) feelings of fear, dread, failure, hopelessness, helplessness, meaninglessness, and despair; (3) lack of closure or reconciliation; (4) loss of faith, dignity, purpose, independence, and control; (5) an inability to experience God's providential care and/or questions about the future after death; (6) concern for family; (7) economic concerns; (8) confusion; and/or (9) fear of pain or fear of deterioration. This is not an inclusive list.

Regardless of the religious tradition of the individual, a prerequisite for effective spiritual care is the identification of the causes of suffering and barriers to integration. With such support, one very distressed woman recognized her need to mend her broken relationship with her daughter and spend the time remaining getting to know her teenage grandchildren whom she had never met. A woman who had refused an amputation was encouraged to communicate to her family her fears of being a burden and of losing the remnants of her prized independence. Following a reassuring conversation, she agreed to move in with her family, who promised that they would respect her need to retain some responsibility for her own care. For a man whose feelings of hopelessness had been overwhelming, conversations about a previous crisis allowed him to recognize the sources of strength that had sustained him then. He realized that he could still count on those same resources—his faith and his neighbors. With the assistance of staff he contacted his next-door neighbors, who were eager to assist him, and he began to make plans to be discharged to his home.

For Viktor Frankl, the human being's ability to identify meaning and find purpose in suffering transforms that suffering and promotes healing. In *Man's Search for*

Meaning, he draws on his own experience in the death camp in Auschwitz and states, "Everything can be taken from a man but . . . the last of the human freedoms—to choose one's attitude in any given set of circumstances, to choose one's own way."[8] Grieving losses, addressing fears, exploring faith questions, recognizing sources of strength and viable hope, as well as finding meaning and purpose in suffering are critical factors in the alleviation of that suffering.

Referral to chaplains or other clergy assists those who suffer in confronting the sources of spiritual and emotional distress. Chaplains and other clergy are trained to address the painful and potentially fragmenting "why" questions. For John, in the initial narratives, verbalizing those questions and wrestling with the meaning of his suffering were therapeutic. He spoke of his life and expressed the belief that he had been a man of faith who had accepted the adversity of debilitating illness and pain. He also focused on the accumulation of losses he had experienced. As a young man John had found strength in the belief that "God would reward the good and punish the evil." Now he felt betrayed by the failure of that mythology. He looked for answers to this predicament and could find none. He turned to scripture and literature for assistance and eventually found comfort in prayer and an awareness that God is faithful and was indeed present with him throughout the complex course of his illness. His identification with Christ's redemptive activity on the cross evoked a sense of purpose and meaning for his suffering. John's almost daily dialogue with the chaplain was instrumental in his experience of healing and the attainment of some peace. No answers were given. Those conversations were characterized by nonjudgmental presence with an openness to, and respect for, John's struggle to make sense of what was happening to him and to find some meaning in his suffering.

Nonetheless, for some people, the journey toward death is one of disintegration, which may be the result of longstanding, unremitting suffering. Caregivers invite the sufferer to address concerns, always respecting the person's right to refuse that invitation or accepting that person's inability to respond. Recognition of the adage "people die as they live" is a reminder of the limits of the caregiving relationship. Caregivers must refrain from imposing their own beliefs or values or attempting to "fix" the other. Either action would be an abuse of power and a violation of the trust implicit in the caregiver's covenant with people who are the most vulnerable.

Family

Families engage in a similar process as that of the dying person as they assimilate and integrate the potential for the death of a loved one. Swigart and colleagues identify specific tasks and processes that facilitate "letting go" for families. These include obtaining and understanding information about the illness; seeing the illness as part of the patient's life story, and reviewing the patient's life to find meaning, especially in this illness; and attempting to maintain family roles and relationships.[9] I supplement this list with the obligations to address unfinished business and advocate for appropriate treatment. When these tasks are addressed, the family often experiences a sense of peace, as they come to believe they will endure as a family, that they have done what they could and that letting the patient go was the right thing.[10] This process allows families to honor their loved one as well as to promote that person's integrity and dignity.[11]

Many family members find it important to tell over and over the person's story and the story of their relationship with that person. This storytelling provides the caregivers with an awareness of who this person is and how they have lived. Storytelling may also be cathartic and provide a mechanism to grieve what and who is being lost and to verbalize the complex emotions associated with that loss. This sharing of memories may occasion celebrations of or the paying of homage to a loved one. Reminiscences often reveal significant aspects of the individual's life, including accomplishments, failures, an understanding of the individual's role in the family, and the nature of his or her relationships with the family. Communication might disclose unresolved conflicts or estrangement and opportunities for reconciliation and healing. During John's lengthy hospitalization, one of his daughters realized that his years of illness contributed to experiences of grief and loss and feelings of anger. The chaplain and other staff members assisted her in recognizing those feelings as well as her own need for healing and for addressing those feelings honestly and compassionately with John.

Often, grieving family members assume the decision-making role for loved ones who are impaired and unable to participate in that process. Such decisions are influenced by the person's previous expressions of wishes or goals regarding quality of life and functional capacity. If none are known, a life review of the patient may reveal what is appropriate and consistent with previous choices. Strong leadership by medical, nursing, and other members of the staff guides family members in making decisions consistent with the patient's values or beliefs. Conferences with the whole family provide an invaluable forum to discuss a loved one's illness, prognosis, and desired quality of life and to make decisions congruent with that person's values and beliefs. Effective person-centered decision-making facilitates the honoring of commitments and relationships and fosters a sense of peace.

Family members benefit from information about what to expect as death approaches. Apprehension can be lessened by explanations as to what happens when the body shuts down, reminding those present of the naturalness of the death process. Such knowledge and the assurance of attention to the patient's comfort encourage family participation in the dying process.

In a hospital setting open visitation is crucial and allows the dying person and family to maintain connection. Creating a peaceful environment may involve dimming lights, minimizing noise, or playing music. The presence of religious or cultural symbols may assist those present to connect with the power inherent in their heritage and traditions. Family members are to be encouraged to engage in comforting activities such as hand-holding, hair brushing, massaging the dying person, singing songs, and telling stories. Religious rites of the patient's faith tradition provide blessing, a connection with the faith community, and significant sources of spiritual and emotional support. Examples include reciting prayers, singing hymns, and reading scriptures. In addition to relevant religious rites, rituals following death might include bathing, or for one daughter (a beautician), cutting her mother's hair. One spouse who was a nurse participated in the removal of IV lines after her husband had died.

Being present may also promote the redefining of hope. Hope may shift from hope for recovery to hope that the dying person will be kept comfortable or will not die alone. As they engage in the tasks of letting go—making plans for the funeral, for the journey home, for the future—family members can begin to experience the hope that the family will go on and will not die with the patient.

These duties and obligations are the road map for the integrative work of the family and contribute to peace for all. A good death involves promoting the dying person's dignity while attending to his or her pain and suffering, supporting the family members in their grief and loss and addressing the spiritual needs of both patient and family.

Challenges for Caregivers

Compassionate, dedicated caregivers fashion effective relationships characterized by honesty, faithfulness, authenticity, and empathy, which support and facilitate the work described before. Such relationships require the capacity to listen deeply to the individual's concerns and feelings, to what is said and unsaid. Reverence for the mystery of that person is made manifest. It is in and through those relationships that life-giving connections are made and a sense of safety is experienced. These healing relationships may empower the individual to address necessary tasks and create wholeness and hope.

Effective communication is also essential. Skills in relaying bad news, in supporting feelings of grief and loss, and in assisting people to examine options and make necessary decisions congruent with goals and values are requisite for this process. With an awareness of how much the individual is able to absorb in any one conversation, caregivers share information about prognosis in language the patient can understand. "Tell the truth and tell it slant," advised Emily Dickinson.[12] Information is repeated, updates given, and questions are answered at significant intervals. Patients and families need straightforward communication about prognosis, including the potential for death, in order to engage in integrative work and prepare themselves for the future. These conversations must not be delayed until the patient is on his or her deathbed.

I have observed that the patient's illness and death may impact the spiritual life of caregivers as well as the patient's family. Being present with and providing care for the dying often results in a confrontation with one's own grief, frustrations, and questions of meaning. Paying attention to one's own spiritual and emotional needs, to feelings of unresolved grief and loss, and to signs of one's own spiritual distress is essential to participate in this sacred work. Engaging in spiritual practices enables the caregiver to maintain balance and to recognize the presence of the Holy in this challenging and rewarding work. Rabbi Abraham Heschel states, "To heal a person one must first be a person."[13] At the same time, healthcare institutions, whether acute care, long-term care, or hospice, must commit to excellent care at the end of life and to support those who provide that care. They fulfill this obligation through the provision of adequate resources and the creation of environments that address the needs of the dying and their families.

Relevant Catholic Teaching

The *Ethical and Religious Directives for Catholic Healthcare Services*, developed and promulgated by the National Conference of Catholic Bishops, are policy for Catholic healthcare services. As a chaplain in Catholic healthcare, I am aware of a continuum of beliefs and various interpretations of Church teaching about the end of life. The Directives provide an authoritative framework on Catholic teachings, including those about life and death. In summary, human beings are created in the image and likeness of God. They find meaning and fulfillment in and through relationships. Destined for union with God, the human finds complete fulfillment only in God. For Catholics, life is a precious gift of a loving God, but it is not the ultimate. God, the source of all life, is alone the ultimate. Human beings are charged with being stewards of their lives. Pope John Paul II stated, "Both the artificial extension of human life and the hastening of death, although they stem from different principles, conceal the same assumption: the conviction that life and death are realities entrusted to human beings to be disposed of at will. This false vision must be overcome. It must be made clear again that life is a gift to be responsibly led in God's sight."[14] Stewardship of life does not imply ownership of that life. Human beings are mortal and will die. Death is thus part of life, and life is preparation for death and eternity. The obligation to preserve life does not mandate needless prolongation of that life. Opportunity for integration and closure occurs as one faces the end of life. Death has the potential to be an active process validating the values and beliefs of one's life.

Illness and suffering are part of the human condition. For the Catholic, suffering may find meaning in relationship to Christ's suffering (Col 1:19-22) and has the capacity to be meritorious and redemptive. At the same time, human beings are not asked to become masochistic. "Patients should be kept as free of pain as possible so that they may die comfortably and with dignity, and in the place where they wish to die."[15] The use of medications to relieve and alleviate the pain of the dying is recommended, "even if this therapy may indirectly shorten the person's life, so long as the intent is not to hasten death."[16] The Church's teaching places a value on one's capacity to prepare for death and on maintaining consciousness in order to do that integrative work.

Decisions about treatment modalities carefully consider the value of human life and the purpose of the proposed intervention. Will their use result in the individual's capacity to strive for the goals of his or her life or the purpose of life itself? Each person is "obliged to use ordinary means to preserve his or her health. No person is obliged to undergo a procedure that the person has judged, with a free and informed conscience, not to provide a reasonable hope of benefit without imposing excessive risks and burdens on the patient or excessive expense to family or community."[17] Ideally, the person or those who know that person's wishes will make treatment decisions. Medical therapies are evaluated as to the potential benefit to the person and viewed as burdensome when they offer no benefit and serve only to prolong physical life. There should be a "presumption in favor of providing artificial nutrition and hydration," but this presumption is subject to the same benefit/burden of scrutiny.[18]

The Catholic Church recognizes the individual's choice to withdraw from life-sustaining technology. However, the taking of a life is never permissible. Withholding and withdrawing therapy with the intention of removing a burdensome treatment is not euthanasia (i.e., taking of a life). At the same time, insisting on aggressive medical care that will only delay death, not providing any realistic hope for recovery, is discouraged.

Catholic Ministry

Ministry to the Sick

For Catholics, the sacraments are a sign of God's presence. They provide connection with the faith community and are a source of grace and strength. The classical definition of a sacrament is "an outward sign instituted by Christ to give grace."[19] All sacraments derive their power from Jesus Christ's birth, suffering, death, and resurrection. The theologians at the Second Council of the Vatican (1962-1965) attempted to reclaim the relationship of sacrament to particular life experience and need.[20] As such, sacraments commemorate significant events in human life and "can be understood only in relation to one another as [an] effective memorial of the mystery of the Cross in the life of the Christian community."[21] The minister of the sacrament manifests God's love and acceptance.

For the sick and dying, frequent reception of the Eucharist provides comfort and strength and is a source of much-needed sustenance, as it was for John (described in the initial narratives). An ordained or lay minister may distribute this sacrament. In many areas of the United States, lay people, known as extraordinary ministers of Communion, make this sacrament accessible to the hospitalized and homebound.

For those unable to receive Communion, a spiritual communion may provide the recipient with a viable alternative. The recipient manifests openness to God's healing while life-giving presence, and prayer is offered for that intention by the one providing ministry. In Catholic hospitals the crucifix is often present in patients' rooms. The crucifix is a cross displaying a figure of the crucified or risen Jesus Christ. In other Christian hospitals a cross (without the figure) may be in evidence. People who are facing illness or death frequently speak of an identification with the "cross," articulating that experience as resonant with Christ's suffering or recognition of his love for them or an awareness that death will be followed by "more." These reflections are often associated with feelings of connection and hope. Praying the rosary may also provide comfort and peace. As my father-in-law was loaded into an ambulance, leaving his home for the last time and unable to communicate, he gestured frantically for his rosary. He had recited the rosary daily for many years and made it clear he did not want to be without it then.

The initial narratives allude to the significance of the sacrament of the Anointing of the Sick, once referred to as the Last Rites. Prior to Vatican Council II, this sacrament was called Extreme Unction. For many years it was performed only close to death, following a deathbed confession, and was thought to expedite the recipient's passage to heaven. Although the Catholic Church has never formally taught that anointing is a "free ticket' to heaven,"[22] that perception continues to influence contemporary Catholics' view of this sacrament as Last Rites, contributing to the tendency for the sick and their families to postpone its reception or to request it again at the moment of death, as Margaret did in the initial narratives.

Historically, this sacrament stems from the early disciples ritualizing the custom of using ointments as a therapy for healing. The New Testament text, found in James 5:13-16, provides the authority for this sacrament. In the rite itself, the priest states, "Through the apostle James, he has commanded us: 'Are there any who are sick among you? Let them send for the priests of the Church, and let the priests pray over them, anointing them with oil in the name of the Lord; and the prayer of faith will save the sick people and the Lord will raise them up; and if they have committed any sins, their sins will be forgiven them.'"[23]

Following the second Vatican Council, the Catholic Church attempted to reinstate the original intent of the sacrament, that is, an experience of strengthening and healing. Administered by a priest, this sacrament combines three functions: reconciliation, Eucharist, and anointing. There are also three components of the sacrament, each rooted in scriptural references to the ministry of Jesus: (1) a "prayer of faith" by the community for the sick person (see James 5:14-15); (2) a "laying on of hands" reminiscent of Jesus' healing action: "They brought the sick with various diseases to him; and he laid hands on everyone of them and healed them," (Luke 4:40); and (3) an "anointing with oil" as demonstrated in the disciples' efforts to continue Jesus' ministry, incorporating the pharmacological therapy of their culture: "They anointed many sick people with oil and cured them" (Mark 6:13).[24]

The sacrament of the Anointing of the Sick addresses the need for both physical healing and spiritual comfort. In the hospital it is offered, if possible, at the onset of an illness. An experience of grace, this sacrament provides the sick with reminders of God's steadfast presence and love while fostering a sense of well-being and wholeness. Ideally, the recipient ought to be alert and actively seeking God's healing and the courage to face illness through reception of the sacrament. The sacrament of the Anointing of the Sick should not be delayed until the individual is unable to participate. It is a sacrament of the living and is not given to the dead.

Sacramental anointing may be repeated when the condition of the sick person worsens or when the individual recovers from an illness and then becomes sick once again. Many Catholic parishes offer this sacrament during special services for those who are struggling with chronic physical or emotional illnesses and for the elderly or frail. The family and friends of the individual, as well as other members of the faith community, are encouraged to be present for the anointing. Whether in a parish or hospital room, this sacrament is to be celebrated within a community.

Ministry to the Dying and the Dead

Viaticum is the sacrament for the dying in the Catholic Church. It is the patient's last communion. Long neglected as a vital form of ministry to those facing death because of the emphasis on anointing as the last rite, an effort is underway to reclaim its role as providing food for the journey. Viaticum literally means "on the way with you" in Latin. The ritual includes scripture reading, renewal of baptismal vows, and an exchange of the sign of peace preceding the reception of communion. The words that follow reception of viaticum, "May the Lord protect you and lead you to eternal life,"[25] bless the recipient of this last Eucharist and provide connection with a familiar ritual at the core of Catholic faith life.

Viaticum does not require distribution by a priest and may be offered by a chaplain or an extraordinary minister of Communion entrusted with the care of the sick. People unable to swallow the sacred bread may instead receive a few drops of the consecrated wine on the tongue. Reception of this sacrament requires a degree of awareness and some capacity to participate.

Pastoral Care of the Sick: Rites of Anointing and Viaticum contains the rituals for the anointing of the sick and viaticum as well as prayer for commendation of the dying and the prayers for the dead. The pastor, chaplain, or lay minister may lead these official prayers of the Catholic Church, and family members are encouraged to participate. In the initial narratives, James' wife joined the chaplain in reciting some of the prayers for the dying as death approached. The Church's prayers comforted her and her family. The prayers for commendation of the dying provide an opportunity for those present to relinquish a loved one to God, to faithfully mark the transition from life on this earth to eternal life. The prayers for the dead are the designated ritual for those who have already died. Participation in the Church's rituals for the dying or dead provides comfort and hope for those present as well as a vital connection with those who have previously died, namely, the "body of saints" as they are described by the Catholic Church.

Hospital chaplains have created prayer services to be implemented at significant junctures, such as for decision-making conversations and for the removal of a ventilator or other life-prolonging therapies. Family members and caregivers may also employ various rituals to support the dying. Relevant hymns, scriptures, prayers, readings, poetry, letters, and blessing with salves or ointments or oils by loved ones serve as meaningful benedictions. These ceremonies pay tribute to the life of the individual and his or her significant relationships. Caregivers may assist family members in identifying and conducting activities that are meaningful. One family shared memories and reflections on their life with their father while each blessed his hands with oil. Two sons draped a quilt with a large purple cross over their mother as they prepared to withdraw the ventilator. That quilt had been made by members of her parish and blessed at the Sunday Mass. For that family the prayers of the members of their church and the reminder of Christ's redemptive sacrifice on the cross provided a much-needed connection with their faith and their faith community.

For another family, the recitation of the Rosary provided a link with a daily practice of their childhood. This meditation on the events of Christ's life and repetition of the familiar words of the Our Father and Hail Mary prayers filled the overwhelming silence with echoes from the past. It also reminded them of the strength of their family, as well as of their belief in Christ's salvific activity in their lives and in the life of their mother who lay dying before them. These rituals acknowledge the presence of the Holy, bless relationships, and foster a sense of security and continuity in the face of an unknown future.

Catholic parishes need to continue to educate parishioners as to the appropriate time for the sacrament of the Anointing of the Sick and the use of viaticum for the dying and to develop support services for those who are facing serious illness and death. Research reveals that 9 out of 10 people want to die at home.[26] Frequent communion, access to sacraments, and the connection with one's faith community are essential to the support of people at the end of life, for their families, and for those who provide care for them. However, parish resources are often stretched. Many parishes rely on deacons, parish nurses, and trained lay ministers to extend parish ministries to those who are homebound. Unfortunately, this practice is not universal, and those discharged from the hospital (after increasingly shorter lengths of stay) to return home to die often do not have access to spiritual or religious support unless they are hospice patients. Healthcare facilities and local congregations are challenged to collaborate in coordinating these essential services, thereby assisting dying people and their families in making this important transition.

Caregivers serve as midwives for the dying process. They skillfully strive to orchestrate a peaceful death while providing spiritual care that is respectful of the unique journey of each person and incorporating practices pertinent to that person's faith tradition. For Catholics, this healing ministry incorporates the Church's prayers, sacraments, and rituals. Compassionate caregivers provide expert leadership in addressing the individual's realms of concern. Knowledgeable about what is intrinsic to a "good death," caregivers of all disciplines collaboratively facilitate this sacred passage from life on this earth to eternal life.

10

Building Bridges
The Protestant Perspective

THE REVEREND NATALIA VONNEGUT BECK

*Ever since I can remember I have been privileged to 'listen' to
people as they proceed through their life journeys. I'm always
amazed—first, that they share so deeply and readily, and second,
how filled with strength and courage they are.*

Rev. Natalia Vonnegut Beck

A Collect for Healthcare Providers

*God, our Healer and Redeemer, we give thanks for the compassion-
ate care N. has received. Bless these and all healthcare providers.
Give them knowledge, virtue, and patience; and strengthen them in
their ministry of healing and comforting; through Jesus Christ our
Savior.* Amen.[1]

This chapter gives an overview of Protestant approaches to end-of-life care. Stories
of the dying and their caregivers show how different people approach the impending
dying process and issues that attend death. Each story illustrates a different type of
death experience and different experiences in attending the dying. Each instance is
different and will expose us to some of the issues that face us as we serve the dying.
In the Appendixes there is a sample of a series of documents that are imperative to a
preparation for death. Preparing these documents, having them notarized and placing copies in the files of members of the family, the physicians, and the church, can
save many hours of anguish, anger, and confusion. I encourage every member of my
congregation to fill them out. A certain Sunday in the fall and in the spring is designated to help parishioners prepare these papers.

    This introduction is a potpourri of ways to ensure preparedness to make the life
transition as peaceful as possible for all concerned. God has given us all what is nec-

essary to attend others and to prepare for our own journey. Often, in these times, we find it hard to realize that God is present. In the Christian tradition, we learn to rely on our faith. As Anne Frank said, "I believe in God even when I cannot see Him."[2] To best access the power that faith can bring, Christians prepare themselves in all ways possible to be open to God's never-failing presence.

Protestants, like most people, want peace at death. In the course of their lives, they have been taught about death and witnessed funerals and other rituals of death, but when death comes to them, they suddenly don't know what to expect and need help. Faith impacts the process, as do trust, the ability to endure pain and suffering, and knowing how to let go. However, many external factors can color the picture of death negatively: perceived and/or real physical and emotional pain; fear of abandonment by loved ones and friends; lack of information about self; low-quality hospital or nursing care facility, and lack of positive interaction with physicians and nursing staff, as well as the lack of a good relationship with clergy or spiritual advisors. These negative influences discourage dying patients and rob them of power and deny them the peace they so greatly desire. This is particularly true if the death is traumatic. In this day of great mobility, it is more imperative than ever that healthcare givers realize how crucial their role is in providing an anchor for the dying, so that they may combat these negative outside forces. Peace requires advance preparation on the part of the dying, especially concerning certain legal aspects and spiritual matters.

The words from the Burial Rite of the Episcopal Church's *Book of Common Prayer* sum up what most Protestants want to believe about their death experience—that the Lord is omnipotent, helps his people, will not abandon his people, and that believers belong with their Lord:

> I am resurrection and I am life, says the Lord.
> Whoever has faith in me shall have life,
> even though he/she die.
> And everyone who has life,
> and has committed himself/herself to me in faith,
> shall not die for ever.

> As for me, I know that my Redeemer lives
> and that at the last he will stand upon the earth.
> After my awaking, he will raise me up;
> and in my body I shall see God.
> I myself shall see, and my eyes behold him
> who is my friend and not a stranger.

> For none of us has life in himself/herself,
> and none becomes his/her own master when he/she dies.
> For if we have life, we are alive in the Lord,

and if we die, we die in the Lord.
So, then, whether we live or die,
we are the Lord's possession.

Happy from now on
are those who die in the Lord!
So it is, says the Spirit,
for they rest from their labors.[3]

For too long, the sacredness of dying has been a secondary consideration in this extremely important passage in life. The act of dying has largely been left in the hands of physicians and nurses. God knows the crucial part these healthcare givers play. But there is yet another imperative that has been largely overlooked—that of the spiritual well-being of the patient in transition.

Being very present with the dying is one of the most rewarding experiences, both for the dying and for the loved ones attending. Holding hands, massaging feet, and wiping the patient's mouth and lips are all acts of kindness and can give the patient a sense of being loved. Many Christians love to hear familiar hymns sung softly. Psalms and familiar sacred passages often initiate memories of warmth, caring, and belonging. I am always amazed at the response to the repeating of the Lord's Prayer:

Our Father, who art in heaven,
hallowed be Thy name,
thy kingdom come,
thy will be done
on earth as it is in heaven.
Give us this day our daily bread.
And forgive us our trespasses,
as we forgive those
who trespass against us.
And lead us not into temptation,
but deliver us from evil.
For thine is the kingdom,
and the power, and the glory,
for ever and ever. *Amen.*

People who have not uttered a word or shown signs of recognition for some time will try to mouth the words along with the attending chaplain, minister, or spiritual caregiver. Out of the depths of a soul still very "alive," in the spiritual sense, comes forth a response to the familiar words. Examples of some psalms which offer peace are the following: 23, 42, 46, 91, 103, 121, 130, and 139.

This time of preparation for the crossing over should be a time devoted to the needs of the patient. It is not a time for family and friends to pour out their woes on the dying. Rather, it is an opportunity for mindfulness and intentionality toward them. Stories with great meaning from the past, moments of joy or fun or intimacy, experiences that meant a great deal—weddings, birthday parties, reunions, secrets shared, occasions recalled—all of these are part of a sacred passage. It may seem that the person cannot see or hear any of these shared moments, but it is known that those who cannot respond *can* receive. Touch and reassuring words are almost always signs of love and affection that can be soothing.

Attending to the Dying

The sacred space in which the dying person resides can be filled with memorabilia, pictures, candles, a small altar, flowers, familiar religious pictures—any icons that were important to the patient are appropriate. What is *inappropriate* is to create an environment that is not familiar or important to the person. Too often, family and friends create such a space in order to satisfy their own spiritual needs. This can be abrasive and agitating to the patient.

Emotional response to the dying process is another integral part of care. If the dying person is important in the lives of the attendees, of course, sadness occurs. However, the release of these emotions needs to be done with some decorum. Certainly, crying is part of the sadness, but the tears should not be out of control. This is crucial, for I have witnessed times when the dying person fails to let go because he or she is afraid to leave the inconsolable alone. I have also seen times when so much love and caring are being given that the dying person will prolong the moment of passage simply because this is such a warm, wonderful time. If this inability to let go occurs, sometimes the dying hold on to life, just in order to see or hear the voice of one dear to them. If this is the case, I suggest the caregivers take a walk down the street, allowing privacy in the dying moments.

It is important to acknowledge the strength of the will of some as they are in the dying process. Caregivers, physicians, nurses, and hospice workers can seldom state a given time when death will occur. The will to live, even for the unconscious and those who have stated that they are ready to die, is amazing. Relinquishing life, even if painful, is not easy for some—and the last days or weeks may be long and exhausting. It is important to gather as many people as possible to take turns being present with the terminally ill person. It is far better to share the end times, so that each caregiver is rested enough to be intentionally present when it is his or her turn at the bedside. If the sharing of bedside care is not a possibility (and often it is not), then personal care for the caregiver is imperative. Some ways to accomplish this follow:

1. Use the relaxation response (a method introduced by Dr. Herbert Benson): This simple tool can allow for a quieting of the inside. Say a word, a phrase, or a prayer on the in-breath, such as, "Lord Jesus Christ has mercy on me," and "Thank you" on the out-breath. If other thoughts, words, or disruptions occur, simply disregard them and return to the breathing and repetition of the phrase on the in-breath and "Thank you" on the out-breath.[4]

2. Relax your body, beginning with the feet. Slowly squeeze the toes, move the feet, and relax the muscles of the legs, buttocks, abdomen, arms, hands, and fingers. Stretch your neck to the right, left, and downward. Relax your jaw muscles, wiggle your ears, and then blink your eyes in an exaggerated fashion. Shrug your shoulders and stretch your entire body.

3. Ask someone to put his or her hands on your shoulders for a few minutes. Breathe deeply and allow the touch to help you calm yourself.

4. Pray—not prayers of petition, but prayers of adoration. Examples are, "God, I love you," or "Lord Jesus Christ, thank you for being with me."

5. Write a story, a poem, or a piece of music. If you are attracted to some medium of art, bring the sketch pad or paintbrushes with you as you tend the one who is dying. One dear parishioner I was with for an extended time loved to read. I read a great deal to her, and when my voice tired, books on tape were a godsend.

It is a special art to attend the dying. It is a sacred privilege, but it can become an exhausting time. Self care becomes so important in order to serve fully. Following are several patient stories that illustrate rituals, beliefs, struggles, and triumphs experienced by believers facing the end of life.

Arturo's Story

The world rushes on over the strings of the lingering heart, making the music of sadness.[5]

Rabindranath Tagore

Typical late summers in Florida are very hot and very humid, and this Wednesday afternoon was no exception. I regularly set aside these midweek days for pastoral care: visits to the sick and shut-in, errand running, accompanying the ill to healthcare appointments, and so on. Visiting Arturo was always on my list. Arturo was barely twenty, tall, dark, and had been ruggedly muscular—a beautiful human being ravaged by AIDS. He had had it for 3 years. He contracted it on a risky one-night stand, urged on by his new teammates at a small midstate university. Arturo had been a stunning young athlete with a promising sports career. His situation in this day of technological achievement is tragic. His torso, covered with a sheet, was often wet with sweat and urine. He was basically a set of bones held together with a very thin layer of human flesh. Conversations with Arturo were limited at that point—mainly he wanted to know about the large wood cross that he held to his chest most of the time. How much did Jesus suffer? Was there lots of blood from his hands? What did his mother say? Did his friends desert him? Who was there with him? All of these questions, asked again and again over the days, held meaning for him. Arturo's mother, aunt, and siblings had left him to die—ashamed and embarrassed, they had not forgiven Arturo for his transgression and had given up all ties to him.

I had first met Arturo in an AIDS house in South Florida at a better time for him. He was well enough for a buddy to transport him, and he began to attend our church. The experience, brief though it was, did offer him some fellowship and an introduction to Christ, hitherto unknown to him. But, good as it was to have a piece of knowledge about Christ, it was also terrifying to him: "Christ died for my sins. I am so ashamed. Jesus should never accept me. I sinned in the worst way. My mama hasn't forgiven me. How could Jesus?" Thus his fixation on the cross. I had offered it to him, saying, "You know the cross experience—you are living it right now. Jesus knows that experience well. Perhaps you can consider sharing prayerfully about this experience." It was important not to take away Arturo's reality, but instead to try to relate it to a similar experience for Jesus. He felt comfortable about that sharing. It was a start in the process of preparing Arturo for death.

Time was short, and Arturo's pain level was getting higher. The medications to keep him comfortable had to be increased, and therefore short, focused periods of time were what I had to work with. The goal was to offer Arturo a strong listening ear, information that might release him from the terror of dying an unforgiven sinner, and possible reconciliation with some members of his family.

To approach the issue of guilt, we read and discussed scripture revealing the forgiving of sins by Jesus and the *acceptance* of that forgiveness by the "sinner." I used the story of Peter's discourse about forgiveness in Matthew (the 18th chapter), and the story of the tax collector, sinners, and God's will in chapter 9 of the same gospel. I made an effort not to persuade Arturo to a different vision of himself, but rather to point out interactions of Jesus, in whom he believed, with others who struggled with similar dilemmas. The scriptures seemed to relieve him some, but they were important in other ways. As a relatively new Christian, Arturo listened to the parables, the healing stories, and the crucifixion with deliberate attention. I spent much of my time simply reading and reflecting on the scriptures that he found powerful. Often his response to a reading was simply, "Again, please." At the end of our time together, Arturo would often reach for my hand and place it on the wooden cross with his. Quietly, I sensed there was a deeper sense of acceptance of what he was hearing and of himself.

The second challenge that Arturo faced was reconciliation with some family members. I made contact several times with members of his immediate family. Initially, they were hesitant to talk—however, gentle persistence opened a door to dialogue. Discussions revealed that, again, guilt was a major part of their rejection of Arturo, particularly by his mother. Guilt again had reared its head and caused a major rejection, first Arturo of himself and then Arturo's mother of him. To dissuade this feeling was more complicated in the mother's case, as faith was not apparent in her philosophy of living. Arturo's mother believed that somehow she had let her son down, that she had not instilled in him her view of morality. It was a weakness in her parenting skills that had caused this tragedy to occur. Again, it was important not to try to dissuade her from her image of what she had been as a mother, but to open her to looking at a larger picture. Was she the only influence on Arturo? Where did his school and his peers fit in his upbringing? Asking questions but not giving answers seemed significant. At this point in the dying process, it's important to open options to those who may feel alienated and to reassure family and friends that what they are feeling is valuable. The conversation *always* revolves around an easier death for the patient. In Arturo's case, he loved his mother and his sister and was deeply hurt by their rejection. Any facilitation I could provide to encourage the family to be present with him was crucial.

It took time and intentionality to open Arturo's mother to laying aside her feelings of guilt and spend her energy with her dying son. Ultimately, this occurred—both the mother and sister came to be with him in his last days. For Arturo, life and impending death had a sense of solace. He had found his faith and had received love from the mother he adored and companionship from his sister. He matured rapidly in the few months he had to live. His maturity helped him to come to his death in peace.

Several lessons can be learned from the journey with Arturo: (1) He demonstrated that forgiveness of self and other is an incredibly important aspect of the dying process; (2) He was able to release his guilt feelings, and this in turn led to new and deeper relationships; and (3) The ability of the caregiver to listen carefully and facilitate change is crucial in attending to the dying.

Forgiving

Of all inner transactions, forgiveness may be the most difficult. It means letting go, taking new risks, and sometimes forcing painful confrontations with ourselves and with others. At many points of crisis in the caregiving role, we may feel the need to be forgiven or to forgive. We may find ourselves faced with tying up old unfinished business, resolving conflicts, struggling to get through our parents' final days, or those of friends or even our children, and discovering that we may even feel angry toward the loved one who is leaving us. Even at the funeral, old hurts and tensions often erupt in anger.

In traveling around the United States in the last 10 to 12 years and talking to many people in many places, I have found that the issue of forgiveness is one element of our lives that is frequently misunderstood and mistaken. We need to understand

and use forgiveness more effectively. But the act of forgiveness, whether we are trying to forgive ourselves or other people, is a very difficult act to perform—it is not easy to forgive truly. To forgive is to understand wrongdoing, to release emotions, and to be ready to risk again—that asks a great deal of us. Forgiveness, however, is the core of the deepest, most fulfilling, most meaningful, and most giving kind of love. We must face the fact that, since we are human beings, real, honest forgiveness is difficult—very difficult, but not impossible. We tolerate most negative situations in our relations with others, but we don't truly forgive. It is ludicrous to throw the term around lightly; however, we say it all the time. I may laughingly say, "Don't worry about it. I forgive you." But when I say something like that, I really mean that I accept the reality of the wrongdoing. I accept releasing my fear, my anger, my ego needs connected with the act, and I cancel my demand that the person change. I work through the levels of anger and pain, challenging them over and over until the ability to risk and trust emerges. I resist demanding an ironclad guarantee that the behavior will not occur again, and I accept the possibility of action again and again and again.

Forgiveness is an act of passion, equally as important in the balance of life as love, faith, and hope. Actually, it's the integral element present in all three that enables us to grow, change, and find inner peace.

The process of forgiveness looks something like this:

1. See oneself and the other as having worth again, regardless of the wrongdoing. See both human beings as unique, beautiful people, even though limited.
2. See self and the other as equally precious again, in spite of the pain being felt.
3. Cancel the demands of the past. Recognize that changing the unchangeable is impossible and accept the reality of the present.
4. Work through the anger and the pain felt by both of you in reciprocal trusting and risking, until genuineness is perceived by both people.
5. Drop the demands for an ironclad guarantee of future behavior and open the future to choice, to spontaneity, and then of course to the possibility of failing again and being present with that person if failure occurs.
6. Touch each other deeply. Feel moved—warmth, love, and compassion. Celebrate it in mutual recognition that right relationships have been achieved. The right relationship may be no relationship at all, other than the acknowledgment of a friendship.

Remember that the bottom line of forgiveness is self-acceptance and self-care. If you choose to feel guilty and alienated for the rest of your life, you choose to stop growing, and you aren't really living. If you choose to forgive yourself and others, you choose to cope with life, to grow, to keep struggling, and to find new behaviors that will serve you in a more positive manner. Remember that forgiveness requires time, space, releasing grudges, confrontation, and a good sense of self-worth—a passion for life.

Now, in working with people and their caregivers at the end of life, what aspects do you see that you need to work on in the business of forgiveness of self and other? It might be helpful to ask yourself these questions:

1. Who still needs forgiveness in a particular situation: you or the other person?
2. What risks are you afraid of in this act of forgiveness? Are you afraid of more rejection, of seeming foolish, of being vulnerable again?
3. What action steps must you take to get yourself ready to be present with the other person openly?
4. What anger or persecuted feelings are you hanging on to, and what needs are those feelings filling for you?
5. What support do you need in order to face the pain of forgiveness, and where can you receive that support?
6. What new feelings of release and freedom can you imagine as you enter into the act of true forgiveness?

It has been my experience that it is far easier to forgive others than to forgive ourselves. Yet to forgive ourselves means we understand the frailties and foibles of others because we understand our own.

Joey's Story

Jesus said, "Let the little children come to me, and do not stop them; for it is to such as these that the kingdom of heaven belongs."[6]

(Matthew 19:14)

Joey was five, bright-eyed, and always moving. It was difficult to believe his recent diagnosis of leukemia. After receiving this news, life in Joey's household changed dramatically. The early months were filled with hopes rising and hopes dashed. As Joey's condition deteriorated, spiritual issues and questions became a mantra for his parents: "This isn't the way it was supposed to be. We are not supposed to have our child die before us. Why is God punishing us this way? We are faith-filled people. Why us? Why Joey? Lord Jesus Christ, have mercy on us—change this scene! Save Joey." From the depths of their faithful hearts came the pleading for mercy.

The death of a child carries a special trauma for family and friends. Nothing feels fair. Nothing seems right. Many Christian families feel abandoned and are angry. Still, many others believe and wait for a miracle. The whole issue of God's will and man's inadequacy becomes central. Caregivers and clergy involved in the situation need to listen carefully to what family and friends express.

Joey's grandfather was a minister. His parents were active members of their parish. The parish had a large, viable prayer chain that alerted the congregation to Joey's plight and gave regular updates on the progress of his illness. All prayers were urgent pleas for help, guidance, understanding, and a miracle. In fact, as time went on, the focus of parish life was this child and his well-being.

I had arrived at this parish just 3 months prior to Joey's diagnosis. At that time, there were some critical parish life issues to be addressed, but when Joey's illness became general knowledge, all the energy of the parish shifted to this tragedy. In fact, for many, the certainty of Joey's recovery defined their proof of faith alive. The questions posed by friends and parishioners had deep theological aspects: Does prayer really work? Is there a difference between healing and curing? Does God make the choice? How can there be faith and belief in a God that allows bad things to happen?

In Protestantism, there can be many answers to these questions, from a strict, biblically based theology to a broader approach to finding "the truth," which uses scripture as a historical base from which to build a faith orientation. In some denominations, many approaches may be present. In fact, in some individual congregations—while the parishioners may believe Jesus Christ is Lord and Savior—many find that beyond that, there can be a great divergence of belief concerning the acts of Jesus and the message he brings.

For the caregivers, it is important to remember the following:

1. The beliefs and feelings of the dying come first. This is not the time to educate or proselytize or allow others to do so.
2. Be as supportive as possible to all involved, with simple "I" messages, such as: "I hear you," "I understand," "I'm here to listen to your dilemma," "I'm sad for you," "I've thought about that," and "I find praying calms me. Would you like to join me in prayer?"
3. Silence is always welcome. The temptation to "deliver the answers" is great. When people are struggling with the hardest questions life can produce, seldom does any caregiver have all the answers for the dying person or loved ones. Intentional silence offers some good help. Here's why:
   (a) It does not interfere with the integrity of the person searching for answers.
   (b) If truly intentional, that is, offered with complete attention and caring, it can give time and peace for the suffering to find that which makes sense to them.
4. In addressing those trying questions about the power of prayer, God's helping us, God's curing, and a definition of God's purpose for us in suffer-

ing, stating the issues in terms of one's own experience is helpful. Some examples are as follows: When has prayer seemed to help you? How did you experience this help? Are you open to that sort of help again? What does healing mean for you? Are you comfortable knowing that one can be healed if not cured? Has God been with you when you felt healed, even though there wasn't a physical cure? Is it okay for you to be angry with God? I sense that you feel you must have done something very wrong for this to happen. I'm here to listen if you want to talk about it. What would help you resolve this guilty feeling?

In Joey's dying process, there were three distinct areas of concern:

1. Comfort and constant awareness of where Joey was in his spiritual journey.
2. Comfort and stability for the grieving family.
3. Being present with a congregation of caring people who had thrown their energies and faithfulness into the curing of this child, to the exclusion of all other community matters.

The art of dying—of making this transition—is a fragile one, and many outside influences that are beyond human control color the natural progression. My experience is that children face this crossing over with a simplicity that is refreshing. They cry when they hurt, they allow comforting, they are open to gentle touch and are grateful for attention. As they begin to slip out of this world, they do so with a special gentleness. Many times, they request good-byes with animals or friends, and when that has been accomplished, they are prepared to let go.

The pain of loved ones present in this journey is indescribable. Added to the spiritual questions heretofore discussed is the overwhelming sadness of losing someone that they have created. For them, the essential offering is for caregivers simply to be a presence in their lives. Trying to get them to be open to alternatives in their thought processes, or even defining issues for them, will most likely fall on deaf, pain-filled ears and will be lost. Helping them find plenty of time to attend to the needs of their child, keeping an orderly number of visitors—enough to be supportive but not overwhelming—and praying with them on a continual basis are helpful. Prayer is a powerful tool in this situation. It helps all involved to move beyond personal anguish into the reality of God's love.

Likewise, the grieving of a congregation can be complex. Aside from the very personal love for the child, the situation often gives people permission to dismiss the usual day-to-day issues found in any church. Instead, a real community has the best of each of its members working as a powerful team on forms of compassionate caring. It is important for clergy to honor and support this effort, while at the same time to bring to the congregation's attention the fact that all the work of the Gospel must continue. After the intensity that the death of a child in a congregation may bring, it is necessary to allow a congregation to mourn; in fact, clergy can lead them in that process. Then remobilization around other crucial issues can be gently reintroduced.

A word to the wise for caregivers and clergy: self-care is imperative at this time. A great deal depends on clergy being emotionally available. The fear that clergy may not be all everyone expects is very real. The answer to that is that perfection is not possible. I find prayer time and using the minirelaxation response often during the day to be lifesaving in these instances.

Lessons Learned

1. Presence is often the greatest gift to give.
2. It is best to facilitate the beliefs of the child and the loved ones, unless asked to give a theological explanation of why this tragedy is occurring. Later, the search for answers can become a more helpful exploration.
3. Encourage the congregation to be available but not overwhelming. Remind them that all energies need to be directed toward the comfort of the child and grief assistance to the family.

Anna's Story

God our Wisdom: Bless the decisions we have made in hope, in sorrow, and in love; that as we place our whole trust in you, our choices and our actions may be encompassed by your perfecting will; through Jesus Christ who died and rose for us. Amen.[7]

Anna's life systems had begun to lose their capacity to function normally. Heart defibrillation and other complications were leaving her weaker and weaker each day. Living alone at home was no longer a possibility—nursing care was needed. Anna's mind, although somewhat stretched, was clear enough to realize that changes were happening in her life—physically and spiritually. Major disruptions were occurring; at times Anna felt confused, and this confusion, coupled with her physical weakness, was becoming an issue that her family needed to address.

Fortunately for all involved, Anna had signed a living will, assigned a power of attorney, and appointed a healthcare surrogate. These documents provided a framework for an orderly, caring environment. (Sample copies of these documents can be found at the end of this book. Please use them as samples only, and refer to your local jurisdiction for help in putting together similar documents.)

Eighty-three-year-old Anna had four children. Two lived close by, the others some distance away. The initial decision to move Anna from her home to a nursing facility was fairly simple. However, Anna's condition deteriorated rapidly after that, and hospitalization was needed in a matter of a few weeks. The two children living far away were summoned to be present with their mother while she could still recognize and appreciate their presence. Enough medication was dispensed to keep her out of severe pain. When one of her daughters asked, "Mom, are you sure you do not want any resuscitation if that time comes?" Anna was aware enough to answer, softly but clearly, "No, I am ready to go." The hospital staff was reminded of this decision and the matter was settled—or so it seemed. However, one of her children was not prepared for this decision. He lived the furthest away and had not been available to spend much quality time with his mother in these last weeks. Even though he had been present when his mother reinforced her decision for a Do Not Resuscitate (DNR) order, he voiced that "she was not prepared for death," and it was apparent that neither was he. The doctor had advised them that she was slipping quickly and ordered the pain medications increased to keep her comfortable. The children and grandchildren were keeping watch over her. The one son was pacing relentlessly outside the door or in the hospital parking lot, talking on a cell phone, trying to obtain more information that would help him stop the process that was in progress. There were some clear issues here:

1. All the legal documents were in place.
2. Anna had verbally reassured her family of her comfort with this decision.
3. The hospital staff and physicians were following her wishes.
4. There was, however, a child who was uncomfortable with these decisions, for reasons not known completely.
5. There now was a split in the family; and
6. A dying mother who probably was aware at some level that her family was in disarray.

From a caregiver's point of view, Anna's mental and physical comfort must be the center of the caregiving needs. To expedite this, I asked the son to talk with me alone. In our conversation, I acknowledged his discomfort with the decision. He responded that he had not felt well enough informed by his siblings as to his mother's condition. He was angry, hurt, and defensive. After some discussion, I asked him if he would like some time alone with his mother, so that he could tell her of his love and caring for her. I stressed the importance of peace of mind for her, so no discussion of his anger toward others would be allowed.

He accepted this proposed time alone and promised to relay only positive messages to her. Although the three siblings were concerned that he might not keep his promise, they did leave Anna and him alone. I suggested 10 minutes initially and a negotiated extension if necessary. As he and his mother spent the time together, I suggested a walk for the rest of us. As we walked in the hospital parking lot, our time was mostly silent. There were a few moments when we recited the Lord's Prayer together. I prayed aloud for Anna and her son, that there be a good sense of closure and that the son could move beyond his pain for now and put his energy into fully expressing his love to his mother. At the end of 10 minutes, I quietly checked the room. At 20 minutes, I entered the room and prayed with the two of them. Although Anna could not say the words to the Lord's Prayer aloud, she moved her lips with us. That was a wonderful sign to the son that she had heard him. I asked the son to invite the rest of the family to join us. As the next hour proceeded, we sang her favorite hymns, told wonderful stories of remembrances, and finally Anna slipped away. In her faith orientation, a blessing is given and the holy oils are placed upon her. Prayers followed this ritual. This being done, Anna's body was prepared for the funeral home.

Planning for Pre-Death and Post-Death

In the appendices at the end of this book there is, in addition to the three legal documents, a predeath planning checklist. It is helpful to have parishioners fill these out ahead of time. This preparation can alleviate much confusion at the time of death. The decision about cremation or burial may have its roots in the religious tradition of the faith denomination. If that is not the case, there may be a family tradition to follow. If there is still no precedent, talk about the practical aspects of expense and visitation access. This discussion may be very difficult. Caregivers and clergy can be helpful at this time by reminding the loved ones that the presence of their departed is still available through memories and through her or his vibrant spirit. Initiating the moment with prayer, a reminder that this is the body that was and that the soul remains very alive with them, can help put a new perspective on the decision at hand. Separation from the body can be a significant moment, for it is a visible sign of the finality of dying. The spiritual awareness of the finality of death is usually strong at this point. The clergyperson who is empathic, yet somewhat distanced from this pain, can offer these ideas for consideration.

Ministration at the Time of Death

When a person is near death, the Minister of the Congregation should be notified, in order that the ministration of the Church may be provided.

A Prayer for a Person near Death

Almighty God, look on this servant, lying in great weakness, and comfort *him* with the promise of life everlasting, given in the resurrection of your Son Jesus Christ our Lord. *Amen.*

Litany at the Time of Death

When possible, it is desirable that members of the family and friends come together to join the Litany.

God the Father,
Have mercy on your servant.
God the Son,
Have mercy on your servant.
God the Holy Spirit,
Have mercy on your servant.
Holy Trinity, one God,
Have mercy on your servant.
From all evil, from all sin, from all tribulation,
Good Lord, deliver him/her.
By your holy Incarnation, by your Cross and Passion, by your precious
  Death and Burial,
Good Lord, deliver him/her.
By your glorious Resurrection and Ascension, and by the Coming of the
  Holy Spirit,
Good Lord, deliver him/her.
We sinners beseech you to hear us, Lord Christ:
That it may please you to deliver the soul of your servant from the power
  of evil, and from eternal death,
We beseech you to hear us, good Lord.
That it may please you mercifully to pardon all of his/her sins,
We beseech you to hear us, good Lord.
That it may please you to grant him/her a place of refreshment and ever-
  lasting blessedness,
We beseech you to hear us, good Lord.
That it may please you to give him/her joy and gladness in your kingdom,
  with your saints in light,
We beseech you to hear us, good Lord.

Jesus, Lamb of God:
Have mercy on him/her.
Jesus, bearer of our sins:
Have mercy on him/her.
Jesus, redeemer of the world:
Give him/her your peace.
Lord, have mercy.
Christ, have mercy.
Lord, have mercy.

Collect for the Officiant

Let us pray. Deliver your servant, N., O Sovereign Lord Christ, from all evil, and set *him/her* free from every bond; that *he/she* may rest with all your saints in the eternal habitations; where with the Father and the Holy Spirit you live and reign, one God, for ever and ever. *Amen.*

A Commendation at the Time of Death

Depart, O Christian Soul, out of this world;
In the name of God the Father Almighty who created you;
In the name of Jesus Christ who redeemed you;
In the name of the Holy Spirit who sanctifies you.
May your rest be this day in peace,
and your dwelling place in the Paradise of God.

A Commendatory Prayer

Into your hands, O merciful Savior, we commend your servant N. Acknowledge, we humbly beseech you, a sheep of your own fold, a lamb of your own flock, a sinner of your own redeeming. Receive *him* into the arms of your mercy, into the blessed rest of everlasting peace, and into the glorious company of the saints in light. *Amen.* May *his* soul and the souls of all departed, through the mercy of God, rest in peace. *Amen.*[8]

11

Spirituality in Palliative Care—
A Hindu Perspective

Physicians' openness, as caregivers, to patients' spiritual experience has tremendous positive influence on interaction with terminally ill patients. This has given me the strength and intensified my faith in God and spirituality. I have realized that if we miss the experience of human spirit, it is like the reader who skips several chapters in a book; they do not truly comprehend the whole because they avoided crucial information.

Uma Mysorekar

Spirituality

Spirituality means different things to different people. It may include faith or what provides a sense of personal meaning in life (and death). When dealing with illness, spiritual issues often come to the forefront of the patient's life, as well as the caregiver's. Sometimes illness disrupts one's sense of meaning, values, and even one's faith. In these situations, the caregiver should address his or her spiritual needs, too, so as to be better able to deal with the illness of the patient.

Palliative Care

"Palliative care is the total care of the patients who are not responsive to curative treatment. Patients may be treated at home, in the hospital or in an inpatient hospice care facility. The goal of Palliative care is to achieve the highest quality of life possible, keep the patients as comfortable as possible and to allay the fear of death."[1]

In addition to standard methods of management of the terminally ill patients, such as pain relief, nutrition, and other support activities, the importance of priests or religious counselors has grown considerably in the care of the sick. Hinduism believes in the rebirth or reincarnation of souls. Death is therefore not a great calamity, not an end at all, but a natural process in the existence of the soul as a separate entity from the body.

According to the Hindu view, *Atman* is the inner essence of an individual. It is Divine, Immortal, Perfect, Omnipresent, Omnipotent, and Omniscient. In the words of Sage Yajnavalka, "The Self (*Atman*) as not this, not that (*neti, neti*), is imperceptible, for it cannot be perceived. It is indestructible, for it cannot be destroyed. Being unfettered, it never feels pain, nor can it be injured. Being unattached, it never attaches to anything."[2] When associated with a body and under the influence of cosmic ignorance, the *Atman* forgets its true nature and mistakenly identifies with the body-mind apparatus.

The ultimate goal of Hindu religious life is to transcend individually, to realize one's own true nature, which is potentially divine and pure. This realization is called *Moksha* or the liberation of the soul from the cycle of birth and death, resulting in union with God.

This chapter will describe some of the principles and practices of the Hindu religion that are important, especially in the care of Hindu patients who are seriously ill and dying.

Hindu Religion

The Hindu religion is essentially a fellowship of all those who believe in the sacredness of the individual, personal experimental realization of the Divine through spiritual practice and moral discipline, preservation and propagation of Dharma (righteousness, complete freedom of thought in religious matters, harmony of religions, nonviolence in word, deed and thought, reverence for all forms of life, and the law of *Karma*).

The Sanskrit word *Atman*, meaning "God within," is usually translated as the soul, self, or spirit. An individual, according to the Hindu view, is the *Atman* living in a human body. Hindus declare that *Atman* is immortal and divine. Whereas the physical body perishes following death, the *Atman* does not. The ultimate goal of Hindu religious life is to attain *moksha*, union with the Divine or freedom from all physical limitations. Hindus believe that life does not end with death. What perishes is the body; the soul is immortal and eternal. When the body dies, the soul assumes a new body in order to experience the fruits of our good and bad actions in the previous life. The theory of *Karma* and rebirth/reincarnation fits in well with the doctrine of immortality of the soul, because "as you sow, so shall you reap."

For Hindus, death is not a fearsome prospect. They know that they have been born and died before, and *Karma* and reincarnation make the inevitable seem natural. "Death is like falling asleep and birth is like waking from that sleep." Some sages have spoken joyously of death as release from bondage, as return to the source: The soul, the Vedas declare, is immortal. Some patients who have had a near-death experience have narrated their encounter with a vision divine in nature.

Theory of Karma

The explanation for any form of human suffering is accounted for in Hindu philosophy by the law of action (*Karma*). It is also said that by surrendering oneself to God, it may be possible to mitigate the suffering—but it cannot be entirely avoided. Hinduism asserts that it is the duty of good people to help relieve the sufferings of others by sharing their pains and sorrows. This view is reflected in a Sanskrit saying: "we have to look upon others as we look upon ourselves."

A Hindu is encouraged to fulfill all his or her obligations and give love, help, and blessings to others so as to accumulate good karma. In addition, his or her attentions turn to God, reading scriptures, attending Temple, and concentrating on meditation and devotion. Sick patients who cannot go to Temple or read scriptures can concentrate on meditation and devotion from wherever they are.

Reaffirmation of Faith

Hindu faith guides our transition from this world, offering solace to the suffering and those facing the foreboding certainty of death. "Lead me from unreal to real; Lead me from darkness to light; Lead me from death to immortality." This famous Vedic prayer from Shukla Yajur Veda Brihandaranyaka Upanishad proclaims the human urge to survive, to conquer death, and to know the joys of illuminated consciousness.[3]

Reaffirmation of one's faith and spirituality has become an integral part of palliative care. No matter what faith the patient follows, he or she should have faith in him- or herself. Men and women live by faith, and when faith is directed toward God, it becomes the cause of liberation of the individual.

A woman who was near death following surgery, but was brought back to life by medical intervention, recalled that she felt an incredible energy going through her and her conscious feeling of something unique. She described the feeling as some superior, indescribable energy around her to protect her. Such experiences affirm what Hinduism teaches—that death is a blissful, light-filled transition from one state to another, as simple and natural as changing clothes.

Fear

The spiritual leader by the side of the patient must make every effort to allay his or her fear. As Malkani has mentioned in his definition of spirituality, that fear is an aspect or primitive urge of self-preservation. It is the source of many emotions. Fear can be the result of many reasons—fear of sickness or death, of leaving behind possessions, loved ones, and so on. It is a fountainhead of emotions, which must be rechanneled if one is to spend the rest of life with a sense of happiness and joy. The less dependence there is on the temporal world for happiness and more direct attention inward, then one can achieve freedom from fear and will find a sense of fulfillment. When one learns to let go, one finds the greatest secret of life for experiencing peace and happiness. This feeling of letting go is always accompanied by a feeling of opening, blossoming, and coming into a new and more encompassing space, devoid of any fear or tension. Freedom from fear is one of the main messages of Gita—Lord Krishna says:

> Sarvadharman parityajnya, mam ekam saranam vraja
> Aham tva sarvapapebhyo, moksayisyami ma sucah
>
> *Leave all else behind; you can come to me for shelter. I shall*
> *free you from all sins. Do not grieve any more.*

The practice of Hinduism makes us fearless of death. Living with fear means living in a world of imagination, with fancy and fantasy and clinging to the things to which we are seriously attached. Rather than facing the fact that everything in life is subject to change, we desperately try to hold on to them and struggle against the basic law of change, which pervades our universe, bringing thereof pain and unhappiness. It is only when we learn not to depend on the temporal world for our happiness but direct our attention inward that we will continue freedom from fear and will find that a source of fulfillment abides within us and is no different from us.

Prayer

Prayer is the basic tenet of Hinduism and is a path by which God can be reached. Man thinks of God with devotion, and prayers are a call from the heart of the devotee, during which he asks for God's help and guidance and at the same time sings his praises. Prayers, therefore, stand for asking, requesting, and appealing. The purpose of prayer is first to cultivate Godly attributes in oneself, secondly to rid oneself of evil thoughts and desires by meditating on God, and thirdly to express gratitude to God. Prayers, therefore, strengthen one's resolve, decrease fear, lead to peace of mind, and set one on the path of righteousness; all of this will eventually lead to introspection and self-realization. To help in this process, one utilizes images of deities, symbols, mantras, japas (chanting), and meditation, and eventually contemplation of the absolute. Prayer elevates the mind and fills it with purity, in tune with God. It can reach a realm where reason does not dare to enter. Most importantly, it frees the patient from the fear of death.

In addition, prayer is the road to fulfillment: Through prayer, one seeks grace from God and gets comfort in time of distress. It also works wonders, and its power of healing is beyond the comprehension of a human mind. All the prayers are equally effective. Some prayers, such as the chanting of *"Vishnu Sahasranama or the 1008 holy names of Lord Vishnu,"* are considered to be the easiest and the best means by which mankind can attain lasting happiness, peace of mind, relief from all bondages and sorrows, and ultimately salvation. Similarly, recitation of *Hanuman Chalisa*, consisting of 40 stanzas praising *Lord Hanuman*, renowned for his strength and courage, will help overcome all obstacles. Following are some of the common prayers:

Universal Prayers

1. ŜUKLĀMBARADHARAM VISNUM ŜAŜIVARNAM CHATURBHUJAM. PRASANNAVADANAM DHYĀYET SARVA VIGHNOPŜANTAYE.

The grace of God has to be prayed for obtaining peace and removal of obstacles. He [God] is omnipresent and has four hands and is attired in pure clothes. He has luster like Moon with benevolent look on his face.

2. YAM BRAHMA VARUNENDRA, RUDRA MARUTAH STUNVANTI DIVYAIH STAVAIH VEDAIH SANGAPAD KRAMOPNISHADAIR GĀYANTI YAM SAAMAGĀH DHYĀNĀVASTHIT TADGATEN MANSĀ PASHYANTI YAM YOGINO YASYĀNTAM NA VIDUH SURĀSURGANAH DEVĀYA TASMAI NAMAH

He who is worshipped by Brahma, Varuna, Indra, Vāyu through divine prayers; whom Sām Ved singers praise by chanting Vedic and Upnishadic Hymns; Who is seen by Yogis, always immersed in His thoughts, through meditation; whose limit is not known to Gods and demons; our salutations to the Lord!

3. TWAMEV MĀTĀ CH PITĀ TWAMEV, TWAMEV BANDHUSH CH SAKHĀ TWAMEV, TWAMEV VIDYĀ DRAVINAM TWAMEV, TWAMEV SARVAM MAM DEV DEV

Thou art my father and mother too, Thou art my kith and comrade too, Thou art my knowledge and my wealth too, Thou art in all, O God of god.

4. OM PURNAMADAAH PURNAMIDAM PURNAAT PURNA MUDACHY-
ATEY PURNASYA PURNAMAADĀYA PURNA MEVASVASHISHYATE.
(Isavasya Upnishad)

*Om! That is absolute; this too is absolute; Absolute arises from the absolute; taking
out absolute from the absolute what remains is Absolute and Absolute only.*

5. ASATO MAA SADGAMAYA, TAMASO MAA JYOTIRGAMAYA, MRITY-
ORMAA AMRITAM GAMAYA

*Lead me from untruth to truth, Lead me from darkness unto light, Lead me from
death unto immortality.*

6. OM SARVE BHAVANTU SUKHINAH, SARVE SANTU NIRĀMAYAH,
SARVE BHADRĀNI PASHYANTU MĀ KASHCHIDDUKIHBHĀG
BHAVET. (Isavasya Upnishad)

*May everybody be happy! May all be free from disease! May all have good luck!
May none fall on evil days!*

Prayer to "Sun" (Isavasya Upanishad)

The face of Truth is covered by a golden vessel. Remove, O Sun, the covering, for the law of the Truth, that I may behold it!

O Pushan (Sun Nourisher), only Seer (sole traveler of the heavens), Con-
troller of all (Yama), Surya, son of Prajapati, disperses the rays and gathers
up Thy burning light. I behold Thy glorious form. I am He, the Purusha
within Thee!

(May my) *Prana* melt into the all-pervading Air, the eternal Sutratman,
and may this body be burnt by fire to ashes. OM! O mind! Remember my
deeds! O mind! Remember, remember my deeds!

O Agni! Lead us on to wealth (Bliss, *Mukti*, and Beatitude) by a good path,
as Thou knowest, O god! All the ways. Remove the crooked sin from
within us. We offer Thee our best salutations!

This prayer to *Surya* (Sun) can be said by one and all, including a person who may be
newly diagnosed to have cancer or a person who is terminally sick. Prayer to *Surya*
(sun) bestows health, long life, vigor, vitality, and *Tejas*, or brilliance. It is believed to
remove all diseases of the body.

Mantra/Japa

A *mantra* is a sacred syllable, word, or verse, which has been revealed to a Sage in deep meditation. A mantra revitalizes the body and mind with mystic power and harmonizes thought and action when it is recited with devotion, concentration, and understanding. A mantra produces a change in one's consciousness depending upon the mystic power associated with the mantra. A *japa* is the repetition of any mantra or name of the Lord. "A *Mantra* is Divinity and it is the Divine power or *Daiva Sakti* manifesting in a sound body. A *Mantra* accelerated, generates creative force."[4]

The positive results from scientific studies on the clinical benefits of mantra, japa, and prayer on health, combined with patients' desires for doctors to acknowledge their spirituality, have led more and more physicians to seek education opportunities that, until recently, were unavailable, according to John M. Templeton, president of the John Templeton Foundation. Hence, physicians caring for the terminally sick can be trained to chant small mantras that would be comforting to sick patients. Hindu temples in the area can depute a spiritual person to hospital or hospice facility where the terminally sick are being cared for.

Helping patients find spiritual resources is another way of providing care. Arranging a meeting with a priest or a spiritual person, or allowing the patient and family to pray and conduct devotional chanting of mantras, or doing japas in a hospital environment can succor a patient at the end of his or her life. An awareness of and respect for common religious practices around death and dying are integral to compassionate care for terminally ill patients.

Following are some of the popular mantras chanted by Hindus, especially those with terminal sickness.

Gayatri Mantra

The *Gayatri Mantra* is the most sacred Rigvedic mantra. *Gayatri* means "the savior of the singer." The mystic power of this mantra is considered so significant that it is called "the Mother of the Vedas."[5] There is nothing higher than the *Gayatri Mantra* in the Vedas. *Gayatri Mantra* is also called *Savitri Mantra*, as it is addressed to Savitri (i.e., the sun as the creator).

OM BHOOR BHUVAH SVAH; TAT SAVITUR VARAYNYAM; BHARGO-DAYVASYA DHEEMAHI; DHIYO YO NAH PRACHODA-YAT; OM.

God is the giver of life, the dispeller of miseries, and the bestower of happiness. Let us meditate upon that Creator, the most worthy and acceptable Almighty God. May He inspire and lead our minds and intellects.

Dhanvantari Mantra

Lord Dhanvantari is an incarnate of Lord Vishnu and is revered as the physician of the devas and of the three worlds (who expounded the Ayurvedic medical science), because at the conclusion of the great churning of the ocean holding a vessel containing *Amruta* or the nectar that conferred immortality on the devas. Worshipping Sri *Dhanvantari* and continuous chanting of *Dhanvantari Mantra* are believed to cure all ailments and confer longevity of life.

> AUM NAMO BHAGAVATE DHANVANTARAYE AMRUTAKALAŜA
> HASTĀYA SARVĀMAYA VINAŜANĀYA TRILOKANATHĀYA ŜRI
> MAHĀVISHNAVE NAMAHA

Maha Mrityunjaya Mantra

This *Maha—Mrityunjaya Mantra* is a life giving mantra and has great curative effects. This mantra should be chanted with sincerity, faith, and devotion. It is not only a weapon against all diseases but is also considered a *Moksha-Mantra*. It is the mantra for Lord Siva and bestows health (Arogya), long life (Deergha-Ayus), peace (Santi), wealth (Aisvarya), prosperity (Pushti), satisfaction (Tushti), and immortality (Moksha)

> OM TRYAMBAKAM YAJĀMAHE SUGANDHIM PUSHTIVARDHANAM
> URVĀRUKAMIVA BANDHANĀN—MRITYORMUKŜIYA MĀMRITĀT.
>
> *We offer our worship to the fragrant, three-eyed Lord Ŝiva who confers ever-increasing prosperity. Please liberate us from the bondage of death like the watermelon (effortlessly separates from the vine); do not let us turn away from Immortality (liberation).*

This mantra is taken from *Rudram,* which is a hymn to Lord Ŝiva. It invokes the grace of the Lord of death. The verse contains a beautiful metaphor. The *urvāruka* is a melon, which grows on the ground, attached to a vine. It takes its time to ripen. When fully ripe, it does not have to be plucked. It detaches itself effortlessly, remaining where it is, but free from the vine. *Amrta* is total freedom from the sense of all inadequacy and limitation. An essential requirement in gaining *Amrta* is emotional maturity, which is gained by the process of inner growth by living a life of values and prayer. This maturing of the mind is likened to the ripening of the fruit. There is another important aspect of this example. Freedom being the essential nature of the self, the mature mind does not have to seek outside itself to gain this freedom. When a mature mind is exposed to the teaching, it effortlessly comes to recognize that freedom. Thus, this is a prayer of a *mumuksu,* a person who desires that total freedom and who makes it his or her main pursuit in life. It is also a mantra that is traditionally chanted by family and friends for a person who is ill or approaching death.

Nama Mahima

Hindus believe that the Name of God, however chanted, is sure to give the desired result. The Glory of the Name of God cannot be established through reasoning and intellect. It can certainly be experienced or realized only through devotion, faith, and constant repetition of the name. Every name is filled with countless potencies or *Saktis.* The power of the Name is ineffable and Glory indescribably great.

Silent repetition of God's Name, *Hari Om* or *Sri Rama,* is a tremendous tonic and potent specific for all diseases. It is like food—spiritual food for the hungry soul. Repeating or even thinking of His name produces a tremendous influence on the mind.

"The Name of the Lord is a sovereign specific, a sheet—anchor, an infallible panacea and a cure for all diseases."[6] This is called "Divine Namapathy," a mysterious power and divine potencies that are hidden in the Lord's name. A spiritual leader can sit by the side of the patient and repeat, with sincere devotion and faith, the name of the Lord, like "Hari Om," "Sri Ram," "Om Namah Sivaya," "Om Namo Narayana," and so on. Singing *Bhajans* (songs in praise of God) or chanting various Namavalis, such as Vishnu Sahasranama (1008 names of Lord Vishnu) or Lalita Sahasranama (1008 names of Divine Mother), which will have miraculous effect and bring peace and solace to the terminally sick.

Yajna

Yajna, literally meaning sacrifice, is used in various connotations, implying ritual worship as well as the principle of sacrifice and surrender. As ritual worship, *yajna* involves offering materials such as clarified butter, grains, seeds, spices, leaves, and branches of certain sacred trees to the sacred fire while chanting special mantras by trained priests, in accordance with scriptural injunctions. It has been stated that the sacred fire is the medium through which the material gifts, offered as oblation, are actually transformed into spiritual substance, which is acknowledged by the Deity that is being worshipped. *Yajna* intensifies one's spiritual power, which in turn helps one to attain supreme well-being in life on earth and thereafter. *Yajnas* are performed by learned Priests; various deities, such as Lord Ganesha, Lord Siva, and Lord Dhan-vantari, are worshipped in this manner for the benefit of the sick.

Yoga and Meditation

Yoga comes from the Sanskrit word *yuj*, which means to join, meet, or come together. Yoga, therefore, represents the union of man with God and embraces the threefold nature of man (physical, mental, and intellectual). Hindus believe that when prayer or meditation is engaged in the soul, one becomes engrossed in thoughts about God. At that moment the soul unites with the Almighty. This is Yoga. The aim of Yoga, therefore, is the realization of God. There are many branches of Yoga, which can be followed according to one's interest and ability. The Rishis scientifically developed these, and sages in ancient times bestowed upon them their spiritual experiences. The following are the four main Yoga systems.

- Raj Yoga—Yoga of Meditation; teaches the control of mind and soul.
- Karma Yoga—Yoga of Action; teaches that one should perform all actions without the expectations of reward.
- Jnana Yoga—Yoga of Knowledge; teaches to discriminate the Real from Transient.
- Bhakti Yoga—Yoga of devotion. Here man is endowed with the feeling of love and devotion, and this takes total refuge in divinity. One performs all actions as an offering to God.

Many research studies indicate that meditation improves health and can ameliorate the symptoms of even serious illnesses. Over the last 20 years, extensive research at Harvard and other prestigious universities has shown that only 20 minutes of daily meditation has dramatic effects on physical health. It improves the immune system and enhances physical response to chronic diseases, boosts energy, increases stamina and emotional stability, hastens recovery, and reduces stress. According to Dr. Herbert Benson, founder of the Mind/Body Medical Institute at Boston's New England Deaconess Hospital, "Meditation can be an important complement to conventional medical treatment for depression, anxiety, hypertension, cardiac arhythmias, migraine headaches, insomnia, and many other conditions."[7]

Dr. Benson firmly believes that practicing advanced forms of meditation "can uncover capacities that will help us to better treat stress related illnesses." Benson, who has been studying Tum-mo, a yoga technique, for 20 years, states "Buddhists feel the reality we live in is not the ultimate one. There is another reality we can tap into that's unaffected by our emotions, by our everyday world. Buddhists believe that this state of mind can be achieved by doing good for others and by meditation."[8]

Summary of Rituals

Recommended rituals for the terminally sick:

1. Offer prayers to the Lord as often as possible
2. Chant common mantras as many times as possible.
3. Chant the glorious names of the Lord.

Recommended rituals performed for the benefit of the sick:

1. Ganapati Homa
2. Mrityunjaya Japa and Homa
3. Ayushya Homa
4. Dhanvantari Homa
5. Navagraha Homa
6. Chanting Vishnu Sahasranama or Lalita Sahasranama
7. Read scriptures such as Bhagavad Gita, Upanishad, and so forth. Sundara Kanda of Ramayana / Bhagavatham

Hinduism believes in reincarnation of the soul and the theory of *karma*. The cycle of birth and death continues until the individual attains *moksha* or freedom/liberation from birth and death by his or her continuous good deeds in the present life. The physical suffering due to illness is the result of one's *karma*, which brings back results in this life.

Spirituality is that which gives meaning to one's life and draws one to transcend oneself. Spirituality is a broader concept than religion, although that is one expression of spirituality. Other expressions include (as narrated earlier) prayer, mediation, interaction with others or nature, and relationship with God or a higher power. Spirituality was cited as integral to the dying person's achievements of the developmental task of transcendence and important for healthcare providers to recognize and foster.

Palliative care is rooted in the affirmation that death is one step in the cycle of life and death. This care begins when a person is diagnosed with a life-threatening illness and continues through the spectrum from anticipating grief right through bereavement. Spirituality is reflected in each person's most precious beliefs, values, or activities. Spiritual caregiving helps a person to live fully until death occurs. Spiritual care includes helping family members in locating appropriate religious support from the community, both during illness and immediately after the death occurs.

12

Faith and Islamic Issues at the End of Life

IMAM YUSUF HASAN AND YUSEF SALAAM

One patient related that all hope of recovery had gone, and all he had left was his faith in God. He said, "It is easy dying, but hard living."

Yusuf Hasan

Principles of the Islamic Religion

A Muslim, whether he or she is in perfect health or struggling with a terminal illness, depends on Islam—the way of peace, purity, submission, or adherence to the will of Allah, God—for guidance and support. The five specific principles of worship and the beliefs of Islam are what support Muslims through the unpredictable circumstances of life.

The basic paradigm of worship among Muslims is the Five Pillars of Islam—*Shahadah*: the spoken declaration that there is no god but Allah and that Muhammad is the Messenger of Allah; *Sala*: pray five times daily; *Zakat*: donate a certain amount of one's yearly earnings, which is shared with the needy; *Sawn*: a 30-day fast from sunrise to sunset, especially during the month of Ramadan; and *Hajj*: the once-in-a-lifetime pilgrimage to Mecca. The Five Pillars of Islam are the basis of the religion. All Muslims all over the world must uphold these principles. The following is a further elaboration of these principles:

1. *Shahadah:* Declaration of faith: There is no God but one God, and Muhammad is his last prophet.
2. *Sala:* The need for constant prayer, to keep life in perspective, which means praying five times a day: before sunrise; when the sun is just off its zenith; at the sun's mid-decline; directly after sunset; and before retiring for the night.

3. *Zakat:* The need to give to the poor, and for the maintenance of the mosque, exemplified by donating 2.5 % of annual earnings.
4. *Sawn:* The observance of Ramadan, the month of fasting, during which able-bodied Muslims are required to fast from dawn until sundown.
5. *Hajj:* A pilgrimage to Mecca, at least once during a lifetime, which serves as a reminder that are all equal before God. During the pilgrimage, all distinctions of rank and hierarchy are prohibited.

The belief system of Islam also shares common beliefs with the other two great monotheistic faiths: Christianity and Judaism. These are as follows: belief in one God and angels; divine scriptures of God and all of God's messengers, including Muhammad, Jesus, Moses, and Abraham; and the Day of Judgment, the Resurrection, and life in the hereafter.

From these principles flows the belief that it is spiritual medicine that heals and gives serenity to Muslims who are terminally ill. The practicing Muslim who faces an end-of-life sickness walks with faith and trust in God.

Muslims believe that the Holy Qur'an contains God's last message to humanity, as revealed to Prophet Muhammad by the angel Gabriel over a period of 23 years, 1,400 years ago. The text of the Holy Qur'an and the authentic Ahadeeth—sayings and actions of the Prophet Muhammad—guide over one billion adherents throughout the world. One of the definitions of faith is belief and trust in God. The Muslim belief and trust in God is not based solely on scientific analysis, logic, or material evidence, but on the absolute adherence to one's faith and belief. This faith serves as a powerful aid for the terminally ill, not only to help face the situation but to face it with one's soul at rest. In other words, *iman* (or faith) is the spiritual healing that the terminally ill Muslim employs to understand and accept the propositions, doctrines, and ways of Islam in relationship to the laws of life and death that Allah has ordained. The understanding and acceptance of faith is not only a mental and physical one, it is also an understanding and acceptance that is sealed in the heart, the soul, and the spirit. "The Qur'an is a guide and a healing to those who believe."[1]

Sincere belief and faith in God guides the heart and soul to submit to his will and is the best balm for the self-doubt, self-pity, anxiety, and grief that too often threaten to beset the psyche of the terminally ill. The case of 31-year-old Abdullah speaks volumes to the above-mentioned discourse about the faith of the believer in Islam. Abdullah was unable to speak because of his illness. When his physician informed him of his terminal prognosis, he requested a sheet of paper and wrote, "We are people of faith, and will continue to have faith until the end." He used the word "We," which indicates that he saw himself as part of a group of believers. Abdullah did not see himself as being isolated, which was excellent psychological support for him. As Muslims would say, "To God we belong and to God we return."

Abdullah indicated his understanding that he had a life-threatening ailment. His abundance of faith enabled him to handle the news with spiritual sobriety, integrity, and maturity. He also understood that God is all-powerful, the Absolute, and the Giver of Life and Death, and he has appointed a time for both. Abdullah humbly accepted that his life had been ordained by Allah, as well as his death, and he kept an optimistic attitude until his demise.

Faith in Times of Distress

The terminally ill Muslim walks in faith, rooted in trust in the Almighty. While Islam offers an abundance of logical proof and scientific evidence in the Qur'an for the seekers of such data, the believer stands on a firm foundation of faith in the seen as well as the unseen—that which is in the grasp of his or her understanding and that which is not. Of course, sometimes a Muslim can lose faith during trials of immense trouble. When such a believer is threatened with spiritual darkness, it often takes the assistance of a chaplain to help bring him or her back into "The Light," as was the case of a mother and her only son.

Kareem, a 17-year-old native of Yemen, was terminally ill. His mother was having a hard time coping with his illness. The teenager was struggling, too, with anxiety, not because of his fading health, but because he was worried that his mother's faith was weakening. He feared not being united with her in the Hereafter if her faith was lost. He was particularly concerned because she stopped offering prayer at his bedside and would leave when the chaplain arrived.

Kareem shared his concerns with the chaplain: "Please help my mother keep her faith in Allah." The chaplain and the mother discussed the situation. The chaplain highlighted Kareem's unyielding faith and that he worried about his mother losing her faith. He advised her on the importance of resuming her prayer, not only for her son's peace of mind but for her own soul. He reminded her that God tells the Muslims that he will test their faith so as to purify them and be worthy of Paradise. He informed her that she must exercise patience, because God rewards those who are patient. The Qur'an states, "He guides to Himself those who turn to Him in patience, those who believe and whose hearts find peace and satisfaction in the remembrance of God. Without doubt, in the remembrance of God do hearts find satisfaction and peace."[2]

The counseling sessions helped Kareem's mother face her denial of her son's condition and refocus her energy on reading the Qur'an, while praying and deepening her faith. The combination of her and her son's prayers and faith eventually rewarded both of them with deep-felt satisfaction and peace of mind.

Faith and Healing

In this example, we see a sterling model of faith and healing. While Kareem thanked his healthcare providers (physicians, nurse, chaplain, etc.) for helping ease the tension and fear that terminally ill patients and their family members experience, he only recognized God as the ultimate healer: God is Al-'Alim (the All Knowing). In the Qur'an, Prophet Ibrahim (Abraham) asserts, "(God) created me and guides me, gives me food and drink, and cures me when I'm ill."[3] Prophet Muhammad is the model healthcare provider for Muslims. In one saying of the Aisha (wife of the Prophet), Aisha related that when Prophet Muhammad sat at the bedside of the sick, he offered this prayer: "Lord of the people, remove the disease, cure him, for thou art the great Cure. There is no cure but your healing Power, which leaves nothing of the disease."[4]

Like Kareem's mother, 49-year-old Lateefa, a lung cancer patient, was very much in despair and confusion. Lateefa's crisis was due to her lack of faith in her prayers. This lack provoked her to say, "I have been praying and praying; maybe I am praying too much, because God is not answering my prayers." A wife and mother of two teenaged children, Lateefa's heart was distressed about her family. The fact that family members visited her often did not calm her agitation.

Lateefa and her chaplain talked constantly about her predicament. The faith-focused sessions concentrated on her need to rely on God's will (qadr) and his promise to rescue the believer in times of crisis and tragedy. The chaplain assured her that God was well aware of her prayers. He pointed out to her that the Qur'an says God's nearness to her is closer to her than her "jugular vein."[5] There was no need for her to overexert herself in her prayers of petition to God for aid, because God is not deaf or absent. He is the All-Hearing, the All-Seeing.

The chaplain and Lateefa conversed about the Qur'an's instructions. God said, "He does not place on us a burden greater than we can bear." He assured her that her anxiety would definitely be relieved. Unlike Kareem, Lateefa did not have the faith that assured her that she was part of the "We" in her faith-based community. She felt lonely and insecure about whether the Muslim community and her family would provide support for her children when she was no longer present to love and care for them.

The chaplain arranged sessions that included Lateefa and her family members, during which they discussed Lateefa's apprehensions. The imam (cleric) of the mosque that she had attended for many years was summoned, and he, too, assured her that the security of her children was a priority for the Muslim community. Persistent discussions centered on her concerns about her family, until her fear was reduced, which gave her space to concentrate on and to develop her own coping skills. As time passed, the long-term goal was completed: Lateefa learned to rely on God's will, which anticipates events before they happen.

The person not based in faith plans his or her life according to his or her perception of the secular world. The practicing Muslim is obligated to balance the secular and the spiritual worlds in his or her plans. The Qur'an advises him or her that Allah is the better arranger of life's directions. The practicing Muslim believes that every event is preordained and that we cannot alter what will impact us.

The Muslim who has faith knows that at the end of life, death awaits. Every human being will taste death, so the faithful Muslim is comfortable that life on earth is a preparation for the life to come—the Hereafter.

The prophet said, "None of you should wish for death because of a calamity befalling him; but if you wish for death, you should say: 'O God! Keep me alive as long as life is better for me, and let me die if death is better for me.'"[6]

The terminally ill Muslim should think "life" in the face of chronic illness. If he or she is able, he or she should utilize the treatment of laughter, enjoyment of recreation, employment, and staying active. Above all, he or she should pray to God to give the vigor to courageously battle the foe that intends to terrorize his or her body, soul, spirit, and faith, which threatens to annihilate his normal lifestyle.

Yusef, a resident of Harlem, was afflicted with end-stage kidney failure and actually embraced his illness. At first he was too fragile to fast for Ramadan, so, as Islam allows, he fed the hungry for each of the 30 days of the fast for 3 years. He nurtured his faith with study, prayer, and improvements in his moral life. He made peace with his past and grew closer to being the type of Muslim he always wanted to be. Eventually, after 3 years of dialysis, 3 days a week, he gained enough strength to return to the fast—thanks to rest, prayer, peace of mind, and a deepened faith. He remarried, and for 2 years he has been teaching English full time at a high school, part time on the college level, and is enjoying his favorite recreation. He has also written a play that was produced off-Broadway.

The significance of Yusef's story is that it reflects the experience of many Muslims born in America. Once Yusef found himself on long-term life support, he began reflecting back on a life that he considered to be misguided from the proper moral and religious life of a good Muslim. His experience of getting on the right track, only to be afflicted with a life-threatening illness, could easily have caused him to give up all hope, but with prayers and faith in God, Yusef was able to regain his strength, face his fears, and move on with his life. Although physically ill, he was spiritually healed.

Islam and Medical Technology

Muslim medical science has contributed for 14 centuries to medical technology, treatments, and remedies for an array of diseases. The Islamic person is thus obligated to seek the blessings of treatments that modern medical technology extends. However, his or her faith must not be in the treatment that modern medical technology extends, but in the Lord of Creation, who created human curiosity and intelligence, which discovers medical ingredients in plants, animals, and other natural resources in the universe. The Islamic treatment for the ill does not depend entirely on medicine but uses other health-giving methods, such as the recitation of the Qur'an. Recitation of the Holy Qur'an, with its beautiful sounds, relaxes the patient and helps reduce anxiety and stress. Prophet Muhammad would recite certain verses from the Qur'an while visiting the sick.

The potent effect of Qur'anic recitation on the faithful is seen in the case of a 27-year-old Muslim male who was struggling with AIDS for 5 years. During his last hospital stay, doctors gave him a few days to live. His mother, against the doctors' advice, signed her weakening son out of the hospital and took him home. The mother, a registered nurse, surrounded the young man with Qur'anic recitation and prayers, causing restoration and extending his life.

The Muslim patient should also seek truth about the nature of treatments offered. Imam Ali, a 63-year-old African American, was a pillar to his family and a highly regarded Imam in the Islamic community. He suspected that his family and doctors were concealing information from him about the nature of his illness (his wife requested the doctors' permission to delay informing her husband about the terminal diagnosis until she believed the time was best). When he finally received the truth, he communicated in writing that it was good news, because he wanted to know the truth. He added in the note his adoration for God and that he felt an enormous psychological relief, now that he finally knew the truth. Imam Ali immediately began to plan as though he was going on a permanent trip. He began to put his obligations in order (will, insurance policies, etc.) and to brace his family members for his definitive earthly demise.

Similarly, the truth did not hurt Saleema, a 60-year-old African-American woman. She was at life's end after an unsuccessful operation to remove cancer. The truth about her prognosis caused her to rejoice in anticipation of going to meet God. During her entire hospital stay, she showed her faith by her good composure and dignity.

Islam and Resuscitation Orders

Treatment is not mandatory for the believer in Islam if there is no hope of a cure. Technical procedures to prolong the dying may be terminated, and the individual is free to choose a "Do Not Resuscitate" (DNR) order. The Prophet Muhammad advised his companions not to force treatment on a patient if that person refuses it. In Islam, there is no requirement or mandate to sign a DNR agreement, nor is there a prohibition against it. The Qur'an states: "Say to every people a term is appointed; when their term has been reached, you can cause no delay nor can you abound in anticipation."[7]

When a Muslim has signed a legal and Islamically applicable agreement in advance concerning his medical care and when he is then no longer capable of making a decision, his wishes or the preference of his surrogate must be respected.

Customs and Rituals in the Healthcare Setting

There are important issues that non-Muslim healthcare providers should familiarize themselves with when they are administering to Muslims. Healthcare providers should be aware of the customs concerning Muslim patients. Females may request to be treated only by female personnel, and Muslim males may request to be treated by male healthcare personnel. Of course, there is always common sense and balance in Islam. In case of an emergency, the patient's life supersedes whether the lifesaving care is given by a male or a female. Because the dominant religious practice for the Muslim is to pray five times a day, a doctor should not think it is strange to see a Muslim patient standing at the sink washing his or her hands, face, head, and feet in a ritual fashion. That ritual is called *wudu* (abolition), which prepares and makes him or her clean for prayer.

Yusef, the teacher who was mentioned earlier, said during an interview that when he needs to do *wudu* for prayer at the hospital, he is usually in the dialysis chair and can't get up. The attending nurse accommodates him by giving him a cup of water to prepare for the prayer as best he can. A nurse should not be shocked if she comes into her Muslim patient's room and sees him bowing. He may be praying in the Islamic way. The proper etiquette when attending Muslims is to knock on the door before entering or announce one's self vocally to minimize the chances of interrupting the prayer. The attending doctor and nurse should try and cooperate with the Muslim patient about the schedule of the daily prayers, so that those times can be integrated into the patient's healthcare program.

As discussed earlier, the Holy Qur'an is of vital importance to the Muslim. Reading it gives the Muslim's soul rest and is his spirit medicine. It should be noted that a patient may prefer to listen to the Qur'an on audiotapes or compact discs, rather than to read it. This may be especially true when the Islamic patient is very ill and unable to read. To avoid conflicts with the patient, the healthcare team could organize a system that respects the patient's reading of or listening to the Qur'an by coordinating a time for prayer with the doctors and nurses, if only 5 or 10 minutes each day.

If the Muslim patient is physically or mentally able, he is required to attend *Jumah* (worship) every Friday, usually at midday. *Jumah* is a congregational service with sermon and prayers. Many hospitals in the United States provide a suitable space for *Jumah*. The staff could work with a hospital imam or an imam of a local mosque to make sure there are no religious symbols—meaning no crosses, pictures of humans or animals, mirrors on the wall, or stained glass with pictures—in the prayer room, when the patient is attending *Jumah*. There should also be a clear space for prayer rugs. If there is not a hospital imam to lead the *Jumah* service, there are usually male Muslim staff members who are qualified to lead.

Like many other faiths, Islam has dietary laws. *Halal* means what is good, pure, clean, wholesome, nourishing, and pleasing to taste—these foods are permissible for consumption for Muslims as prescribed in the Holy Qur'an. In the case of meat, this specifies the way the animal is raised, slaughtered, and prepared by Muslims, under the supervision of an imam and the slaughterer, who must say the words *bismi-llah . . . allahu akbar* (with God's name . . . God the greater) at the time of each animal slaughter, to ensure that the blood has been properly drained from the animal. All Muslims are required to eat *halal* meats for health reasons. All meat, but absolutely no pork, consumed by Muslims must be *halal*. Meat is only *halal* when it is raised and slaughtered in the Islamic way. Healthcare workers can consult a hospital imam or a local imam of a mosque to ascertain the nearest source of *halal* food. The majority of the other hospital foods, such as grains, vegetables, fruits, pork-free desserts, and seafood, are *halal*.

There are religious items that Muslim patients need and should be in supply according to demand in the hospital. Specifically these objects are Holy Qur'ans (books and tapes), prayer rugs, and *dikr* beads (used to count the number of times that the believer chants various supplications to Allah).

Care of the Dying

The Muslim patient is acutely concerned about not becoming unconscious or in a drugged state during prayer. The Holy Qur'an instructs: "Do not approach your prayers in a befogged state of mind."[8] The Muslim patient, therefore, might not want to take medicine that induces sedation or lack of clarity, especially near prayer time.

The primary reason that a terminally ill Muslim patient insists on not being sedated is that he or she wants to be as sober-minded as possible to make the declaration of faith when the angel of death comes. Islam teaches that when a Muslim proclaims the declaration as he or she is taking his or her last breaths—"There is no god But God, and Muhammad is his last prophet"—he will go immediately to paradise. This Islamic principle is a potent motivation to be in possession of one's faculties and speech when death approaches.

Yusef, the dialysis patient discussed earlier, once wrote a memo to his doctor stating, "My sickness is a sign of my eventual demise, and I warmly embrace it like a friend." In other words, Yusef is saying that life is his friend and so is death. He is enjoying the life that God has given him, but, now that his life is threatened with sickness and is no longer enjoyable or tolerable, God will bring that great and merciful friend, death, in His time, just as in the beginning, He issued in that great, merciful friend, life, in His time.

Dying and Funeral Rituals

When it is medically evident that the patient is near death, an imam or family member may recite *Yasin,* the 36th chapter of the Holy Qur'an. When a Muslim who is terminally ill returns to God, the body should be cared for by a funeral home that has experience in handling the remains of a Muslim. Muslim men wash the body if the body is a male, and Muslim women wash if the body is a female. Then the remains are enshrouded in three white sheets. Both male and female Muslims are permitted to wash and shroud deceased children (before they have reached puberty).

The Muslim funeral is very simple. The deceased is placed in a plain pine box or the least expensive casket. The body, unembalmed, is interred for 3 days after death. Flowers, organ playing, and singing are not a part of the Islamic funeral service, because they are not a part of the tradition of the Prophet Muhammad. The Islamic funeral is only about 5 or 10 minutes long. Funeral goers may dress formally or casually, but always in a manner that shows respect to the occasion. An imam gives an oration regarding the deceased and leads the *Janaaza* (funeral prayer.)

Needs of the Family

As stated previously, it is natural for the terminally ill to be worried about the welfare of the family that he or she will be departing. That patient, male or female, may have been the source of economic security for the family. The chaplain or social worker should approach the patient with honesty and sensitivity when discussing the needs of the patient's family in his or her inevitable absence. This verse from the Qur'an is an excellent source in such a situation and can be used to begin a discussion about the patient's fears: "And those who believe and whose families follow them in faith—to them shall we join their families. Nor shall we deprive them (of the fruit) of aught of their works: is each individual in pledge for his deeds."[9]

The living will or healthcare proxy is of utmost importance to the terminally ill Muslim. Indigenous Muslim-Americans are not only concerned about the distribution of their estate to family members, but also they want to make sure their living will or proxy mandates that their remains be buried in the proper Islamic manner. Sometimes, decision making about the funeral of an indigenous Muslim-American can be chaotic if his or her will or proxy does not stipulate an Islamic funeral, because the family normally consists of individuals of other faiths, and they may want their now-deceased family member to be buried in the manner of their specific faith(s). Muslims who have emigrated from predominantly Muslim countries usually do not have this problem, because most of their family members are Muslim.

The two major authorities in Islam are the Holy Qur'an and the sayings and actions of the Prophet Muhammad. They determine the thinking and attitude of the faithful Muslim; therefore, most Muslims do not view illness and death as a bad thing. Death is considered a natural part of life, because the Holy Qur'an says: "To every people is a term appointed; when their term has been reached, not an hour can they cause delay, nor an hour can they advance it in anticipation."[10] As quoted above, the Prophet Muhammad said, "None of you should wish for death because of a calamity befalling him, but if he has to wish for death, he should pray: 'O Allah! Keep me alive as long as life is better for me and let me die if death is better for me.'"[11]

Because of these very important sayings, most Muslims will not think of being angry with God because of illness or impending death. Illness, in the life of most Muslims, is not considered suffering but rather a hardship and an opportunity to get close to Paradise, because the Prophet Muhammad said illness helps erase sins. Therefore, when a Muslim feels good or bad, most will say, "Praise be to God." Most Muslims see death as a good thing, especially after living a good Islamic life—praying five times a day, giving of charity, fasting during Ramadan, and making pilgrimage to Mecca—and would welcome death as the way to enter Paradise. A Muslim having practiced his or her religion to the best of his or her ability, as the end of life approaches, will welcome death as a friend and not as an enemy. It is said that if a person's good outweighs his or her bad, then his or her chance of entering paradise is excellent. Therefore, for Muslims, death is welcomed.

13

Spirituality, Suffering, and Prayerful Presence within Jewish Tradition

DAVID J. ZUCKER AND BONITA E. TAYLOR

A wheelchair-bound resident had a variety of hats that she wore with great flair. One day I remarked how much I "loved" her different hats. She looked up at me, cocked her head, and with a wink, said, "Better you should love me than my hats."

David J. Zucker

Spirituality

"At the beginning of God's creating of the heavens and the earth . . . God's spirit (*ruah*) hovered over the face of the waters . . . and God formed the human . . . blew into the human's nostrils the breath of life and the human became a living being."[1]

The Hebrew word used in this passage from Genesis to refer to God's "spirit" is *ruah*. When God wants to connect with us, God does so through God's *ruah*. The biblical prophet Isaiah refers to God's spirit that will be poured upon humans from on high,[2] and likewise the prophet Joel speaks of the divine promise to pour forth God's spirit on all people.[3] When we want to connect with God, we do so by claiming God's *ruah* as a part of us, as in Numbers, where Moses addresses God as the spirit of all flesh: *Elohey ha-ruhot l'khol basar.*[4] An individual who has received God's spirit is said to be inspired, much as Joshua was when Moses described him as a *ruah bo*, an "inspired man."[5] The definition of "inspire" is "breathe into" and "connect to spirit."

Today, the Hebrew word for "spirituality" is *ruhaniyut*, a variant of the word *ruah*. *Ruhaniyut* "refers to an intense, personal, awe-based concern for questions about life and meaning, as opposed to religion, [which is] a traditional collection of institutionalized and canonized doctrines, rituals . . . and creeds about those same questions. . ."[6]

Ruaḥ refers to one of the dimensions that are inherent within the soul.[7] According to Jewish mystical tradition, the "Jewish soul" has several dynamically interactive dimensions, each of which has a purpose. Our ruaḥ bridges heaven and earth.[8] It is also our soul-dimension, which mobilizes when we engage experiences that stir our emotions.

Our emotions are indeed stirred when we—or our loved ones—are ill or infirm. From a Kabbalistic perspective, when we feel well, our physical and spiritual dimensions are integrated. If our health fails, the connection between our bodies and our souls weakens to greater or lesser degrees, depending upon our distress. If our condition worsens and our souls are no longer able to express themselves fully through our bodies, our physical and spiritual dimensions continue to separate. When we die, our souls separate from our bodies, although they maintain a tenuous relationship as long as our bodies retain their form. This connection loosens further as our bodies decay.[9] In our finality, we become one with God. (See the subsequent section on Jewish views of the Afterlife).

When we are ill or infirm, we feel the beginning of this disconnection, particularly from the selves that we have known and cared for. We also begin to distance ourselves from our previous lifestyles and from our colleagues and loved ones. Although we may have faith, we also begin to feel disconnected from God—at the very time that we need to feel God's Presence the most. Often it comes as a shock to us that the relationship that we thought we had with God—one that would protect us and our loved ones from pain and suffering—is not the one that we have. We may feel anger, abandonment, betrayal, isolation, loneliness, or other emotions that we may never have expected to feel toward God. We enter a spiritual crisis. The more serious our infirmity, the more we want to feel connected to God and the more we go looking for a God with whom we can connect, a God who elevates rather than judges, loves rather than intimidates, who helps rather than hovers in distant skies.[10]

When we are infirm, we want to feel that God will aid us. For some of us that means to cure us, either through medical science or a miracle. For all of us, including those approaching death through aging, that means to heal us. "Healing ... is the transmission of energy and the emanation of spiritual light. It is not meant as a cure for disease but as an aid in assisting [us] toward [our] destiny."[11]

At the point of what may be no return to our former, more desirable way of life—whether because of illness or aging—we want to know two things. The first is that despite our transgressions, God will forgive us and receive us in heaven. The second is that we made a difference, that our lives mattered. If we are the one who is infirm, it may be hard to experience these two goals without assistance. Fortunately, there is a tradition within Judaism that God can work through angels.[12] "Since the beginning of time, there have been people who kindle their inner light, are generous in sharing the energy that flows through them, and are available as vehicles of God for healing others. . . . The energy that kindles the inner light originates from God and may come through you or another who willingly offers to be a vehicle for healing."[13] These stages are difficult to go through alone. Loved ones and/or chaplains can serve as angels during times of disconnecting.

"Think about it. We are blessed with *ruah Elohim*—God's own breath—flowing directly into us to enliven us. Take a deep breath . . . now another even deeper breath. . . . If you take your time and breathe with intention, you will be able to feel God's Presence and, with it, God's vitality traveling through each and every part of your body, bringing healing to parts that are wounded, energy to parts that need healing, and inspiration to activate you. Sense yourself awakening by this infusion from—and of—God. Imagine what it's like to feel the spirit of God moving inside you."[14]

Suffering

No words can address fully the fear and anguish that course through our veins when we receive grim news—either about ourselves or our loved ones. No explanations can soothe our troubled thoughts in moments of deepest torment. The heartache that we feel within may—or may not—eventually ease.

We can ask: "Why?"; "Why me?"; "Why them?"; or "Why now?" but there are no simple responses to these laments, these existential cries from our souls. Whether we like it or not, the light of life is a finite flame. It burns, glows, and grows, but in time, as with all things finite, it ends. Unfortunately, the flame doesn't always finish in a moment. Instead, it diminishes in size, dims, flickers, and in its time, it dies.

We are born into a finite life. We know this and still we suffer when we learn that we—or those we care about—are seriously or terminally ill.

We suffer when our lifestyles are perpetually interrupted by the way that we experience tribulations. Dr. Eric Cassell[15] says that suffering occurs "when an impending destruction of the person is perceived." Writing extensively on this subject, he further explains that suffering "continues until the threat of disintegration has passed or until the integrity of the person can be restored in some other manner."[16]

Suffering is subjective. The diagnosis of a terminal illness may shock someone aged 35 more than someone 95 or older. In our beauty-conscious society, an individual who has visible scars may suffer more than one who has scars in less observable areas—unless disclosure of these "imperfections" seems imminent. On the other hand, an individual with similar scars from military battles may be proud that others know that these scars exist.

Often, suffering is linked with pain, although it is a different phenomenon. Individuals who ail from migraines, back problems, cancer, or other conditions associated with prolonged pain may experience less pain in later weeks of their ordeal—but more suffering. For example, by the third week of facing ordeals such as these, the way that a person lives and interrelates with colleagues and loved ones may have been seriously curtailed. With no end in sight, he or she often feels emotionally exhausted and excluded from life's more fulfilling and joyous aspects. On the other hand, acute suffering sometimes can be mitigated if we value a contribution to someone else through medical research or, perhaps, through organ donations.

Trying to reconcile suffering has long intrigued Jewish sages. The biblical view is that suffering comes from God. "Is it not from the mouth of the Most High that good and bad come?" asks the book of Lamentations.[17] This disturbs many individuals, who would like to believe that God represents only "good" and never "bad." The idea that our suffering emanates from God is often easier to accept when we believe that we have done something to provoke God. When Jeremiah asks, "Why have all these things come upon me?" God answers that "It is for your great iniquity."[18] This view was appealing to a community that rejected the idea of vicarious suffering but rather believed that individuals were responsible for their own suffering. In Judaism, individuals are personally responsible for all of their actions. This includes taking personal responsibility for misdeeds. Jews do not seek salvation through the intervention of others who suffer for them. As Trude Weiss-Rosmarin explains, the "idea of 'vicarious atonement,' that is to say, the payment of the penalty not by the sinner but by a substitute, is irreconcilable with Jewish ethics."[19]

Concepts of vicarious suffering and vicarious atonement were known in Judaism and surfaced periodically in Judaism's history. By biblical days, they already had been rejected by mainstream thought. In the biblical period, the opposition to vicarious suffering and vicarious atonement is most pointedly articulated by the prophets Ezekiel[20] and Jeremiah,[21] as well as in Deuteronomy, where it states that "parents shall not be put to death for children, nor children put to death for parents: [persons] shall be put to death only for [their] own crime."[22]

Most unsettling, however, is the Book of Job. It wrestles with the concept that suffering can be without provocation. In fact, it implies that sometimes the righteous may suffer worst of all. In the end, Job accepts that God cares enough about us to provide a response, even if that response is not satisfying.[23]

Like the Hebrew Bible,[24] the Talmud[25] and Midrash[26] present varying views about suffering. In these rabbinic writings, our sages express the idea that because even the righteous were imperfect, all people needed to purge themselves of some wrongdoing. They encourage us first to examine our own acts, and then, if we believe that we are blameless, to consider our difficulties as "*yesurin shel ahavah*—chastisements of [God's] love." In their view, God "reproves the one [God] loves."[27] As another form of consolation, the ancient rabbis suggested that suffering in this world brings rewards later in the World to Come.

Yet not all chose to benefit in the Afterlife by suffering in the present. Witness this sacred story from the Talmud:

> In an age where pain was thought by some to be "precious," and where the pious were expected to accept suffering willingly because they would receive their reward in the World to Come, Rabbi Hiya bar Abba fell ill. His colleague, the famous Rabbi Yohanan, visited him and said, "Are these sufferings acceptable to you?" Rabbi Hiya replied to his colleague, "Neither they nor their reward." Rabbi Yohanan then said to his ill colleague, "Give me your hand." Rabbi Hiya gave Rabbi Yohanan his hand and Rabbi Yohanan cured him.
>
> Next, we learn that the same Rabbi Yohanan, the man who had effected his colleague's cure, fell ill. A third colleague, Rabbi Hanina, visited him. Rabbi Hanina asked Rabbi Yohanan the same question, "Are these sufferings acceptable to you?" Rabbi Yohanan replied to Rabbi Hanina, "Neither they nor their reward." Rabbi Hanina then said to his ill colleague, "Give me your hand." Rabbi Yohanan gave Rabbi Hanina his hand and Rabbi Hanina cured him.[28]

The idea that suffering brings rewards in the World to Come is reiterated in the Middle Ages. Medieval Jewish thinkers also taught that—given free will—we suffer because of the choices that we make. Ultimately, they withdrew from the discussion by stating that the answers to questions such as "Why does God allow suffering?" are beyond human understanding and will be revealed at the end of days.

In contemporary times many continue to support the idea that "human suffering may be the terrible price that we pay for moral choice and freedom."[29] Still others hold that God "is limited . . . by laws of nature and by the evolution of human nature and human moral freedom. . . . God does not cause our misfortunes. Some are caused by bad luck, some are caused by bad people, and some are simply an inevitable consequence of our being human and being mortal, living in a world of inflexible natural laws."[30]

An explanation for why we suffer, which engages those with an interest in Kabbalah, emanates from the writings of Isaac Luria, a sixteenth-century mystic from Safed.[31] He begins before the beginning of time, when God was everything and everyplace. In order for anything and anyone else to exist, God contracted in an activity that the mystics called *Tzimtzum* (Contraction). However, God still wanted the world to be filled with Divinity, and to this end, God created vessels to hold Divine Light to infuse our world. When the infinite light of God entered these finite vessels, they shattered, and Divine Light splattered across the universe. Much of it returned to

God, but some entered vessel shards and remained in our world. These broken fragments tore the fabric of our universe's soul. Jewish Kabbalistic traditions invite us to believe that it is primarily these rips in the universal soul's fabric that cause the fragility, brokenness, injustice, and deterioration that we experience. It is the Divine Light that is diffused within our world that allows for the possibility of repair, but only through our actions. We partner with God to bring about healing.

A great strength of Judaism is that, with exceptions, it does not insist that its members adhere to one doctrine. One of the few points which all Jews, across the denominational spectrum, *do* accept as true is the following: "God" always means the totally unified, indivisible God, who possesses absolute sovereignty and is supreme over the entire world. Individual Jews may differ in how they understand God's attributes or God's Presence—and some may even choose to deny God's existence—but all Jews agree that God has never walked the earth in human form. We are still waiting for the Messiah to come—the first time.

Each Jew is religiously and spiritually free to choose the view that offers the most consolation. As the Talmudic story cited earlier demonstrates, we can find respected Jewish sages who espouse value in suffering and others who do not. More to the point, Judaism teaches us that we can believe one thing in principle and another in practice. In other words, even though most Jews believe that God is all-powerful (omnipotent) and all-knowing (omniscient), these are descriptions of God in principle and not in practice. In practice, there are two main Jewish views about how God acts in our world today. Both views agree that in an earlier time, God intentionally withdrew. However, from that point, many Jews today believe that God can intervene and end suffering but chooses not to in order to sustain human choice, while many others believe that God cannot now intervene.

Whether God can—or cannot—now intervene in human affairs continues to be a subject of debate. It is not disputed within mainstream Judaism, however, that God is involved in our lives. Jewish tradition teaches that when the Israelites were enslaved, exiled, and weeping about their plight, God suffered with them.[32] Similarly today, God suffers with us when we suffer. In addition, God responds to suffering by empowering us to find ways to react effectively to the trials that confront us. Jews learn to pray as though everything depends on God and to act as though everything depends on us. Both are essential, because central to Jewish theology is the belief that the world can be a better place when we participate and partner with each other and with God.

In our attempts to deal with our suffering, we often look to God to explain our woes. It is commonplace for chaplains in hospitals, geriatric centers, hospices, or during home care visits to meet with people who search for "a reason"—something in their own past that they've done—that made "it" happen, for which they are now being punished.

We suffer unbearably when something happens to those of us who feel that we have led "good" lives. The more wronged we feel, the more we suffer. We suffer immensely when something happens to our children, who have not had time to be "bad" during their short lives. We suffer excruciatingly when we conclude that the relationship that we have with God is not the relationship that we thought we had. It tears our souls, and we suffer.

In our attempts to deal with our suffering, we also look to each other. It is important to our healing process that others validate the full impact of our suffering upon the integrity of our lives. In fact, suffering is intensified when others try to minimize our experience or "cheer us out of it." We may put on a happy face for them, but it makes us feel more burdened and alone. Suffering also is intensified when loved ones try to persuade us that there are lessons to be learned from our suffering. Although it may resonate for some, many believe that the only lesson learned from suffering is that it is insupportable. The only ones helped by these practices are those who offer their comments, who are understandably trying to feel less helpless in the face of unrelenting suffering by someone they care about.

Suffering is further intensified when onlookers encourage sufferers to search for their culpability. Frequently, the first question asked upon hearing of another person's plight is: How did it happen? Which really means, what did you do or fail to do to allow (or cause) this to happen? Although it's an understandable question, it has less to do with the sufferer and more to do with onlookers trying to assure themselves that "it" won't happen to them. Despite our societal protestations against blaming the victim, we are more comfortable doing so than considering that we live in a chaotic world where injurious events randomly happen and may befall us. We are more comfortable believing that if we are "good" people, our goodness will safeguard us and may even protect our loved ones. When we can't find something that we've done to deserve our situation, we turn to—or away from—God.

The most valuable assistance that you can offer someone who may be feeling abandoned by—or angry with—God is to allow and encourage him or her to speak his or her own truth. Inviting spirituality into our lives means being open to a full relationship with God, a relationship that sometimes includes awe and praise and, sometimes, anger. The Hebrew Bible portrays many examples of individuals expressing anger at God. Not only is God able to take it, but sometimes God is moved to change a rendered verdict.

In Judaism, we speak of being created in the "image of God," *B'tzelem Elohim.*[33] You can invite spirituality into your life and into the lives of your suffering loved ones by imitating God. Just as God always is "present" with us during our time of need, so too can you be present, to help someone feel less alone at a time when loneliness or isolation make a sad situation worse. Just as God is willing to listen to cries of "Why?"; "Why me?"; "Why her/him?"; or "Why now?" as laments of sorrow, angst, and anger at an unjust situation and an unfair world, so too— without giving advice—can you. Just as God is a witness to the depth of a sufferer's experience and the impact of the situation upon the integrity of his or her life, so too can you. All you need to do is to validate the enormity of his or her experience and its impact upon his or her life. You do not need to fix the situation—indeed, it is probably impossible for you to do so.

Every time you praise someone for never complaining about his or her adversity, you are sending the message that you don't want to hear the story of his or her sorrow. And indeed, you may not. But just consider: It is the spiritual equivalent of telling someone with an infection that you don't want to help him or her get rid of the infection. You can choose to offer those sufferers extraordinary gifts that will assist them in their spiritual healing (and maybe even their physical healing) by letting them lament, even if doing so makes you uncomfortable.

If you can't offer this kind of companionship, see if a chaplain is available and/or look for an accessible support group. Speaking with, and listening to, other individuals who are suffering—even if the "why" of their suffering is different—often has a cathartic affect upon a sufferer. It's one of the reasons why the adage "misery loves company" is so popular. It reflects real-life experience. It's also one of the reasons that some individuals feel consoled upon hearing that God is suffering with them.

Whether you've thought about God's interaction in our lives, you probably have prayed for something—even if it just was for passing an exam. You've also probably prayed in your heart for loved ones when they've been in danger. Think about praying aloud with—and for—the one who is suffering. You can pray for a diminishment of suffering and loneliness. Indeed, at times you can assist in that effort. (See subsequent suggestions for ways you can help through prayer.)

It is noteworthy that Judaism continues to preserve, present, and accept many historical and contemporary thoughts and debates. Today, they are all available for us to choose from while we are trying to cope with our share of suffering. As you think about suffering and spiritual healing, we invite you to think about being in the midst of brokenness and injustice and not in the midst of sin. Think about being in the middle of sparks of holiness that are ready to infuse our lives, if only we let them in. Think about participating and partnering with others in such a profound way that each of us actually mends some of the brokenness in our own souls as well as some of the rips or gashes in the fabric of the soul of our universe.

Dying and Death

"An old woman visited the cemetery and gazing at the peaceful graves, she commented: 'Holy souls! How happy is your lot! How soothing is your sleep! And yet, I have no wish to be with you.'"[34]

Judaism asks us to honor and respect life, including the dying process and death itself. There are varying denominations within Judaism. Each engages the same or similar texts but may yield very different interpretations. The discussion about the dying process and death itself, "while text-centered, is hardly univocal. Different authorities read the same texts in diverse ways. They offer different opinions as to which texts provide appropriate analogues for understanding a contemporary situation . . . the interpretive process is nuanced and variegated . . . judgments that emerge from such an approach are often multivalent."[35]

A person who is on the verge of death is categorized as a *goses*. Although Judaism speaks about stages of dying, in the reality of today's modern medicine, it is difficult to know for certain where an individual is in the dying process. Generally, Jews turn to texts to understand what may or may not be done on behalf of a *goses*.[36] Usually these texts are derived from ancient sources that have been interpreted in *responsa* written by respected members of each Jewish denomination.[37]

If an individual is suffering from a disease or condition for which there is no known cure, nor reasonable hope for improvement, many Jewish ethicists would consider the possibility that these individuals are at the end of their lives. One of the questions often posed is, "Are we prolonging life or prolonging death?" When there is no reasonable hope of cure, any intervention that prolongs the dying process may be rejected or discontinued. If that person is also in pain, their pain must be treated as aggressively as necessary.[38] There are situations in which acceptance of death is in the best interest of the individual.

Whether a person dies at home, in a hospital, hospice, or a nursing home, the body is removed to a mortuary. If an individual dies on the Sabbath (Friday sundown through Saturday after sundown) or on festivals (from sundown through after sundown the next day), many Jews will request that the body not be moved until after the sacred day, so that its holiness is not compromised.[39]

It is commonplace to hold funerals within 24 hours of death unless they fall on a Sabbath or other holy days. This has been the standard practice, in part because loved ones lived within a few miles of each other and it was simple both to inform them of a death and for them to attend a funeral. Now that so many families are separated geographically, perhaps requiring many hours of driving or air travel to attend a funeral, this period before burial is often extended by a few days.

In death we are all equal. Jewish tradition suggests that a loved one be buried in a plain wooden box. Burial in a Jewish cemetery, in land that has been consecrated for that purpose, is standard practice. Burial returns the body to the earth, reflecting the biblical tradition: "For dust you are, and to dust you shall return."[40] However, today some Jews choose cremation as the form of their funeral. In some communities these ashes may be buried in a Jewish cemetery; others forbid this.[41]

Rabbi Abraham Joshua Heschel calls Judaism "the theology of the common deed."[42] The Jewish predilection toward "doing" dates back at least as far as Mt. Sinai, when, following God's revelation of the Torah, the assembled Israelite community unanimously responded to God with the words, "All that [God] has spoken we will faithfully do."[43] Consequently, it is standard practice to highlight a person's life and accomplishments during his or her funeral service with a eulogy. Flowers are not generally a part of Jewish funeral ceremonies. Oftentimes the family designates a favorite charity to which well-wishers may make a donation in memory of the deceased.

Mourning Practices

Following a funeral, some Jews wash their hands in a special place near the cemetery office or exit gates. Some wash again in a basin placed for this purpose just outside the residence that has been designated as the mourning home. "Official" mourners are one of eight different relationships: mother/father, sister/brother, wife/husband, and daughter/son.

After the funeral, official mourners "sit *shiva*." *Shiva* is a Hebrew word that refers to the first 7 days of mourning, counted from and including the day of the funeral. It is a time-out period that permits mourners to grieve without having any other responsibilities. Some mourners wear a cut black ribbon to symbolize their grief, while others tear a garment that they wear during this period. This cut symbolizes the rupture that they feel within.

Many mourners sit *shiva* for 7 days. In mystical Judaism, the number seven is associated with Divine Presence, holiness, and mystery.[44] Some mourners, particularly those with responsibilities that cannot go untended, grieve intensely for the first 3 days. In mystical Judaism the number three is a potent symbol of balance, reconciliation, holiness, and completeness.[45] The next 23 (or 27) days complete the period of *Sheloshim*: literally, "thirty." This less restricted time-out period allows mourners to continue to grieve while gradually reengaging their normal activities. After *Sheloshim*, mourners return to their normal schedules.

During these mourning periods, friends and family visit to offer condolences. In fact, consoling the bereaved is one of the precepts for which we receive spiritual credit both in our here-and-now lives and in our afterlives. Generally, loved ones, friends, or members of the congregation provide food. The first meal eaten usually includes hard-boiled eggs. The roundness of the egg is a reminder of the circularity of life and death.

Jewish mystics conceive of the body as an encumbering garment, which falls away at death and leaves the true person free to rise into the light of the heavenly life.[46] To assist loved ones in their ascension, many mourners, including those who are not regular synagogue-goers, attend services for the 12 months following the death of their loved one. In some Jewish mystical traditions, mourners discern that their loved ones lived such exemplary lives that they need only 11 months of prayer to ascend. Traditionally, mourners stand while they recite the Mourner's *Kaddish*, a prayer that concludes the synagogue service. The *Kaddish* prayer acknowledges God's constant presence in our lives, at times of joy and sorrow, light and darkness, life and death. In many Jewish communities mourners are joined by the congregation, who stand and pray for those whose names are unknown, who have died among all Jews, in the Holocaust, and in the aftermath of 9/11, tsunamis, hurricanes, and such. At the end of the 12 months and thereafter, on every anniversary of the death of a loved one, many mourners commemorate the *yahrzeit* (year's time/anniversary) of their loved one. They attend synagogue services to recite *Kaddish*, and they light special 24-hour *yahrzeit* candles at home.

Euthanasia

Jewish tradition forbids any direct action that will result in a life being shortened, even if the person is expected to die soon.[47] It is, however, permissible to remove external causes, which may prevent the departure of the soul. Two stories illustrate this.

> When Rabbi Yehudah was dying, the rabbis declared a public fast and offered prayers that God would show mercy so that Rabbi Yehudah would not die. Rabbi Yehudah's handmaid [who knew how great his pain was] ascended to the roof and prayed [for Yehudah to die]. The rabbis, however, continued to pray for God's mercy. She took a jar and threw it from the roof to the ground. Startled, they stopped praying, and the soul of Rabbi Yehudah departed to its eternal rest.[48]

> A very old person came to Rabbi Yose ben Halafta and said, "Rabbi, I wish to live no longer. I find no taste in food or drink; my limbs are heavy, and I should rejoice to take my departure from this world." The Rabbi asked: "Have you no interest left in life?" The woman replied, "I go daily to the synagogue; this is my sole interest in life." The Rabbi then replied, "If you feel too weary to continue living, try giving this up." The woman ceased going to synagogue and on the third day she sickened and died.[49]

In Judaism, doctors are not obliged to resort to extraordinary measures to keep the incurable alive.[50] How do we pray for the life of someone who is suffering from an incurable disease and is in great pain? Our sages teach that to pray for the impossible is disgraceful.[51] Our sages further teach that it is permissible—indeed obligatory—to pray for someone to be released from agony. That said, at present, rabbinic authorities debate whether physicians should administer a drug that would eliminate extreme pain, when in the process the result might be shortening someone's life.

Transplants

In Judaism *pikuah nefesh* (saving a life) is a paramount value. We respect the enormous strides that medical science has made over the past years. The harvesting of organs once dreamt of is now a reality. The general ruling on these issues is that transplants—whether donated or received—are instances of *Kevod Hamet* (respect for the dead) because they offer the deceased an opportunity to save a life. They also offer the near-dying an opportunity to live.

Autopsies

In general, autopsies are not permitted, because they would be *Nivul Hamet* (disgrace to the dead); they would mutilate the deceased. Nevertheless, if medical authorities claim that new knowledge derived only from an autopsy would help to cure others, it may be permitted. Likewise, an autopsy is permitted if secular law requires it to determine the cause of death.

In today's high-tech world, authorities from all Jewish denominations are faced with questions that simply were unknown in ages past. Where is the line between prolonging dying and continuing life? What constitutes appropriate intervention? Jewish ethicists honestly debate these questions. As is true throughout Judaism, no one answer fits all situations or all denominations.

Jewish Views of the Afterlife

Death is a particularly delicate subject—my death, your death, and the deaths of people close to us. "Death transcends human comprehension. No one has ever had an 'experience' of death. Even those who claim that they have 'died' and 'come back' again can, in truth, speak only of a 'near-death experience.' Because of the limitations of the human mind, a genuine understanding of death will inevitably elude even the wisest of us."[52]

Indeed, anyone's death poses all kinds of questions for the living, such as: Do all the dead go to the same place? If so, just where is that place, and what is it like? When we die, can we communicate with others who are deceased? Can the dead communicate with the living? Do we continue to know what is happening here on earth? Is the Afterlife a safe place? In our Afterlife existence, is there pain? Are we at peace? Is the Afterlife the same for all people? Do we see those who have died before us? Further, what of those people we do not wish ever to encounter again? As explained earlier, Judaism does not have a single "party line" when it comes to these questions. Although Judaism does have much to say about the subjects of death,[53] the Afterlife, immortality, and resurrection, the ideas about these subjects have changed enormously over the centuries of recorded Jewish thought.

The Biblical Period

The biblical period does not have a well-developed idea of the Afterlife. Often the Bible states that when people die, they join those who have gone before them.[54] They go to *Sheol*,[55] which is an underground locale, where eventually you simply cease to be. *Sheol* is a land of forgetfulness, where there is silence.[56] For the longest period of biblical history there was neither a concept of immortality of the soul nor of physical resurrection of dead bodies.[57]

The Rabbinic/Talmudic Period

In the next era, the Rabbinic/Talmudic period (about 2,000 years ago), we first find concepts concerning immortality of the soul and ideas about resurrection of dead bodies. According to the rabbis, death may be painless or painful.[58] Some say that angels record all our actions, good and bad, and that when we die there is a kind of life review, the outcome of which determines whether one attains heaven.[59]

The rabbis introduced the concept of the World to Come, *Olam ha-ba*.[60] "Better is one hour of repentance and good works in this world, than all of the World to Come, but at the same time, better is one hour of bliss in the World to Come, than all the life in this world."[61]

"In the World to Come, there is no eating or drinking, nor procreation nor commerce, nor jealousy, nor envy, nor rivalry. Rather, the righteous sit around with crowns on their heads and enjoy the radiance of the divine presence, the *Shekhinah*."[62]

They also suggested that the dead can converse with the living.[63]

The rabbis of the Rabbinic/Talmudic period were very interested in *Gehenna*, the Jewish form of hell. In their view a number of deeds will earn you time there: incest,[64] idolatry,[65] those who lead the masses to sin,[66] and (not surprisingly) speaking ill of a scholar after the scholar's death.[67] Ways to avoid *Gehenna* include giving to charity[68] or visiting the ill.[69] Time in *Gehenna* was generally limited to 12 months,[70] but exceptions exist: Some are there for eternity—people who committed particularly horrible crimes.[71]

Some rabbis say that Paradise (*Gan Eden*/Garden of Eden) was your destiny if you studied Torah; if you did not, it was *Gehenna*.[72] Some said that Paradise was a present reality; others said that it would come in the future.[73]

For the rabbis, resurrection of the body was a cardinal doctrine of Judaism.[74] "Through the process of homiletical textual exegesis, the Rabbis continually validated and reasserted the primacy of their belief in resurrection."[75] They taught that this idea had been part of Jewish life since time immemorial.[76] The rabbis did this through reference to biblical verses, taken out of context, but which supported the rabbis' views. They were able to do this because in their minds, all of Jewish teaching—past, present, and future—had been revealed to Moses on Mt. Sinai. There were no new teachings—there were no new concepts in Judaism—just new ways of understanding more fully what God had intended from the beginning of time and had revealed to Moses.

> The Rabbis believed not only that the Torah given at Mount Sinai anticipated all that would happen in the course of history, but that all new interpretations are an implicit part of the original text. They taught that whatever students will teach in future generations . . . was already given to Moses on Mount Sinai. . . . Therefore, the written text [of the Bible] and its interpretation [by the rabbis] are not viewed as totally distinct entities. On the contrary, they were thought to be part of the same revelation. What is deduced from the biblical text is not separate from it, but rather a latent part of it. It is the text within the text.[77]

The rabbis believed that resurrection would take place through the Land of Israel. That is the reason for the custom, followed by some Jews, to bury a person with some earth from Israel. The rabbis debated when resurrection will take place. Answers include the End of Days, or the Coming of the Messiah, or some indeterminate future time.

There also were debates about who would—or would not—be resurrected.[78] A popular view was that only the righteous would attain this status;[79] others said that all people would know resurrection.[80]

The Middle Ages

In contrast to these views, Moses Maimonides, the great Jewish philosopher, physician, and scholar of the late twelfth/early thirteenth century, argued that it is the soul, not the body, that is immortal. While there may be resurrection of dead bodies in the World to Come (*Olam ha-ba*), which only the righteous will earn, "there is nothing corporeal, and no material substance, there are only the souls of the righteous without bodies."[81] Further, Maimonides says that life in the World to Come is beyond human understanding.[82]

Other thoughts were developed by the Kabbalists about 500 years ago in the later Middle Ages. These Jewish mystics described several stages that the soul goes through after a person dies. The Kabbalists embraced the idea of the soul's immortality and accepted something that is akin to reincarnation. It is part of the tradition of *gilgul,* or circularity, that we die and are reborn again.

In this Kabbalistic postmortem journey our souls continue to progress through a variety of heavenly domains as they advance toward increasingly lofty and transcendent spiritual heights. Primarily this occurs in a seven-stage process: In the first stage of our postmortem experience, our physical bodies die. Many believe that with our final breath, we recline into the loving embrace of the wings of the *Shekhinah,* God's earthly "Presence." Kabbalistic images speak of a River of Light and of some sort of life review that goes on at this early stage.[83] In the second stage we surrender our attachments to our physical bodies.[84] The third stage is kind of like a prolonged and deeply intensive psychotherapy session.[85] The fourth and fifth stages feature a series of transitional steps between Lower and Upper *Gan Eden.*[86] The sixth stage brings us to transcendental bliss. Finally, in the seventh stage, we begin the process of returning to the earth, reborn into another body. Others hold that in the seventh stage our souls reunite with God.

Some Modern Approaches

Contemporary Orthodox prayer books speak of the resurrection of dead bodies. In the *Amidah* (one of the central prayers), it states, "Blessed are you, God, Resurrector of the dead." Many Orthodox believe this, but many do not. The Conservative prayer book modifies this language. The Hebrew remains the same, though the English is rendered, "Praised are You, Lord, Master of life and death." Probably the majority of Jews associated with conservative synagogues do *not* believe in a physical resurrection of dead bodies, though this is what they pray when they pray in Hebrew.

In the Reform prayer book, both the Hebrew and the English are changed at the conclusion of this prayer to "Blessed are You, Eternal, who renews all life." Reform Judaism stresses individual autonomy in practice and belief. Most Reform Jews do not believe in the resurrection of dead bodies. Most Reform Jews would speak of immortality of the soul as the normative state of the Afterlife.

In the Reconstructionist prayer book the words are: "God who gives and renews life."

Today, Jews continue to hold a variety of beliefs and ideas, which range from immortality of the soul to resurrection of dead bodies to some kind of belief in transmigration of souls. In Jewish sacred literature, be it biblical, Talmudic, medieval, or contemporary, whether it is liturgical or philosophical writing, there are several Hebrew words that are translated as "soul." Because Judaism does not have one systematic theology, sources often use these words inconsistently and even synonymously. The Bible uses three different words for soul: *ruah*, *nefesh*, and *neshamah*. It is our understanding that *ruah* and *nefesh* are connected to a person being physically alive. Our *neshamah*, our eternal soul, lives within us, and then, some time after we die, our *neshamah* returns to God. To offer an analogy, we are like an ocean wave that for a brief moment in time has a separate identity. Then, when its time is passed, it reunites with its source and becomes part of the ever-flowing eternal ocean.

We can influence how we will be remembered after we die. We do this in three ways: biological immortality, immortality through influence, and immortality through deeds.[87] *Biological immortality* takes several forms. This may mean having children. Another way is to associate with a group—for example, the people of Israel. Through this connection we are linked with our historical forebears. Secondly, there is the *immortality through influence*. This may mean adopting children. In addition, we all have been influenced by our teachers, friends, and colleagues. We ourselves influence other people, knowingly or not. Immortality through influence can have as much of an effect as biological immortality. Thirdly, there is *immortality through deeds*, for our actions allow us to live on through their impact on the minds and hearts of those who come after us.

A Brief Guide to Prayerful Presence

"Miriam was shut out of the camp . . . and the people did not march on. . . ." (Numbers 12:15)

Pastoral Visitation

Unlike our biblical ancestor Miriam, most of those who are seriously or terminally ill encounter the reality that, increasingly, the world goes on without them. Even when family and friends are attentive in the beginning, if distressed individuals do not become well within a reasonable period of time, sooner or later their visitors will return to the normalcy of their own lives. In large part this is because visitors feel helpless when they repeatedly hear about the lack of improvement—or worsening plight—of loved ones without being able to help them heal. This is intensified when loved ones are dying.

Perhaps we need to redefine what it means to help someone during the times that we "shut [them] out of the camp," in hospitals, nursing homes, hospices, and home-care facilities.

The Talmudic story cited earlier begs the question: If the healer, Rabbi Yohanan, had the power to cure other people, why could he not cure himself?[88] The Talmud provides this response: just as prisoners cannot free themselves from their incarceration, so prisoners of wounded bodies, ailing spirits, and devastated souls cannot heal themselves. If even the healer, Rabbi Yohanan, needed another person to facilitate his healing, so do we.

The wisdom of Jewish sages challenges those of us who think that we are strong enough, resourceful enough, and centered enough to endure various stages of infirmity without some assistance from at least one other person. God heals, but we may often be the essential intermediaries through whom God's will is accomplished, whether that means a curing of the body or a healing of the spirit, whether we are medical practitioners, chaplains, or loved ones. This means that each of us has a responsibility as well as a response-ability.

Of course, unlike Rabbis Yohanan and Hanina, we may not be able to heal others simply by touching them, but—like those ancient rabbis—we can offer compassionate caring, an empathetic ear, a hearing heart, a gentle gesture of concern, a wise word, and, yes, a helpful hand during moments of distress. Of course, it isn't possible for one person to make everyone's life better; nevertheless, each of us can assist another person during at least one traumatic experience.

Visiting individuals during their times of vulnerability and apprehension are sacred tasks. These visits impact upon the health of the souls of everyone involved. They are so significant that they are among the activities for which we receive a reward in our own "World to Come"; they are so significant that our morning prayer services (Shaharit) feature a Talmudic passage that reminds us that visiting the ill, generally acting in a kindly manner, and attending funerals are essential to the well-being of our own souls. This last is considered particularly meritorious, because there is no way for the deceased to repay the kindness.[89]

Visiting individuals who are infirm is not always an easy task. The following are general guidelines when working with someone who is ill: Be there. Be present. Be respectful. Be gone. Bless. And be blessed.

Be There

Continue to include individuals in your life who are infirm. Visit with them, even if it makes you uncomfortable. Bikur holim—literally, "visiting the sick"—is regarded as an important mitzvah (religious obligation or blessing, depending upon where you are along the Jewish denominational spectrum). Each Jew[90]—not only those in care-giving professions—is expected to partner with God in attending to those who are unwell.[91] To reinforce this concept, Jewish tradition teaches that each visitor carries away 1/60th of the beleaguered individual's illness. In response to why 60 people cannot cure someone, our ancient sages replied that the first visitor takes away 1/60th of an ailing person's existing condition. The second visitor takes away 1/60th of that person's remaining illness, ad infinitum.[92] We understand from this that the very presence of a kind and caring visitor brings comfort.

Be sensitive to the physical realities of the infirm, such as medical needs and routines, meal times, signs of fatigue, and so forth. If you schedule a visit at a specific time, respect that commitment. Not to do so may disappoint someone who is looking forward to your being there. At the very least, it conveys the message that you don't consider their time as important as your own, when in fact their time may be extremely limited and, therefore, precious. You tell people that you value them by being on time.

Be Present

The purpose of a visit—for nonprofessional visitors—is to help the infirm feel comfortable by attending to their needs, cheering them, assisting them in continuing to feel connected to the world at large, and praying for mercy on their behalf.[93] An additional—and extremely important—goal for those visiting the dying is to help them feel that they have made a difference—that their lives mattered.

During your visit, make eye contact, fully focus upon them, and interact with them compassionately, emotionally, empathetically, and mindfully. Listen carefully to what they are saying and—by taking notice of their body language and gestures—to what they are *not* saying.

If others are present, visit with them *later*. Your undivided presence with the person who is suffering makes a difference. When appropriate, so does your touch. Often, individuals who are infirm are physically touched only when they are being medically probed or palpated. Your touch may provide the only warm and caring connection from one human to another.[94]

Be Respectful

Use judgment and tact when dialoguing with those who are infirm. Encourage them to talk about their difficulties but do not offer false hopes or cause them to despair.[95] When you visit with individuals who are unlikely to recover, don't pray for their complete recovery. Pray for a diminishment of their suffering or a lessening of their anguish or sorrow. To pray for something that may be unrealistic may leave them more disappointed—in themselves, about their situation, in the medical team for failing them, and/or in God for abandoning them. This is spiritually harmful at a time when they may be contemplating the possibility of "going to God" sooner—or differently—than they had anticipated.

Honor the truth of the individual who is infirm, even if it differs from your own reality. When you visit with people who are suffering from the ravages of dementia, try to remember that it doesn't help to explain to the afflicted, who may be looking for, say, a parent, that their parent died decades ago. Rather, be sensitive to the distress that they are experiencing, irrespective of the facts involved. Finally, be respectful of confidences and do not share privileged information in open spaces, like elevators, where information may be overheard and transmitted inappropriately.

Be Gone

It may have taken a long time for you to travel to make this visit; nevertheless, please be mindful that the physical and spiritual health of the individuals that you are visiting is compromised, so keep visits brief. Remember, they are not there for you, you are there for them.

Bless

We said earlier that one of the essential purposes for visiting an individual who is infirm is for the visitor to pray to God to be merciful to the one being visited. It may surprise you to learn that Jewish tradition further teaches that visitors—including nonprofessional caregivers—who leave without praying have not fulfilled their responsibilities.[96]

Be Blessed

God wants us to visit those we have shut out of [our] camps. God is so pleased when we do that we receive a reward in the World to Come. To further increase the possibility that we will observe this *mitzvah* and go where God wants us to go, Jewish tradition teaches that when we bless someone, God blesses us.[97]

Prayerful Presence

In Jewish belief, each person—clergy and laity alike—has a personal and direct relationship with God. Judaism does not place any special sacramental status upon Jewish clergy. Rabbis or cantors may serve as priests, but that is only one of the many facets of their roles. Most Jewish clergy would say that they are not inherently more holy or even potentially more in touch with God than their congregants.[98] In fact, although rabbis and cantors usually lead synagogue services, Jewish laity may also lead them. Consequently, visitors may offer to pray and to do so in whatever language the compromised individual understands. You do not necessarily need to pray in Hebrew.[99]

If saying a prayer aloud feels daunting, consider that Jewish tradition teaches that the heart's cry to God is the highest form of all prayer.[100] Prayers can be custom made for each individual.[101] They don't have to be fixed prayers that you read from a book (that you may have forgotten to bring) or words that you memorized (and are afraid of forgetting). God wants the prayers that you compose to reflect the moment. Simply talk to God, speak aloud the words in your heart when you wish the best for those you care about. In fact, you probably already are praying to God to grant the one that you care about relief from suffering, strength to endure, companionship, and the like. You just need to say your prayers audibly and in a more intentional way. You might also scan a book called *Talking to God*, by Rabbi Naomi Levy. Her book is filled with many spontaneous prayers. She points out that it is quite "remarkable to see what can emerge from us when we stop trying to pray to God and start *talking* to God instead . . . talking to God is a very natural and intimate experience."[102]

If spontaneous prayer feels too intimidating, then we suggest praying aloud the five words that Moses prayed when he entreated God to heal his sister Miriam. In Jewish tradition, they are believed to be among the most powerful of prayers: *El na r'fa na la*—Please God: heal her now, I pray.[103] It is becoming increasingly common to hear visitors chant these words softly and repetitively, like a mantra, in hospital rooms.[104]

If you are shy about praying out loud, please consider the prayer known as *Mi Shebeirach*—literally the "One who blesses." Here, the "One who blesses" refers to God. This prayer asks for God's blessing for greater health or for the strength to deal with pain and suffering. You may recite this prayer at the bedside—although typically it is recited during synagogue services by the rabbi, cantor, or service leader, who has collected a list of names of those congregants who are in need of an infusion of healing spirit. Ask those you care about if they would like their names read in synagogue along with the others who are infirm. In recent years, Jewish singer/songwriter Debbie Friedman composed an English/Hebrew song called *Mi Shebeirach* that has been incorporated into many Jewish religious and spiritual services, including Healing Services. Today, it is not unusual to hear this song chanted in the synagogue. It is also becoming more frequent for visitors to sing it during visits and to sing it for each other.[105]

Finally, we have *Vidui* (formally, *Vidui Sh'-khiv mey-ra*)—the "confession of one seriously ill." This prayer, or confessional, may also be spoken on behalf of a dying person. The words acknowledge that all life and death are in God's time and that none of us knows the time of our leaving this world for the World to Come. In *Vidui*, we place ourselves in God's power, ask for forgiveness from those we have hurt (both knowingly and unknowingly), and ask to be able to forgive those who have hurt us. We also ask that our death be an expiation for our transgressions. *Vidui* ends with the *Shema*, which is the central affirmation within Judaism—*Shema Yisrael . . .* "Hear, O Israel! The LORD is our God, the LORD alone."[106]

Reciting *Vidui* neither hastens nor prevents death. Sometimes *Vidui* is said for a person who then recovers. The *Vidui* can be said again on another occasion. In fact, most Jews have prayed a form of *Vidui* each year during the High Holy Days, and they return the next year to pray it again. *Vidui* may be read—or its essence recited—by the individual who is in jeopardy or by a visitor on behalf of that individual. It may be said in English, Hebrew, or any other language that the individual understands.

If you can't quite get yourself to pray, chant, recite, or read and you don't feel comfortable asking a synagogue to add the name of the one that you care about to their *Mi Shebeirach* list, find out if the hospital, geriatric center, or hospice has a chaplain. This is probably a good idea in any event. Often, individuals who are infirm are unable to unburden themselves to loved ones, who feel their plight too intensely. Moreover, it can be a cathartic experience for compromised individuals to share their existential angst with professionals who are trained to work with individuals experiencing life and death issues. This is especially true because these "strangers" symbolize a visit by God's representative, much as our patriarch Abraham was visited by God when he was unwell.[107]

We said earlier that visiting individuals during times of vulnerability and apprehension is a sacred task. To achieve the ends of holiness, it is important that visitors be religiously—and spiritually—respectful of the one that they are visiting. This means that visitors may have to withhold their personal religious beliefs when the beliefs of the individual who is infirm differ from their own. For example, it is inappropriate—and spiritually harmful—for visitors from liberal religious backgrounds to ignore religious traditions of the more orthodox—if they are meaningful to the orthodox person visited. It is equally inappropriate and spiritually harmful for visitors from orthodox religious backgrounds to suggest to a religiously liberal person that there is "only one way" that God wants them to go forward—if that orthodox system is not meaningful to the liberal person visited. Of course, it is also most emphatically inappropriate for non-Jewish visitors to impose their religious beliefs upon a Jewish person who is physically compromised and emotionally defenseless.

Today, most institutions have chaplains who can pray with sensitivity and respect, using spiritual language with those whose belief systems differ from their own. To ensure that individuals who are infirm receive the spiritual care that they may need, institutions are increasingly requiring chaplains to engage in extensive education to enhance and refine their pastoral care skills.[108] Ask the one that you care about if they would like a visit from a chaplain, and ask the nurses to tell you how to contact the Chaplain's office.

When we visit those who are infirm, we partner with God in providing for the welfare of the spirit, mind, and body of the one that we care about. Many millennia ago, God charged our biblical parents, Abraham and Sarah, to "Go forth . . . to the place that I will show you . . . and you shall be a blessing, and I will bless those who bless you."[109] Go forth, bless—and be blessed.

Resources

In addition to the Notes listed at the end of this book, for relevant articles on issues of Jewish spirituality and health, please refer to the following.

Flam, N. (1996-1997). Healing the spirit: A Jewish approach. *Cross Currents, 46*, 487-496.

Taylor, B. E. (2004). The healing power of chanting. *PlainViews*, July 7, 2004. See www .PlainView.org (the international chaplain's electronic news magazine). To subscribe, info@plainviews.org.

Taylor, B. E., and Zucker, D. J. (2002). Nearly everything we wish our non-Jewish supervisors had known about us as Jewish supervisees. *Journal of Pastoral Care and Counseling, 56*, 327-338.

Zucker, D. J. (2001). Answering "why me, why now:" Empowering the elderly through response-ability. *Annals of Long-Term Care, 9.5*, 61-63.

Zucker, D. J. (2002). Family of resident's support group: A safe place to vent and lament. *Annals of Long-Term Care, 10.5*, 36-40.

Zucker, D. J. (2002). Family of resident's support group: Sharing disappointments and coping with anger. *Annals of Long-Term Care, 10.9*, 23-25.

Zucker, D. J. (2003). You lift us up. *Healing Ministry, 10.1*, 43-44.

Zucker, D. J. (2005). Para-chaplaincy: A communal response to the ill and suffering. In Dayle A. Friedman (Ed.), *Jewish pastoral care: A practical handbook* (2nd ed., revised and expanded). Woodstock, VT: Jewish Lights.

Zucker, D. J., & Taylor, B. E. (2006). The muse of visiting. In Jack H Bloom (Ed.), *Jewish relational care a-z: We are our other's keeper*. Binghamton, NY: Haworth.

14

Ojibwe Beliefs and Rituals in End-of-Life Care

ROBERT CHI-NOODIN PALMER AND
MARIANNE LESLIE PALMER

For Eugene Begay and Frank Perez

I realize death is not the enemy but the ultimate healing.
Robert Chi-Noodin Palmer, MD

EDITOR'S NOTE: *This chapter details the spiritual traditions of the Ojibwe Tribe, one of many Native American tribes in North America. Native American spirituality is a broad umbrella, under which there is a rich diversity of beliefs, rituals, and practices. This chapter presents one tribe's spiritual beliefs and traditions in depth, rather than a more broad overview of multiple tribes. The author writes from his experience with this tribe, and, per Native American beliefs, it would not be appropriate to discuss spiritual practices of other tribes. For additional information on Native American spirituality, refer to Appendix A. The resources on Native American spirituality listed in the appendix have been selected by the editor.*

Introduction

The traditional belief system of the Ojibwe (O jib' way) tribe of North American Indians, primarily located in the Great Lakes region, identifies life and death as continuous segments of individual spiritual existence. Nonphysical spirit exists before, during, and after incarnation in human form. Therefore, death does not inspire fear, and end-of-life care represents one part in a lifelong practice of respectful care for individuals and community. Ojibwe spiritual practice consists of daily prayer, ritual offerings of gratitude, honoring elders, and looking forward seven generations. In addition to these ongoing practices, special ceremonies provide support at important times, such as during illness. This chapter introduces the basic beliefs and rituals of the Ojibwe and their various applications.

Ojibwe Beliefs

Ojibwe spiritual beliefs and practices derive from embracing the organization inherent in nature, a pattern beyond human ability to comprehend. Human beings play but a small part in a vast, interconnected web. Everything that happens to one member of the community affects the whole. Ojibwe pointedly honor every aspect of life, whether a log for a fire, the hands we use to chop wood, or the fire itself.

Ojibwe teachings encourage awareness of human dependence on—and indebtedness to—the many different elements contained in the world. Recognizing humans exist only in community highlights the ever-widening ripples of consequence following individual action. Living with gratitude and respect for the unseen, unheard, and unrepresented strands in the total fabric of existence teaches conscientious action. Taking nothing for granted and no more than needed decreases personal entitlement and feelings of manifest destiny. Ojibwe teach that humans have the right to use plants, animals, and minerals for sustenance, provided each time we do so we pray for permission, take only what we need, and give thanks for what we have taken.

Ojibwe teach by oral tradition; different levels and variations pass between regions, groups, families, tribe members, and elders and their students. The ideas presented here represent some of what I have learned from my elders in age or wisdom. As a student, I humbly acknowledge the vast richness of the Ojibwe traditions as yet unknown to me.

Gitchi Manitou

Gitchi Manitou translates as the unlimited Great Unknown, Great Mystery, or "All-Giving Spirit," corresponding in some ways to familiar concepts of God. Gitchi Manitou represents the creative source of all existence. Faith in Gitchi Manitou manifests as untroubled acceptance of interconnectedness beyond human understanding. For example, if presented with a windfall of apples, gather only those necessary for survival, and leave the rest for use by other people, plants, animals, and microbes.

Faith broadens understanding of the human position in the many levels of community and sets a course of ever-increasing personal accountability. Before receiving a life-threatening cancer diagnosis, I had discovered two beautiful serpentine boulders near our homesite. A year and many prayers later, driving a backhoe, I delivered these large grandfather stones as sentinels on either side of our entranceway. Soon thereafter, I found one of the perfect boulders split in two. A rush of grief and anger made me want to run out and find the workman responsible. Fortunately, my daily practice of prayer paid off: My focus shifted from impulsive action to reflection. In that moment, I saw the image of a scarred, half-blind, beatific face of an old warrior serenely at peace with himself and the world. I realized perfection, too, exists only in the eyes of the beholder. My anguish evaporated: I confronted no one, and no worker came forward to acknowledge responsibility. My broken grandfather's stone remains, a monument to the perfection inherent in imperfection—our very imperfection providing an unending spiritual path.

Hierarchy of Respect

Age, knowledge, and experience command respect and determine rank in the Ojibwe spiritual hierarchy. Length of time on earth determines age; therefore, minerals rank above plants, with animals next. Rather than placing humans at the pinnacle of God's creation, we occupy the lowest position in the Ojibwe spiritual hierarchy. As infants depend upon their parents for survival, humans depend on minerals, plants, and animals. In contrast, these elders need nothing from humans but respect.

Elders possess patience and wisdom, a deeper acceptance of the implications of coexistence. Honoring elders extends to the human members of the community. For example, during a traditional feast, the youngest offer to fill the plates of the oldest before feeding themselves. For Ojibwe, the elderly deserve respectful treatment independent of perceived merit: Younger members lack the frame of reference necessary for judging their elders. A special respect for age counterbalances today's preoccupation with youthfulness and increases patience with the elderly—and therefore the quality of end-of-life care. Care given with respect, even reverence, allows the recipient greater dignity, despite physical helplessness.

Living in a Body; Living in Balance

Living in a physical body places us in community with all existence. Living in balance means active promotion of physical, emotional, intellectual, and spiritual health. The requirements of physical survival clearly underscore human reliance on a healthy environment. Humans must breathe air, drink water, eat food, and find and build shelter. Every action unavoidably affects the whole. Individuals bear responsibility for maintaining balance within and between community members.

Ojibwe teach that the body serves as a vehicle for spirit. Living in balance confers individual rewards; looking forward seven generations takes care of community and the future. Activity level and focus adjust over the life span as needs, capabilities, and bodies change. Ojibwe help each other face challenges, especially those hardships occurring at the end of life. Listening with open ears, eyes, hearts, and minds indicates how to effectively support others and ensure that no one suffers alone.

Warrior Instinct and Honoring the Enemy

Warrior instinct describes a fierce will to survive and overcome obstacles. A warrior's strength is derived from an unshakable recognition of this quality in others. Respect for all means respect for other, even if threatening. Honoring the strength of an opponent leads to fighting with respect. Fear and hatred undermine strength; honoring an enemy prepares for battle. Utilizing the warrior instinct increases confidence, strength, and a sense of mastery during times of challenge, giving us a fighting chance whether against a human aggressor or inoperable cancer. Caregivers may use this internal resource to combat fears before unintentionally affecting a person facing pain, illness, or death. Honoring an opponent, balanced with acceptance of forces beyond human control, conveys comfort and peacefulness.

Practical Applications

Practical applications of Ojibwe spirituality include daily prayer, learning traditions from elders, and periodic rituals and ceremonies. Ritual involves an established procedure using natural materials such as plants, water, fire, and stone. An attitude of prayerful respect underlies spiritual practice. Familiar patterns of ritual provide an anchor in the face of events beyond human control. Ceremony, performed individually or in a group setting, uses several rituals in a larger sequence for a specific purpose, such as healing. For example, a sweat lodge ceremony performed on behalf of an ill or dying person combines ritual prayer, singing, and use of natural materials. Each of the practices described below adds meaning to end-of-life care, whether performed by or for a person facing death.

Prayer and Forethought

Enter into prayer like an empty cup ready to be filled
rather than one half full of questions.

Paul DeMain

Forethought ranks high on the list of human responsibilities as coinhabitants of
the planet. Prayer connects and communicates between the material dimension
and the spiritual dimension. The discipline of daily prayer increases awareness of
interconnectedness, humility, and gratitude. Praying helps plan actions and gauge
consequences. Praying for guidance at the beginning of a hunt, for example, asks
permission to kill an animal willing to volunteer its life. After a successful hunt,
prayers of thanks and offerings of tobacco help fulfill the responsibility to give back
after receiving.

Praying in words furnishes an outlet; learning to listen with a quiet mind during prayer may supply answers. Routine daily prayer yields spiritual sustenance and
emotional comfort. Performing rituals during prayer requires concentration and focus, an effort similar to flexing a muscle. Opening the mind into a receptive mode
requires expanding attention, as when stretching a muscle. Staying in good shape
spiritually requires as much discipline and effort as does staying in good shape physically, emotionally, and intellectually.

Tobacco Offering

Tobacco, used in prayer and ceremony, represents the initiation of contact between
the material and spiritual worlds. During daily prayer, traditional Ojibwe use a
pinch of tobacco in the palm of the hand or in their personal pipe. Acknowledging
the sacrifice the tobacco has made, Ojibwe return the tobacco to a natural setting
after prayers.

Spirit Plate

Many Native Americans offer small portions of each dish served at mealtimes to
give thanks for plants and animals used for sustenance. Similar to saying grace, the
spirit plate graphically illustrates our dependence on others, human and nonhuman.
Overconsumption dishonors the delicate balance that affords human nourishment.
Offering a spirit plate honors both the foods eaten and the ancestors who have
passed before us.

Smudging

Some plants have healing properties, and when respectfully collected and dried, become medicines. Traditional smudging rituals use sage, cedar, and sweetgrass. Lighting the dried leaves and extinguishing the flames to expose smoldering embers provide smoke for smudging. Silence and prayer accompany the medicinal smoke washing over the body, the group, or place in need of balance. Which medicines are used in smudging depends on the purpose of the ritual. Sage, the most commonly used, helps decrease the impact of unwanted burdens by dissipating negative memories, thoughts, feelings, and sensations. Cedar smoke lessens negative impact, invites positive influences, and promotes balance. Sweetgrass smoke promotes the value of cooperating for the greater good, enhancing the sweetness of life. Especially during times of stress, smudging with sage, cedar, and sweetgrass provides comfort and relief for both caregivers and receivers during end-of-life care.

Healing Stones

Stones possess remarkable strength and endurance and may help heal and restore balance by absorbing fear or pain. The Ojibwe word *mishomis* may refer to a healing stone but literally translates as "grandfather," indicating the essence of the oldest living things on earth. Many have had the experience of becoming acutely aware of a particular stone, as though it had called out for notice. Stones communicate and volunteer their services in this manner. With tobacco in hand, one may respectfully request permission to remove this stone from its natural environment, wait for a sense of agreement, and pick it up while putting a pinch of tobacco in its place. Ojibwe ceremonial healings only use stones gathered and cared for in a respectful manner.

Stones respectfully gathered on behalf of others provide a service for those without access to stones in a natural environment. A recipient blindly touches an offered group of stones until one in particular conveys a unique sensation, indicating which stone has volunteered. Caregivers often feel burdened as well and may appreciate the help of a healing stone. To cleanse and balance a healing stone, place it in pure water and hold it up to the moonlight.

Naming Ceremony

A naming ceremony honors the arrival of new members to the community. Certain elders possess the ability to identify spirit names, often from dreams or ceremonial experiences. The spirit name helps guide an individual through life and back into the spirit world.

Pipe Ceremony

Performed individually and in groups, the pipe ceremony plays a fundamental role in Ojibwe spiritual practice and healing. A ceremonial pipe represents union and family. Prayer, accompanied by ritual pipe smoking, gives thanks, seeks direction, or addresses specific concerns. Designated pipe carriers perform this ceremony when petitioned by, or on behalf of, those in need. Participating in a pipe ceremony for end-of-life issues benefits all involved.

Drumming and Song

Songs accompany Ojibwe ceremonies. Drumming represents communication between the drummer and Gitchi Manitou. Some songs use Ojibwe lyrics; others use vocal sounds without specific meaning. Songs may arise spontaneously or pass from teacher to student; others have specific ceremonial applications.

Making and Using a Medicine Wheel

A medicine wheel symbolizes the cycle of physical life. Traditional Ojibwe see spiritual life as a continuously revolving wheel. Life in the body represents one revolution. A medicine wheel divides into four quadrants, corresponding to physical, emotional, intellectual, and spiritual development. Full balance requires attention equally distributed within and between these four aspects of individual and community life.

To make a medicine wheel, draw a circle with two lines intersecting at the center and adjoining the circle at 12 and 6 o'clock and at 9 and 3 o'clock. The 3 o'clock position represents both the point of entry into physical life and its end point.

A more detailed medicine wheel requires four colors: black, white, yellow, and red. From the center of the circle to 3 o'clock, draw or paint a yellow line. The color yellow and the eagle symbolize the eastern direction. East represents both development through infancy and childhood, and physical life. As the area between 3 o'clock and 6 o'clock occupies one quarter of a clock face, the energy required to maintain physical health should account for about 25% of our time and energy. Overemphasis on appearance, sensation, or physical activity results in imbalance, exemplified by people with eating disorders. Understanding physical needs and limitations, eating a healthy diet, and engaging in moderate exercise lead to balance in the physical quadrant.

A red line connects the center of the circle to the 6 o'clock position. Red indicates the southern direction, also represented by the wolf. South symbolizes adolescence and emotional development. Emotional outbursts such as verbal abuse, or apathy resulting from suppressed emotion, indicate imbalance in the southern portion of the medicine wheel. Discussion, therapy, and anger management courses may help those in need of balance in this direction.

From the center of the circle to 9 o'clock, draw a black line. Black indicates the western direction, represented by the bison. West symbolizes adulthood and intellectual development. Spending too many passive hours in front of the TV creates imbalance arising from underutilization of the intellect. Conversely, overinvestment in this quadrant may result in multiple academic degrees yet produce the inability to communicate with our own children. Challenging interaction with others, reading, and evaluating new information may help keep the intellectual quadrant in balance.

From the center of the circle to 12 o'clock, a white line indicates the direction north, represented by the bear. North symbolizes the wisdom of maturity, and higher spiritual development. Inconsiderate proselytizing or deep, unrelenting fear of death may indicate imbalance in this area. Caregiving provides an opportunity to help a person focus on spiritual needs, by initiating discussion of concerns for family members, performance of a ceremony, prayer, or working with a medicine wheel.

The reflection in a mirror placed at the center of the medicine wheel serves as a reminder of who controls the balance in our lives. The visual aid of a medicine wheel helps individuals see how they distribute their energy and where changing emphasis may help. Using the medicine wheel, caregivers may help assess life satisfaction by discussing physical, emotional, intellectual, and spiritual values and expression.

Sweat Lodge Ceremony

Ojibwe elders often say one cannot heal oneself; healing ceremonies embrace the community as a source of healing and strength. Many Native Americans engage in sweat lodge ceremonies, and sometimes refer to the lodge as their "church." The structure itself symbolizes the womb. Stones removed from a fire occupy the center of the lodge and provide the heat needed to sweat. Ritual smudging of stones used in a sweat lodge ceremony acknowledges the stone's sacrifice. Prayer in a sweat lodge may seek help for self, loved ones, or the larger community. Each lodge leader conducts the ceremony differently. A sweat lodge ceremony may be requested for oneself or on behalf of another, even if both are unable to attend personally. Some have found it uplifting to sit beside the lodge as the ceremony proceeds.

End of Life

Using the phrase "passing over" instead of "passing away" reinforces understanding death as material transition, gradual change, rather than disappearance. Access to the spiritual dimension increases as death approaches; focus on living in a body decreases. Death represents the culmination of a shift over time rather than an abrupt change in condition. Caregivers must attend to physical, emotional, or spiritual suffering. Both caregivers and individuals approaching death walk a fine line between taking care of the body and accepting the spirit's journey toward home. The ongoing nature of spirit deflects attention from physical suffering to the relief of homecoming. Death of the body allows spirit to fully rejoin a greater family independent of time and place. Thus, death does not inspire fear.

Living with honor demands working to give more than we take; listening provides both the caregiver and the dying with a means of giving. Toward the end of life, traditional elders feel compelled to add value to the lives of others, including caregivers. The wisdom shared allows a dying person the dignity necessary for peace of mind. As the time of his death drew near, a beloved Apache elder grew anxious to tell us everything he had learned over the course of his life and made certain that his suffering did not burden us. Reassuring words, singing, prayer, and ceremonies provide comfort and safety; even while unconscious, asleep, or in a coma, words and actions have consequences for the person cared for.

Although approaches to the logistics of end-of-life care differ among Ojibwe individuals, families, and bands, primary objectives include providing physical comfort, unobtrusive company, and reassurance. The possibility of remaining at home during the dying process offers immense security and relief, promising familiarity of place and presence of family. Caregivers shoulder the burden or responsibility for tending to their own needs as well as those of the cared for and must remain alert to possible conflicts of interest. Comfort of the dying must supercede comfort of the caregiver; feelings of helplessness, loss, or incompetence may cause suffering and distort thinking. Performing a ritual burning of a fear bundle (tobacco and sage wrapped in written concerns) helps ease psychological distress, increasing acceptance and peacefulness, benefiting both caregiver and recipient.

Burial Ceremony

Burial occurs on the fourth day after the death of the body. Elders counsel the family during these four days. A small symbolic lodge, a spirit house, stands beside the burial site. For three days family members light a small fire at sundown and place a food offering beside the spirit house. On the fourth day after burial, a communal feast commences.

Personal Experience

Several years ago I received a diagnosis of aggressive prostate cancer. I underwent further tests at Stanford University School of Medicine. The results confirmed my worst fears: My cancer could be managed for the rest of my life but not "cured." My Ojibwe elders referred me to a Blackfoot elder experienced in treating cancer. My elders did not use the word cancer; I had "a condition" requiring specific traditional medicines and ceremonies. In Canada and at home, elders performed sweat lodge, pipe, and healing ceremonies to fight the disease and help me prepare for Western medical treatment. My Blackfoot and Ojibwe elders assured me I would recover; Western medical statistics indicated otherwise.

I felt an intense determination to take my healing into my own hands. I became proactively responsible for every aspect of my health. My greatest challenge lay in distancing myself from the passive mentality seemingly prevalent among medical patients. I did not want to feel like a victim or to act like one. I expected my doctors to help me—but not heal me. I paid strict attention to any reliable information I could use on my own behalf, whatever the source. When appropriate, I asked for help from family, elders, friends, colleagues, doctors, acquaintances, and other patients. I relied on my wife as my main caregiver.

We made certain of my comfort in all areas, physical, emotional, intellectual, and spiritual. For example, I kept traditional Native American medicines, music, and healing stones with me during each radiation treatment. In the waiting room, I beaded leather medicine bags to give as gifts and listened to my Pow Wow music; this helped me relax and kept me engaged in constructive activity. I turned off flores-cent lights or waited in a garden setting whenever possible. I tried to cheer up other patients and overworked staff members. After each treatment, I smudged as soon as possible—in my car if necessary.

I fought to remain alert at all times to the various assaults on my body, to trans-mute fear into the will to survive. At least once a day I prayed, gave thanks and offer-ings—honoring the strength of my adversary, my spirit, and Gitchi Manitou, the "All-Giving Spirit." I took great comfort and guidance from my Ojibwe spirit name, Chi-Noodin, translated: Strong Wind. When faced with a particularly overwhelming situation, I prepared myself with hidden war paint. While exercising, I visualized cancer cells giving way to healthy cells. I realized the necessity of continuing my work and being of service to others. I learned a tremendous amount during this time of adversity.

After 7 1/2 weeks of treatments, my wife and I returned home. I conducted a sweat lodge ceremony, thanking Gitchi Manitou and the human beings, minerals, plants, and animals for having helped me. During the ceremony I felt my spirit thank me for my efforts to keep my body alive and healthy! To this day, I remain so: My cancer is undetectable.

I feel strength and reassurance from winning each battle thus far. Each day I face the renewed challenge to stay engaged in my lifelong struggle to remain healthy. Not facing this battle alone lets me know I have won—whatever the physical outcome.

Conclusion

Respect for all underlies Ojibwe belief systems. Ojibwe spirituality embraces and celebrates life, accepts the limits of human understanding, and inspires responsible action toward self and community. Ojibwe beliefs, practices, and rituals may provide insight and comfort to those facing end-of-life issues themselves or as caregivers. Care offered with respect affords dignity; listening provides a means of both giving and receiving. As part of the process of ongoing spiritual transition, rather than as an unknown, death does not inspire fear.

Acknowledgments: We would like to thank Maryellen Baker, Eugene Begay, Paul and Karen DeMain, and Rufus Goodstriker for sharing their teachings and wisdom: Miigwetch. Thank you, Nancy Forger and Merianne Liteman, for editorial suggestions. Special thanks go to my spiritual brother, Robert Blackwolf Jones, for introducing me to Ojibwe culture: Chi-Miigwetch.

PART III

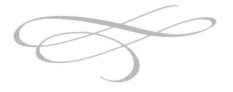

Applications and Tools

15

Spiritual Care

Practical Tools

CHRISTINA M. PUCHALSKI

The other day I sat with one of my patients, Phyllis, as she struggled to express her deep pain and sadness. After years of dealing with debilitating chronic arthritis, she now was faced with a stroke that had left her aphasic. Her words came out slowly, barely audible. For a woman who was verbal and highly expressive, this was the ultimate loss. I sat with her, holding her hand, trying to connect with her spiritually so that I could intuit what she was trying to say. In the midst of that connection, I felt her despair; her will to live was waning. Her daughter struggled as she heard her mother's pain and suffering. As she and I tried to offer some hope in the midst of sadness, we were both struck by Phyllis' amazing courage in the face of yet another setback in a life of challenges. She had courage to face the darkness and to own it yet reach within her to find some light to go on and keep trying. Life is filled with struggles and setbacks. I am continually awed by my patients' inner strength and courage. It gives me hope that within all of us lies a place of hope and courage. We just need to find that place; friends, family, and God can help us do that if we are open to it and willing to look within ourselves.

Christina M. Puchalski

I am often asked, "Who should provide spiritual care?" and I answer, "Anyone who deals with the ill and dying." This includes the family, physician, nurse, aid, social worker, counselor, chaplain, clergy, volunteers, and friends. As seen in Chapter 3, spiritual care is about loving others and being present to them in their time of need. All of us, regardless of our relationship to the ill and dying person, can and should do that. But of all the people listed, there are some professionals who are trained to be professional spiritual care providers. Chaplains, pastoral counselors, spiritual directors, clergy, and trained lay spiritual companions are all trained in different ways to counsel people on spiritual issues. Furthermore, yoga teachers, meditation teachers, Reiki masters, and others are also trained in specific spiritual practices. Healthcare professionals, such as physicians, nurses, and social workers, have varying degrees of training in spiritual care but for the most part are not regarded as trained spiritual care providers.

Increasingly, though, healthcare professionals are recognizing the important role spirituality plays in the lives of patients and, consequently, are including training for spirituality and healthcare in their curricula. For physicians, more medical schools and residency programs are teaching physicians why spirituality is critical in the lives of their patients and how they as healers can incorporate a patient's spiritual needs in the therapeutic plan.[1]

In 1992, there were three medical schools with elective courses on spirituality and health; a course I developed at George Washington University School of Medicine was one of these courses. Today, more than 80 schools have specific material in their curricula on spirituality and health, with many of these being required elements of the curricula. There are several reasons why this has occurred. First, patients began complaining about the harsh, technically oriented system of care that medicine had evolved to in the last half century. Consequently, the Association of American Medical Colleges (AAMC) led an initiative to focus medical education on a more patient-centered, as opposed to disease-centered, model of care.[2] Second, a program I direct, funded by The John Templeton Foundation, gives competitive awards to medical schools and residencies for developing and implementing curricula in spirituality and health. The AAMC, through the efforts of M. Brownell Anderson, Senior Vice President for Medical Education, recognized our efforts as complementary and as enhancing their efforts in humanizing medicine. Through her collaboration with me, there has been support and encouragement for medical educators to develop spirituality and health as a viable discipline in medicine. I also work extensively with physicians and other healthcare professionals, training them how to integrate spirituality, both their patients' and their own, into their professional and personal lives.

Students, residents, physicians, and other healthcare professionals learn:

- The basis of compassionate care and being a compassionate presence to others
- The role of spirituality in health and illness
- How to do a spiritual assessment
- How to collaborate effectively with spiritual care professionals, such as chaplains, clergy and others

- How to incorporate a patient's spirituality into the therapeutic plans
- How to reflect on their own spirituality as it relates to their professional calling as healers

Ethical Obligations

That physicians should be attentive to all dimensions of a patient's suffering, including the physical, emotional, social, existential, and spiritual, has been recognized by the American College of Physicians Consensus Panel on End-of-Life Care.[3] The consensus panel concluded that it is an ethical obligation for physicians to address all dimensions of a patient's suffering.[4] I further believe that it is critical for physicians and other healthcare professionals to address spiritual issues with their patients, because spirituality affects the patient's clinical care in a direct manner. It is integral to healing. Spiritual issues can impact clinical care in a variety of ways:[5]

- *Spiritual beliefs may be a dynamic in patients' understanding of their illness.* Patients come to understand their health, illness, and dying through their beliefs, cultural backgrounds, past experience, and values. Chaplains are trained to understand the differences in the roots of these beliefs, and they are trained to help patients resolve these types of conflicts. In addition, the physician can be helpful by listening to patients, giving patients the time to resolve conflicts, and respecting patients' rights to their own beliefs.
- *Religious convictions/beliefs may affect healthcare decision making.* Patients' cultural, religious, and spiritual values can impact on end-of-life decisions: use of feeding tubes, ventilator support, and blood transfusions. Furthermore, rituals can be a very important part of how people face important events in their lives, including dying.
- *Spirituality may be a patient need.* Studies, as described in Chapter 1, indicate how spirituality for many patients is an important need.
- *Spirituality may be important in patient coping.* Studies, as described in Chapter 1, demonstrate that many patients use spirituality to help them cope with stress and illness.
- *Spirituality may be integral to whole-patient care.* The mind-body connection is becoming well-established in studies. What one believes can have a powerful impact on how one feels, on his or her health outcomes, and on his or her well-being. Therefore, it is important to address all dimensions of a patient's health, including the spiritual.

⌒ Tools of Spiritual Care

The following tools can be applicable to all people who care for the dying. Specific professionals can adapt them to their roles with patients. Spiritual care, as we have seen in Chapter 3, is at its essence relational. There are several relationships involved:

- The relationship of the patient with the transcendent (God, Divine, Higher Power, Energy, or Other);
- The relationship of the patient with his or her family, friends, and loved ones;
- The relationship of the patient with the physician and other members of the healthcare team.

Spiritual care has several practical elements, as shown in Table 15.1

Listening and Presence

The most important skill is listening to the patient. In doing so, we need to put aside all the distracting thoughts and expectations of outcomes from our minds. In essence, we become receptacles into which the patient pours out, heart and soul, all of his or her fears, anxieties, despair, and pain. We then hold that suffering with our patients as we connect with them to help them. Fully present to our patients, with compassion in our hearts for them, we can partner with them to help identify the source of suffering.

TABLE 15.1
Spiritual Care

- Practice of compassionate presence
- Patient-centered communication—Listening to patient's fears, hopes, pain, dreams
- Attentiveness to all dimensions of the patient and patient's family: body, mind, and spirit
- Obtaining a spiritual history
- Assessment of spiritual issues
- Spiritual Care Plan: Incorporation of spiritual practice as appropriate
- Chaplains and other spiritual care providers as members of the interdisciplinary healthcare team

---

Being fully present to another means bringing ourselves in totality to the other person. Physically, we are fully attentive to the person. Our body language is one of openness, reflecting a willingness to listen to all concerns.

We have eye contact with the patient, indicating sincere interest in the other person. We sit close to the person. We may touch the person (hug, hold the person's hand, place a reassuring arm on the shoulder) as an expression of concern and love. Emotionally, we are open to feeling the person's pain and also to not be afraid to acknowledge our own emotions of sadness or helplessness. My students will often ask me if it is permissible to cry with a patient or to touch them. Showing emotion is appropriate as long as the physician's or other caregiver's emotion does not become the focus of the visit. Touching another on the arm or hugging someone shows a sign of support and can help the person feel less alone. It is important to use one's intuition as to whether the person would be offended by touch or an embrace. One can always ask permission to hug or embrace the patient. We need not be afraid to show our emotions to the patients and acknowledge our feelings of care, concern, and sadness to them. We are human beings as well, and to relate from a place of humanity can only serve to enhance the connection and the professional relationship with our patients.

Spiritually, we are present by allowing the connection between ourselves and our patients. This spiritual connection underlies the commitment that we as healthcare professionals have to our patients, which stems from our sense of calling to serve our patients. In this spiritual connection we relate from the spirit within ourselves—however we define that—to the spirit within the other. This transcends the physical and the emotional. It can be experienced often in the midst of the silent moments with our patient or loved one. Letting go of intellectual explanations and emotional fears, as well as raising one's awareness to intuition, helps with experiencing the spiritual connection or presence.

My greatest lesson on presence came from my mother, who has dementia that is quite advanced. Recently, she and I went to the Self-Realization Fellowship Shrine in Los Angeles. I sat next to her, holding her hand, overwhelmed by the awareness that she no longer had the memories of all we had done together. In some way, I felt that our actions together were what defined our relationship. We sat in silence, and I wondered what she was getting out of the visit. Was she aware? Was she thinking? About what? As if sensing my angst with uncertainty, she turned to me, took my hand, and said, "Look around you—it is so beautiful here, the flowers are rich in color, the birds are singing so sweetly." In that moment, I saw her wisdom and the truth. For it is not what we do so much as who we are that matters. My relationship with my mother is not predicated on our memories of the actions we take, but rather on the connection that we share on a deep, spiritual level of being. That connection is limitless. Once I let go of my intellectual ramblings and my emotional tension, I was able to be present to her and to all the beauty around us in a very profound way. Her ability to be fully present in the moment is a gift her illness has enabled her to appreciate fully and share with me. That is what presence speaks to; that is what embracing mystery is all about. So when we are with our patients and loved ones, by letting go of worries or an agenda to get a certain amount of information or the stress of needing to see people in a brief amount of time, we become more fully aware of the other person, and we are open to a fuller, more complete picture of who that person is and what the relationship is predicated on. It is the act of two human beings connecting to each other's humanity and spirit.

In today's medical environment, physicians, nurses, social workers, and chaplains are often overburdened and short staffed and often under a time pressure. It is therefore even more important that we hone our listening skills to be able to be effective and compassionate within a brief amount of time. Compassionate care is not time dependent; it is intent dependent. As I walk into the room of my patient, I have a ritual I perform, to remind myself of my purpose and calling as a physician. As I pick up the chart and have my hand on the doorknob, I take a deep breath in, which for me is the breath of God, and say silently to myself that I am there to serve and help the person in the room for his or her good. That triggers me to release all my frustrations, worries, and pressures and to be as present to my patient as much as possible in whatever time I have.

There are many spiritual practices and exercises that help people learn how to be present to another. Meditation helps one focus on the breath or a word or phrase. By doing so on a regular basis, one learns how to let go of distractions and emotions that might otherwise interfere with the present moment. These skills can be extended to the moment of interaction with another. The person becomes the focus of all attention, and any distraction—noise, thought, feeling—is let go of, so that all the attention can be on the other person's being. There are exercises that help people learn to listen fully. For example, one such exercise is to sit with another person for 5 minutes and not talk at all but listen intently to another without trying to comment or engage in mental dialogue about the content of the other person's talk. Another exercise is for two people to sit and simply look at each other in silence and try to know the person in the silence through nonverbal communication. Practicing intentionality is helpful. Try spending time looking at a flower and trying to see it in its full beauty. Take a few minutes to be aware of all the dimensions of that flower—its fragrance, its form, the way it sways in the wind, how the petals are folded. Next time you walk on the beach, take time to stop and listen to the waves, focusing all your attention on them. And the next time you see your patients in the clinic or the hospital, take whatever time you have to fully attend to them. Focus on their eyes and what the expression in those eyes is telling you. Listen to their words and the pacing of their breath as they talk to you. Are they comfortable, anxious, happy, or sad? Feel their being, and connect to them with the intent to serve. If distractions come up for you, or anxiety rises about your schedule and time, remind yourself of the reason you are in the room and also of your meaning and purpose in your professional life of service.

Patient-Centered Communication

The care of all patients should come from a patient-centered rather than a disease-centered focus. This means that the patient comes first and that our understanding of what is happening to the patient is in the context of the patient and his or her story. The AAMC, in its first report of the Medical School Objectives Project, a study undertaken by the AAMC to evaluate and change medical school education, notes that the most important attribute of the physician is to be compassionate: "Physicians must be compassionate and empathetic in caring for patients. . . . In all of their interactions they must seek to understand the meaning of the patients' stories in the context of the patients' beliefs, family, and cultural values."[6] The patient's story is the important framework, in which the partnership and communication with patients and their families take place. Part of that story is the patient's beliefs and values, which can be elicited in the spiritual history.

In communicating with patients, it is useful therefore to use the biopsychosocial and spiritual model as the basis for communication.[7] The care of the patient involves all the four dimensions: the physical, emotional, social, and spiritual. See Table 15.2 for an explanation of the four dimensions.

In talking with patients and recommending a particular course of action, the physician needs to take into account not only the biomedical aspects of the illness but also the other aspects of a patient's life. Two people can have exactly the same illness but have very different treatment recommendations. This is because the patient's state of health might impact which particular treatments would be tolerable, and the patient's previous experiences with treatments might alter a particular course of action. Depression and anxiety can also affect what a patient might want to

TABLE 15.2
The Dimensions of the Dying Experience

Physical	pain and other symptom management
Psychological	anxiety and depression
Social	social isolation and economic issues
Spiritual	purpose and meaning, relationships with the transcendent, search for ultimate meaning, hope, reconciliation, and despair

do. It is important to evaluate someone for depression, as someone might choose a course of action that is not the most appropriate because of his or her depression. Ideally, a choice should be one the patient freely chooses, not one affected by another illness, such as depression. Socially, a patient may feel like a burden to his or her family and may want to give up. By uncovering that dynamic, the physician can encourage patients to talk with family members about giving up and help them see that there are other solutions to the situation than opting to die out of a sense of being a burden. In addition, the patient's values and beliefs might impact the decisions he or she would make. Values and beliefs can affect decision making as well. For some patients, quality of life, even with the risk of a shortened life span, is more important than extending life. For another person, the importance of living longer to spend time with family or finish a goal might influence him or her to ask for additional treatment to "buy a little time." Spiritual or religious beliefs have a profound influence on decision making.

In caring for patients, all of these dimensions of care are important. So, providing the appropriate care for physical symptom relief and treatment for depression and anxiety is crucial, but equally important is providing the opportunity and care for spiritual distress and suffering, as well as providing the resources to help with social and financial concerns. As an example, I counseled John, Miles' son, about Miles' condition and what we were doing to help him. The discussion went as follows:

> For the physical, we are awaiting recommendations from the radiation oncologists to see if we can use radiation to help your father's back pain, which is caused by his cancer and which has spread to his back. Your dad's emotional state is so much better now that you are here. We will continue to talk with him and listen to all his concerns and fears. We would also encourage you to spend time talking with your dad. Socially, we recommend that your dad be transferred to a nursing home, where he can have 24-hour care. He is unable to care for himself and would benefit from round-the-clock care. He would be surrounded by others and involved in group activities, which might help him. He likes people and tells me that he enjoys "making buddies." He will have that opportunity in the nursing home. Spiritually, your dad has told me that he is not religious but is a Christian. He finds prayer helpful and has benefited from talking with the hospital chaplain. The nursing home has chaplains who work there daily and would be available to visit your father.

I was able to recommend a palliative care approach to Miles and his son based on my conversations with Miles, learning about his life—who he is as a person, what his values are, and how he would like to live and die. Integral to this conversation is the ability of the healthcare professional to talk about spiritual issues. Taking a spiritual history is one way to initiate a conversation about spiritual beliefs and values.

Spiritual History

Communicating about spiritual issues can be done in several ways. One can follow the patient's lead if the patient brings up a spiritual topic. For example, if a patient says "God would not do this to me," one can follow up with, "Tell me more about what you mean by that." Or, if a patient is wearing a religious symbol or reading a religious or spiritual text, one can comment or ask questions or one can ask direct questions about the patient's spiritual beliefs—for example, "Are you spiritual?" I advocate asking a direct, open-ended question, because it gives patients the indication that the physician or healthcare provider is interested in this area. Patients don't automatically think that "nonmedical" issues are welcome in the exam area. Thus, a spiritual history is a necessary part of the overall patient history in order to afford the patient the opportunity to discuss spirituality, if that is what is important to the patient.

The main elements of a spiritual history that have been developed for physicians and other healthcare professionals can be recalled by using the acronym FICA© (see Table 15.3).[8] This acronym was developed with the help of three of my colleagues—Drs. Daniel Sulmasy, Dale Matthews, and Joan Teno—as well as myself, based on a spiritual history I developed while I was a medical student.

The spiritual history is that part of the patient encounter when the patient can tell his or her story and share his or her values. It is that part of the exam that is less technical. Many feel that it is the place where compassionate care can be a felt experience. It is also the time that helps reveal what sources of strength, hope, and meaning the patient has and what kind of coping mechanisms the patient has. The spiritual history can also be done with family members as a way to find out what resources of spiritual strength the family members have, as well as to learn more about the family's values. It also helps one to connect to the family. Spirituality may enhance well-being in a person's life by providing one with the language of hope, meaning, and purpose; offering social support or integration within a religious or other community; or through enhanced coping mechanisms. Thus, the assessment tool asks the person about these areas of his or her life. In talking with people about ultimate meaning in their lives, it is helpful to realize that meaning can come from many sources. People may have found meaning and purpose in their work, their relationships, their avocation, and their attendance at church, temple, or mosque. Now, with aging or dying they may no longer be able to work or do their hobbies or even attend their place of worship. Family and friends may have died or may not be very supportive. Where is the meaning now? How does the patient make sense of a world that does not seem

TABLE 15.3
FICA

F—Faith and Belief
I—Importance
C—Community
A—Address/Action in Care

---

to be intrinsically reasonable? How can that patient continue to feel valued when the things he or she thought made her or him valuable no longer are possible?

Meaning can come from many different sources in life. There are activities and relationships that are meaningful but do not ultimately define one's meaning and purpose or what I call meaning with a small 'm'. When people face their dying, it is then that they must confront what gives them ultimate meaning or meaning with a large 'M'. That meaning comes from values, beliefs, practices, and experiences that lead one to an awareness of God/Divine/Holy/Transcendence and a sense of ultimate value and purpose in life. In terms of James Fowler's sixth stage in faith development, termed universality, this sense of meaning may lead to the reflection upon older, more concrete values and beliefs, a relocation from dependence on other's beliefs and values to a stronger sense of one's own beliefs and values and a move from self-dependence to a dependence on other or God/transcendence. Thus, the universal values of love, justice, peace, and acceptance become prominent. So people may move from meaning with a small 'm' to meaning with a large 'M' to connote this transition. The goal in treatment is to help patients find that deeper intrinsic meaning and value of himself as a person.

FICA©

F—Faith and Belief

"Do you consider yourself spiritual or religious?" or "Do you have spiritual beliefs that help you cope with stress?" If the patient responds "no," the physician might ask, "What gives your life meaning?" Sometimes patients respond with answers such as family, career, or nature. If the patient responds affirmatively to having a spiritual belief, it is important to ask if that belief system gives the person meaning and purpose in life. If not, what does give that person meaning?

I—Importance

"What importance does your faith or belief have in your life? Have your beliefs influenced how you take care of yourself in this illness? What role do your beliefs play in regaining your health?" One can ask about advance directives as related to beliefs. For example, "It sounds as if those beliefs are important to you. In the event that you are unable to speak for yourself, who would you ask to represent your values (healthcare proxy)? Do your beliefs influence you in how you view care at the end of life (resuscitation, feeding tubes, etc.)?"

C—Community

"Are you a part of a spiritual or religious community? Is this of support to you, and how? Is there a group of people you really love or who are important to you?" Communities such as churches, temples, and mosques or a group of like-minded friends can serve as strong support systems for some patients.

A—Address/Action in Care

The physician and other healthcare professionals can think about what needs to be done with the information the patient shared—referral to a chaplain, another spiritual care provider, or other resources, such as yoga, meditation, spiritual direction, or pastoral counseling. Some patients use rituals or journaling as a spiritual intervention. Prayer, sacraments, music, art, and solitude are other types of action plans.

FICA© is not meant to be used as a checklist but rather as a guide for knowing how to start the spiritual history and what to listen for as the patient talks about his or her beliefs. Mostly, FICA© is a tool to help physicians and other healthcare professionals know how to open a conversation about spiritual issues and issues of meaning and value. In the context of the spiritual history, patients may relate those fears, dreams, and hopes to their care provider. The spiritual history can be done in the context of a routine history or at any time in the patient interview, usually as a part of the social history (see Table 15.4).

In addition to religious or spiritual beliefs and values and other aspects of the spiritual history, the social history should address: lifestyle; home situation and primary relationships; other important relationships and social environment; work situation and employment; social interests/avocation; life stresses; and lifestyle risk factors, such as tobacco and alcohol and/or illicit drugs. As with any part of the his-

TABLE 15.4
Social History/Patient Profile

- Lifestyle, home situation and primary relationships
- Other important relationships and primary relationships
- Religious preferences or other important belief systems
- Work situation and employment
- Social interest/avocation
- Life stresses
- Lifestyle risk factors: tobacco, alcohol/illicit drugs

tory, sometimes issues come up that require more attention. For example, if a patient shares symptoms of depression, it is likely the visit will center on that and, therefore, the depression assessment will take longer. For some patients, the spiritual history may take a brief amount of time; for others, spiritual issues may be the predominant part of the discussion for that visit. In patient care, spirituality is part of ongoing spiritual care, both in the context of the caring relationship as well as in active conversation about spiritual issues. As part of the history, the conversation might be lengthy or be something the patient shares at the first visit and then brings up only at subsequent visits, as appropriate to the circumstance.

The spiritual history is patient-centered and family-centered, not physician-centered. One should always respect patients' and families' wishes and understand appropriate boundaries. Physicians and other healthcare professionals must respect patients' privacy regarding matters of spirituality and religion and should avoid imposing their own beliefs onto the patient.[9]

The following case illustrates how FICA© can be used. A patient who died of metastatic malignant melanoma was an Episcopalian. Her religious beliefs were central to her life and, in fact, the way she came to be at peace with dying. During her last hospitalization, the house officers caring for her were apprehensive about discussing advance directives and dying. However, during the spiritual history, the patient told them how her religious beliefs helped her come to terms with dying and how she was ready to die naturally. She handed them her living will. She also asked that her church members be allowed to visit her often. She later told me that being asked about her beliefs helped her feel respected and valued by the physicians, and she felt that she could trust them more. The physicians stated that once they conducted the spiritual history, the nature of the interaction between them and this patient was changed. It felt more natural, more comfortable, warmer, and more honest.

Another case illustrates the variability encountered in practice. When asked "Do you have any spiritual beliefs that help you with stress," a patient undergoing a routine examination answered that she found meaning and purpose while sitting in the woods near her house—that nature brought her peace. This was very important to her, as she noted that on days when she did not meditate near the woods in the morning, her day would be scattered and tense. Her community was a group of like-minded friends who shared her beliefs. She asked that her medical record indicate that when she became seriously ill or was dying, she would want to be in a room in a hospice that had a view of trees and nature. She also asked to learn basic meditation techniques. In a subsequent visit, many months later, she reported that she had stopped meditating, with negative results—but when she resumed meditation, she coped better with her stress.

Ethical and Professional Boundaries

These are guidelines that physicians and other healthcare professionals should follow when addressing spiritual issues with patients. Table 15.5 outlines some of these guidelines.

Physicians and other healthcare professionals should strive to discuss patients' spiritual concerns in a respectful manner and as directed by the patients. A physician or other care professional should always respect patients' privacy regarding matters of spirituality and religion and must be vigilant in avoiding imposing his or her beliefs on patients. Coercing patients to talk about their beliefs or coercing them to have certain beliefs is unethical. The relationship between physician and patient

TABLE 15.5
Ethical and Professional Boundaries

Spiritual History: patient-centered

Recognition of pastoral care professionals as experts

Proselytizing is not acceptable in professional settings. Addressing spiritual issues should not be coercive.

More in-depth spiritual counseling should be under the direction of chaplains and other spiritual leaders

Praying with patients:

- Not to be initiated by physicians or other healthcare providers unless there is no pastoral care available and the patient requests it or in circumstances where the physician/healthcare provider and patient have a long-standing relationship or share a similar belief system.

- Physician/healthcare provider can stand in silence as patient prays in his/her tradition.

- Referral to pastoral care for chaplain-led prayer.

---

is not an equal one and, in the professional setting, neither is the relationship between other professional caregivers with their patients. There is an intimacy in the relationship, but it is an intimacy with formality. The patient comes to the physician/healthcare professional at a vulnerable time of his or her life, often looking to the physician as a person of authority. The physician/healthcare professional should not abuse that authority by imposing his or her own beliefs, or lack of beliefs, onto patients. A vulnerable patient may adopt a physician/healthcare professional's beliefs simply because the patient is fearful and assumes that the physician/healthcare professional knows more.

In terms of spiritual intervention, physicians/healthcare professionals can recommend a variety of interventions: chaplain referral, meditation, yoga, prayer, or other spiritual practice. But the decision to recommend these comes from the patient. For example, the physician/healthcare professional can recommend religious and spiritual practices to their patient if these practices are already part of that patient's belief system. However, an agnostic patient should not be told to engage in worship any more than a highly religious patient should be criticized for frequent church attendance. Thus, if a patient states that prayer helps with stress, the physician/healthcare professional could suggest that prayer might help in dealing with a serious diagnosis. Or if a patient finds meaning and purpose in nature, a physician/healthcare professional might suggest meditation techniques focused on nature.

Patients may ask their physician/healthcare professional about the physician/healthcare professional's beliefs. Given the unequal relationship between patient and physician/healthcare professional, it is important that the question be handled carefully and with the same guidelines that are used when addressing other sensitive issues, such as sexual history or domestic violence questions. Patients sometimes ask personal questions of their physician/healthcare professional to take the attention off of themselves. Sometimes it is to see if they can connect with the physician/healthcare professional, by reassuring themselves that the physician/healthcare provider has the same beliefs as they have. In general, when asked about his or her own beliefs, the physician/healthcare professional could ask the patient why it is important for them to know that information. The physician/healthcare professional can reassure the patient that the focus of the time in the encounter is on the patient's needs and issues, not the physician/healthcare professional's issues.

In some cases, patients will still feel the need to know the spiritual background of the physician. A patient of a certain religious belief may want to work only with a physician/healthcare professional of that same religion. In some cases, it may not be possible to accommodate the patient, but at least the physician/healthcare professional can explore with the patient the reasons for his or her request. Some patients want to know that their beliefs will not be ridiculed. A response from the physician/healthcare professional that they respect and support a patient's beliefs might serve to reassure the patient. In general, it is best to avoid sharing one's personal beliefs unless one already knows the patient and is comfortable that this sharing would not coerce the patient into adopting the physician/healthcare professional's beliefs or intimidate the patient from sharing more about his or her own beliefs. A physician/healthcare professional should not do anything that violates his or her own comfort level. Many physicians/healthcare professionals prefer to keep their private lives private in the professional context of their relationship with patients.

Patients may ask physicians/healthcare professionals to pray with them. It is not inappropriate to allow a moment of silence or a prayer if the patient requests this. In fact, walking away and not showing respect for the request may leave the patient with a sense of abandonment by the physician/healthcare professional. If the physician/healthcare professional feels conflicted about praying with patients, he or she need only stand by quietly as the patient prays in his or her own tradition. Or, alternatively, the physician/healthcare professional could suggest calling in the chaplain or the patient's clergy person to lead a prayer. Physician-led prayer or healthcare professional-led prayer is generally not recommended, since that is usually the role of a clergy or chaplain. In addition, having the physician/healthcare professional lead a prayer opens the possibility of having the prayer be of the physician/healthcare professional's belief, not that of the patient's. Furthermore, clergy and chaplains are trained specifically in techniques of leading prayer in ecumenical and healthcare contexts. However, there is disagreement among experts in this area. Some say that physician-led or healthcare professional-led prayer may be permissible if the physician/healthcare professional and patient share a longstanding relationship, have similar beliefs or religious background, or if the patient requests it. It is still recommended, however, to be mindful of respecting the patient's belief system and avoid any possibility of coercion or imposition of beliefs.

Spiritual Care Plan

The "A" in FICA© stands for address and action. This is the section that enables the physician and other healthcare professionals to develop a spiritual care plan with the patient. The first part of the spiritual care plan is being present and compassionate to our patients and loved ones. Listening to our patients' concerns, fears, beliefs, and emotions is the first step to good spiritual care. Providing a safe environment for our patients to share their feelings, as well as assurance that we are genuinely interested, is critical. The sharing of deep emotions is frightening for many people, and knowing that feelings and beliefs will be respected is very important. For me, hearing my patients express their inmost feelings and beliefs is sacred. It reflects a deep trust that I will honor and value what is shared. My responsibility to my patients

TABLE 15.6

Different Spiritual Care Options or Interventions

- Listening to the concerns, feelings, and beliefs of the patient
- Providing a safe environment and an attentive ear so that the patient can express feelings and experiences associated with illness, stress, and dying
- Providing opportunities for the patient to express grief, anger, despair, sorrow, happiness, joy, and confusion
- Suggesting important relationships that might help the patient (sharing feelings with family/friends, chaplains, counselors, clergy)
- Referring to professional spiritual care providers (chaplains, pastoral counselors, spiritual directors, clergy)
- Spiritual practice (yoga, meditation, prayer)
- Rituals, sacraments
- Worship and other spiritual services
- Sacred reading (scripture, other spiritual texts)
- Reflective readings from poetry and literature
- Journaling
- Reading groups (bible and other texts)
- Nature walks with meditation and reflection
- Joining spiritual support groups
- Time for solitude
- Listening to music and guided imagery
- Expression of spiritual beliefs in art

is that I honor that trust. As we listen to our patients we need to assess what is being shared and then develop a plan with the patient. The plan may be to encourage sharing the feelings with a loved one or a professional, such as a chaplain or clergyperson. The plan may be simply more listening and assessing at subsequent visits until the issues become clearer. Or, there may be specific spiritual practices, readings, or rituals that might be appropriate (see Table 15.6).

For each person, the spiritual care plan will be different. Depending on the issues that come up in the clinical encounter, some patients may need to simply talk more with their physician or healthcare professional at followup visits, some may need more in-depth counseling with a chaplain or pastoral counselor, and others may need to talk with a spiritual director. One of my patients, Lou, was seeking to deepen his relationship with God. I referred him to a spiritual director, who assisted him in his search for a greater intimacy with God. The director listened to my patient's spiritual concerns and guided him in his spiritual practices. Another patient had conflicts about what his religion said about resuscitation and about what he wanted to do. A chaplain worked closely with this patient and helped him come to a decision about care that did not conflict with his deeply held religious beliefs. Another patient, Kate, whose mother had recently died, suffered deeply from depression. While medication helped her with her symptoms, she still suffered from grief and benefited from work with a pastoral counselor who was able to integrate a spiritual approach in counseling. In another case, my patient, Julie, had deep concerns about acceptance by her faith community. She had HIV and felt that her community would reject her because of her perception that she had sinned. Julie felt comfortable with her pastor, however, so I encouraged her to talk with him about these issues. He was able to show her that she was welcome in the community and was very supported by her faith community.

The spiritual care plan, therefore, can include referrals to spiritual care professionals, such as chaplains, clergy, spiritual directors, or pastoral counselors. It can also include personal spiritual practices, such as meditation, prayer, yoga, journaling, chanting, and singing psalms. For some people, walking or meditating in nature can help them feel the spiritual presence in their lives.

Rituals are very important in people's lives. Every culture has developed rituals to guide its members through significant transitions in their lives, including dying.[10] Rituals reaffirm the person's role in society. For example, as people are dying, they may feel they are a less-than-adequate functional member of society. A ritual, however, reminds them that they are going through a normal part of living and are respected and honored by others. Religious ceremonies or rituals allow people to express symbolically their spiritual beliefs and values in a communal sense. Sacraments, such as anointing of the sick or receiving communion, sharing the Sabbath rituals, or sacred ritualized bathing, all have significance for many people. Finally, at the time of death, ritualized bathing of the person's body or special prayers may be very important to people.[11]

Community activities, such as attendance at worship, can provide support to many people and can be the primary way to experience spiritual practice. Communities can provide social support as well as shared experiences. Some religious places of worship offer support groups for patients with illness. There are also national support groups whose focus is spiritual. Jewish Healing Services is one such program.[12] One of my patients joined a Jewish Healing Service support group. The relationships she formed with others in that group provided a "circle of love," as she called them. While she was dying, members of her group read poetry and spiritual readings to her. They were her companions on the journey. Another patient joined a support group in her church, which met weekly to pray as a group. During the other days in the week, the members of the groups would remember each other in prayer. This strengthened her ability to face the stages of her chemotherapy and eventual dying. The group also attended all critical transition points with her: bone scans that determined she had metastasis; chemotherapy sessions; and, finally, seeing her and praying with her at home, where she died.

Developing a Spiritual Care Plan

A plan can be developed in the clinical setting as part of the discussion with the patient. The important part of generating this plan is to recognize that the therapeutic relationship is a partnership and that the plan that is generated is done together as part of the partnership. The plan is patient-centered and comes from the patients' belief framework. I would never, for example, recommend prayer to a person for whom that is not part of his or her tradition and is important to them. In the spiritual history, or during discussions with the physician or other caregiver, there may be spiritual issues or questions that come up. Based on this information, the caregiver can think about the various options for a plan and what would be appropriate for the patient. More in-depth discussion with a trained spiritual care provider, such as a chaplain, pastoral counselor, or spiritual director, may be appropriate, depending on the issue. Some patients may want more information on yoga, meditation, or other spiritual practices. The spiritual care plan may be a meditation program that is developed. I sometimes ask my patients to record the time spent in meditation relative to the target symptoms. For example, for patients with hypertension, the target symptoms are their blood pressure readings. For patients with irritable bowel syndrome, the target symptom may be frequency of diarrhea. Both the patient and I can then measure the effect meditation has on their symptoms. Prayer may be an important part of a plan for patients for whom prayer is part of their spiritual practice. I have often written a plan with a patient where the patient commits to a certain course of action—for example, 20 minutes of daily prayer and 30 minutes of quiet meditation each day.

Trained Spiritual Care Professionals

Appropriate referrals to chaplains are important to good healthcare practice and are as appropriate as referrals to other specialists. Chaplains are clergy or lay persons certified in a pastoral training program designed to train them as chaplains, as described further in Chapter 7. Chaplains work in hospital settings, hospices, outpatient clinics, businesses, schools, and prisons. They are trained to be spiritual care professionals, working with people in exploring meaning in life, coping with suffering, and accessing their beliefs in helping them cope with illness, stress, or dying.

Chaplains work with people of all faiths and with nonreligious people as well. I have referred many patients, including atheists, to chaplains. Clergy are trained to provide religious care usually only to people of their specific denomination.

Pastoral counselors are trained mental health professionals with a focus on spiritual issues as related to mental health. They have a degree in counseling as well as training in pastoral care. Spiritual directors are trained to focus on the person's relationship with the divine or God. Spiritual directors guide people on their spiritual journey but do not do counseling. Patients and any of these professionals do not need to be of the same religious backgrounds, nor do patients have to have any religious background or belief to benefit from of these professionals.

Where are the boundaries between what chaplains do and what physicians/healthcare professionals do? Some would argue that discussions with patients about spiritual matters should be initiated solely by chaplains.[13] Physicians/healthcare professionals can use spiritual histories as a screening tool. By inquiring about a patient's beliefs, the physician/healthcare professional can evaluate whether the beliefs are helpful or harmful to the patient's health and medical care. If a patient has beliefs that support him or her and give meaning and peace of mind, the physician/healthcare professional can encourage those beliefs. If patients struggle with meaning and purpose, further discussion with the physician/healthcare professional, as well as referral to chaplains or other spiritual care providers, may be indicated. In cases in which spiritual beliefs interfere with a patient's getting needed therapy—for example, a patient who thinks an illness is a punishment caused by God and therefore refuses medicine or treatment because of a feeling that the punishment is deserved—a referral to a chaplain would be very helpful. Patients have the right to refuse medical treatment. However, it is important that that choice be made with full, informed consent. Therefore, if a patient refuses treatment based on a religious or spiritual belief, it may be appropriate to refer the patient to a chaplain so that the chaplain can explore these beliefs with the patient.

Sometimes refusal of treatment is based on accepted religious tenets. Other times, the patient may attribute his or her reasons for refusal to religious beliefs, but it actually stems from other concerns, such as lack of self-esteem or depression. The chaplain is trained to explore the beliefs with the patient further and help that patient differentiate between the two. Physicians/healthcare professionals generally do not have the type of training needed to explore these issues in depth. In one case, my patient, an elderly woman who had had a major heart attack, was found to have multisystem organ failure after 2 weeks in the ICU. The medical team approached the family about withdrawing care (i.e., turning off the life-support system), since she was clearly dying. The family, however, believed that God would perform a miracle and cure their mother and wanted to continue aggressive medical treatment indefinitely. In situations such as this, Brett and Jersild suggest that physicians might offer alternative religious interpretations of miracles that might help the family see that turning off the life support system was appropriate and in line with God's will.[14] This could be seen, however, as a conflict of interest on the part of the physician, as the physician has a particular therapeutic goal in mind. Utilizing religious explanations to achieve that goal might be the means to achieve the desired end but may be unethical for the physician. Referring to a chaplain is the appropriate next step, since the chaplain is not only trained in spiritual assessment and helping patients arrive at a decision for themselves but is also not the person making the recommendation to terminate life support. What the physician can do is explain why turning off the life support is the appropriate medical recommendation but do so in a way that is respectful of the beliefs of the patient and family. The physician and chaplain together can offer the patient the information and support needed to make the decision that is in the best interest of the patient.

In the preceding case, the physician is giving the family the necessary information to make an informed medical decision. The chaplain is giving the family the information needed to make an informed spiritual decision. This way the patient and family can have enough medical and spiritual information to make a fully informed consent decision—medically and spiritually informed consent. Physicians in general are not trained to explore the theological aspects of belief, but they can listen and learn about the beliefs from the patient and support them as they make decisions for themselves. Sometimes, simply listening to a patient in a nonjudgmental fashion and asking a few open-ended questions, such as "Tell me more about your belief," can help the patient resolve issues of belief and treatment for him- or herself.

While many studies suggest that spirituality can be helpful, there are also circumstances in which spirituality can have a negative effect on health. It is important for healthcare professionals to recognize this dynamic. For example, a person who interprets his or her illness as a punishment from God may attempt to refuse treatment. In such a scenario, a chaplain or other religious advisor could perhaps work with the patient's belief, to help him or her work through the guilt issues. The patient may accept treatment or may refuse it, but at least the decision wouldn't be motivated solely by guilt. It will be a more informed decision. Some people who feel guilt in their relationship with God may also relate to others in their life in a similar way. Counseling may also be helpful in these cases.

Some religious beliefs forbid certain medical practices, such as Jehovah's Witnesses' refusal to accept blood transfusions. It is important to recognize the difference between refusing treatment based on an established religious principle versus refusal of treatment stemming from depression, unwarranted guilt, or a misperceived sense of punishment from God. Some patients may have complicated ethical and spiritual issues. Physicians/healthcare professionals need not feel that they must solve these dilemmas on their own. Chaplains, members of ethics committees, and counselors often work with physicians/healthcare professionals in the care of patients.

It is important to recognize that spirituality in the healthcare setting is not in any one person's domain. Physicians, nurses, social workers, and chaplains all can deal with patient spirituality. It also is true, however, that most physicians/healthcare professionals are not trained to deal with complex spiritual crises or conflicts. Chaplains and other spiritual caregivers are. Therefore, it is important that physicians and other healthcare professionals obtain a spiritual history as a way of inquiry about spiritual issues that might impact a patient, but that physicians and other healthcare professionals also recognize when to refer to the spiritual care specialists.

Lay Volunteers

As any of us journey through life, we experience many challenges. Chronic loss and dying are perhaps two of the most intense of these challenges. Faced with these challenges, people frequently start questioning their purpose, the meaning of their lives, and dying processes. These questions are the essence of a spiritual journey. Sharing that journey with others is so important. Insight from those who are trained in spiritual care can help others gain insight for themselves. The aloneness one feels in the midst of confusion can be alleviated by another who extends his or her care for that person. The people that help others along their spiritual journeys can be friends, professionals, and families. Everyone needs this connection to others in the midst of confusion and searching.

People who have more specific training, such as chaplains, spiritual directors, clergy, and pastoral counselors, are able to provide advice and direction that comes from a professional base of training that the rest of the healthcare team and family and friends do not have. However, professional spiritual care providers are also not always as available to provide the frequency and intensity of spiritual companionship that a person might need. Currently, the need far exceeds the supply of chaplains and other professionally trained spiritual care providers. Religious communities similarly are faced with a greater demand for services and support than they are able to handle. Thus, the role of the lay volunteer spiritual companion becomes important. The lay companion has some training but also is available to people on a more regular basis; for example, once or twice a week. In the Stephen's Ministry model,[15] companions generally do not take on more than one or two clients. Professional spiritual care providers, as well as others on the healthcare team, care for large numbers of parishioners, clients, and patients. So from a practical point of view, the lay companion is more accessible to the patient and his or her family.

Many organizations have training programs for volunteers, including hospitals, hospices, and nursing homes. Faith-based organizations also have volunteers who visit the ill and dying. Some of these have formal training programs as well. In training programs, volunteers learn how to be present to others, how to address their own spiritual, grief, and loss issues and how to discuss these issues with clients. Depending on the program, some volunteers use peer-support groups to help them deal with issues that are useful in their work with ill and dying clients.

FICA© for Spiritual Self-Assessment

In recent years, many of my patients and colleagues alike have utilized FICA© as a self-assessment spiritual tool. As described in earlier chapters, it is critical for all care providers to be in touch with their own spirituality before helping others. Caregivers and patients alike can use FICA© as a tool to help them begin to look at spiritual issues in their own lives and then as a follow-up tool to continue evaluating and self-assessing. Following is a description of how to use the FICA© tool in self-assessment:

F—Faith and Belief

Do I have any spiritual beliefs that help me cope with stress and with life? Am I spiritual? Religious? What gives my life meaning and purpose?

I—Importance

Are these beliefs important to me? How? Do they influence me in how I care for myself? Should my beliefs be more important or less important? What are important priorities in my life? Do these coincide with my spiritual beliefs? Is my spiritual life integrated into my professional or personal life? If not, why not?

C—Community

Do I belong to a spiritual community? What is my commitment to that community? Is it important to me? Do I need to find a community? Do I need to change my community?

A — Address/Action in Care

Do I need to do something different to grow in my spirituality? To grow in my community? Do I have a spiritual practice? Do I need one? What should I do in my practice in order to grow spiritually? Do I need to do something different? How should I better integrate my spiritual life into my professional or personal life?

Spiritual care ultimately is not only for the ill or dying person but is for all of us who are privileged to walk the journey with another. There is a paradigm shift in medicine, which encourages the recognition of spirituality as central to health but not separate from it. The changes in medical education reflect this shift of focus from attention to only the physical to attention to whole-person care. This encourages the partnership between patient and physician/healthcare professional, and a more integrated healthcare system as a whole. As we partner with our patients and loved ones through their illness and dying, it is through the spiritual connections we make that healing is possible. We enter into relationships that are filled with profound sharing of pain, joy, hope, and sadness. By being present to our patients and loved ones, listening to them, and walking with them in the midst of their pain and suffering as well as their joy, we have a chance to open ourselves up to the emotions our patients experience. By taking the risk to allow these deep and sometimes difficult feelings to awaken within us, we open the door to the possibility of healing and well-being, not just for the patient but for ourselves as well. The journey is not an easy one, but it is one that ultimately enriches everyone's lives, because the basis of that journey is centered in love of another and care for a fellow human being. This chapter gives some tools that one might use along this journey.

Reference

Fowler, J. W. (1981). *Stages of faith: The psychology of human development and the quest for meaning.* New York: Harper and Row

16

Caring for Patients at the End of Life
Honoring the Patient's Story

JOHN D. ENGEL, LURA PETHTEL, AND JOSEPH ZARCONI

The first sign of leukemia came out of the blue. I was sitting in a business meeting one Sunday night at church and was reading a financial report and all of a sudden I couldn't see half of it.

Max

Stories and the End of Life

We tell stories. We listen to stories. We are a storied species. Stories are fundamental to human life and are precipitated by what Bruner[1] has referred to as a *breach of the commonplace*. In clinical contexts, the commonplace of a person's life is breached by illness episodes, as is illustrated by Max's experience of the sudden change in his health.[2] As a patient senses the manifestations of a life-threatening disease, the ordinary or commonplace events of everyday life are breached and transformed to a story of illness and suffering.

> He [the doctor] came back and said, "I have good news and bad news. You don't have diabetes. The bad news is I think you have acute leukemia." I was by myself—my wife hadn't taken off work to come with me because we thought it was just a usual blood test. Well, I immediately knew what this meant. I had pastored with three parishioners with leukemia and I had walked through the last few years with them to the end. I was utterly shocked!

Speaking about patients, Kleinman[3] has recognized that patients are storied persons, telling and listening to illness stories that often constitute daily life. As you have already heard, Max is a storied patient—he represents his life-world through the telling of his story. Throughout the first part of this chapter, we will share Max's story, as he told it to us, to illustrate how clinical narratives construct the personal meaning of illness and provide a framework for the transaction between patients and caregivers.[4] Max's story opens a window to his life, his feelings, and his spiritual being.

When we first met Max, he was 41 years old and had been diagnosed 3 years previously with chronic myelogenous leukemia. Max was married and had two children, a 14-year-old daughter and a 9-year-old son. At the time of diagnosis he was placed on disability from his job as a minister and also from his work as a volunteer fireman/EMT for his town. Because of his situation, his wife returned to work as an educator.

The relationship between a patient and a caregiver exists within a context of stories. Illness stories are the means through which both the patient and caregiver understand, create, and recreate their identities. Consider these three episodes from Max's illness story.

> It's not always easy to stay upbeat about this. The most difficult part was that for years I pastored and shepherded people and cared for people as a caregiver—giving them spiritual comfort and advice. Now the shoe is on my foot. I've got to deal with people giving that to me, and I find that very difficult. I thoroughly enjoy being a server—it's difficult being served. But I found the only way I was going to get through this was to find the strength of friends, faith, and family and to rely upon them.

> I've gotten much closer to God. I established a relationship with God when I was in high school. It was sort of on and off in college, and then when I went into the ministry, it became stronger. I found that my relationship, a lot of times during ministry, was kind of a business relationship. Can you help me, God? Can you help me do this? Give me strength to do this—rather than a personal, loving, caring, nurturing type of relationship. It's just the opposite now. I don't plough through books and devotionals and things. I spend a lot of time in quiet places, just listening and watching and seeing God in operation, and sitting and listening to people talk about their experiences, and that's been very uplifting to me.

> I take care of a lot of the business in our family. My wife is very capable. She could, too, but I fear that if I were to die, she would not know what to do. So we talked about it. She cried; I said, "That's okay. I'm not hoping for it or anticipating it, but we have to think about it. I won't be able to continue taking care of things."

As Max's life and illness unfold, his identity changes as he interacts with others and/or reflects on his situation. In the first story episode, Max moves from caregiver to being cared for. In the second, his identity in relationship with God changes from a distanced "business" one to a personal and uplifting one. In the third episode, he recognizes the identity transition from active family provider to nonexistence.

Illness Stories

Illness narratives portray signs, symptoms, and treatment aspects, as well as various ways of suffering. For the caregiver, it is impossible to interact effectively with a suffering patient without attending to the illness narrative. Because of the storied nature of suffering and how it provides the framework for relationships among patients, families, and caregivers, there is a moral obligation to attend to the patient's illness story as a part of that person's broader life narrative.

> When my vision got blurred, I went to an eye surgeon. He said I had a retinal hemorrhage. There is a history of diabetes and heart disease in my family. I don't have those problems, but my mother died of diabetic complications and had retinal hemorrhages. I also have a brother with diabetes. So the eye doctor asked me all kinds of questions, and asked me to go to a doctor to get checked soon. Well, I'm not fond of doctors, so I didn't go until several months later. I exhibited all the symptoms of diabetes—weakness, weight loss of 40 pounds, thirsty all the time, frequent urination, hungry a lot. Soon I started getting bruises all over my body— big ones, not just little ones. These didn't hurt to the touch and I didn't remember bumping myself. Two nurses in my congregation noticed all this, and that I was getting weaker and weaker and sick and short of breath. So they wanted me to get to the doctor and get blood work. So I went. My general practitioner was away at the time, so I saw his partner. He came back and said I've got good news and bad news. You don't have diabetes. The bad news is I think you have acute leukemia. I was utterly shocked! They sent me to the hospital immediately. After a bone marrow biopsy, they decided I had chronic leukemia, which was a little better—but still the same outcome if I wasn't treated. That's how it started.

In this portion of Max's story, we hear him talking about his symptoms in the broader context of his family's medical history, in the broader context of a relation-

ship with two nurses in his congregation, and in the broader context of his understanding of death from leukemia, based on his experience with three of his parishioners who died from the same disease. This experience serves to meaningfully
influence Max's construction of his illness story. What we don't know is how (or
whether) the physician, the partner of Max's regular general practitioner, placed the
discussion of a tentative diagnosis of acute leukemia in the fabric of Max's life story.
However, we do hear Max describe his reaction to this encounter as being utterly
shocked. It is in this joint construction of Max's illness story, Max from his particular sociocultural position and the physician from his particular biomedical position,
that the caregiver should be able to understand the personal meaning of the diagnosis in the full context of Max's life and, with Max, to construct a meaningful story of
his present and future life. In the next portion of Max's story, we hear about his suffering as a result of his treatment.

> I get treatments daily by mouth—it makes me sick to my stomach, gen-
> erally. It was supposed to make me lose my hair—for 3 years I haven't, but
> all of a sudden last month (*laugh*) it's all fallen out (*laugh*). After 3 years
> now I'm not prepared for it. I kinda don't like it now. I kinda like my hair
> (*laugh*). I get injections of interferon nightly at the hospital and it gives me
> pain—joint and bone pain—a moderate level of pain. Most recently, I've
> had to come to grips with bouts of acute pain, which is a bit unnerving, to
> say the least. I just had an episode last month and was hospitalized for 4
> days. Generally, it's related to the interferon. Painkillers won't touch it.
> They discovered that I have some stenosis in my back, some arthritis and
> deteriorating discs in my lower back. The pain I dealt with for a month
> was unbearable. Now it's fine, it's gone. But it just flairs up and that's been
> difficult. You just never know from month to month when it's going to
> happen—it just flairs up! Occasionally, I get pain for a day or two, and I
> can manage it. But then it flairs up and I have to be hospitalized.

The Substance of Stories

What is it about storytelling that matters in the intimate engagement between
patient and caregiver? Or, to put it another way, what is it about stories and storytelling that make them especially appropriate for the understanding of the patient's
situation and for the direction of therapeutic practice? In thinking about these
questions, we have been guided by the recent work of Mattingly,[5] Mattingly and
Garro,[6] and Mishler.[7] Mattingly's work shows that narratives are event-centered.

They concern action, more specifically human action, and even more specifically, human interaction.

In Max's case, his story centers on interactions with the nurses in his congregation who urge him to see his physician and have blood work done; on interactions with his physician around the diagnosis and his subsequent hospitalization; and on interactions with his wife about her taking over the business functions of the family—his narratives are experienced-centered. They do not merely describe what someone does in the world, but what the world does to that someone. They allow us to infer something about what it feels like to be in that story world.

Max's story centers on the shock of the diagnosis; on the results of his disability—no longer pastoring; on many identity changes; and on the infliction of pain from his treatments. Narratives do not merely refer to past experience but create experiences for their audience (the listener).

Max's narrative refers to his past experiences with three parishioners who die of leukemia, and how this forms his own reaction to the diagnosis and prognosis. For some who listen to Max's story, it has triggered a reexamination of their own spiritual relationships.

Mishler[8] has noted that, in addition to narratives being socially situated actions, they are *identity performances.* Here, Mishler's idea focuses our attention on stories as a way of expressing who we are and who we want to be. On this point, Bruner[9] argues that "we constantly construct and reconstruct ourselves to meet the needs of the situations we encounter, and we do so with the guidance of our memories of the past and our hopes and fears for the future."

> My disease runs in about 10-week cycles, according to my white blood count and chemo treatments. I have about 2 weeks in between, when I'm pretty much normal again. So I do things. I've been able to preach occasionally. I ride with the fire department as I'm able to. I drive. It makes me feel important, like I'm doing something. I have been able to visit people. I've developed a ministry of phone calling and letter writing—something I did very little of before. I'm a face-to-face people person—I can't always do that now. But I can still have contact by phone. I haven't mastered the e-mail yet. I'm not sure how to turn that machine on yet (*laugh*). My 9-year-old son sends e-mail for me.

Here, Max tells us how he reconstructs himself to serve again in both his ministry and his community. Finding new ways to serve helps Max sustain his self-esteem and regain some measure of control over his life.

Further, the sociocultural and emotional embeddedness of stories is an important issue. It is critical to remember that each person tells and hears stories from his or her unique social position. Max's story often shows how his sociocultural background as a pastor and as the son of a father who denigrates the ministry as life work influences how Max tells and understands his life and illness. In the next episodes, we hear Max's reflection on several emotional issues that frame his suffering. First, Max reflects on his relationship with his father. Then, Max talks about the connection between pain, suffering, and spiritual strength.

> My parents were divorced when I was 19. When he left, he left completely. I had no contact with him for 3 years. But then when he came back he made fun of me because he thought going to be a minister was a wimpish type of thing. My mother died 7 years ago, and since then I have a dad again. He takes me to chemo and we talk and cry together—that's been a real joy—something I never experienced my whole life with my father, and now when I need help he comes to help me—that's been a great strength for me.

> I don't think we're born with strengths, necessarily. They come through a lot of struggle. For instance, the last bout of pain, I was in so much pain that I began questioning whether God had abandoned me. I'm presently a member of the church I pastored. The minister came to visit me. We had an hour conversation about whether God had left me. I knew in my heart of hearts that was not true, but that's how I felt. So struggling through the suffering I was dealing with was such a dark cloud I couldn't see the light around me. Once I got through that—that was a positive thing. So going through experiences and learning through them and using those experiences to be strong—I've actually come to believe that pain is a good thing and that suffering can be very motivational. I would never have said that before my disease. I always saw disease as a terrible, awful thing to ever have to deal with or suffer.

The Dynamics of Stories

As narrative time moves, the patient, the family, and the caregiver enter into a routine characterized by revising interpretations, changing prognoses, judgments, hopes, expectations, and therapeutic actions. In this context, the resulting story episodes recast the patient's life in relation to the unknown—the daily, weekly, monthly surprises; the extraordinary; and the breach of the commonplace. This situation stimulates the patient's reframing the narrative plot, often with the help of the family and caregiver. This activity, this *emplotment*, attempts to return coherence to the trajectory of the patient's illness story. The extent to which the patient judges that a better story is in place will depend on how the patient, the patient's family, and the patient's caregiver treat the incoherent narrative. For the patient, a better story results from reframing the incoherent episode to take into account the strong sense of temporal ordering characteristic of the patient's life as a journey. In the process of this emplotment, both patient and caregiver become readers of the patient's life journey. Listen to how Max struggles and only partially succeeds in replotting the anxiety within his family. Because there is only partial replotting, this would signal to the caregiver that Max and therefore Max's story need further work or treatment.

> There have been several episodes of crisis with my family. My son developed bed-wetting again. His psychologist feels it's all related to this situation. Particularly when I've been extremely sick, when I get home I hug my kids a lot, and then they get worried that daddy's going to die. My daughter takes the quiet road—although recently she's been developing a relationship with her mother and she's been opening up. So that's been a good feeling for me to see that blossoming.

Now listen to Max as he replots his story to help return coherence to his lifeline.

> We can't choose a whole lot of what happens to us. We make choices that make decisions on what happens to us, but a lot of what happens to us, we don't choose. I wouldn't have chosen this disease, although now it's okay that it happened. I think a lot of life is perceiving what is given to you and then dealing with it the best you can. I've been trying to change this [illness] for years, but I can't change it. The struggle set me back in my mind and spirit a lot, so I'm just going forward. I'm taking each day and allowing the strength I have to live it.

> I do a lot of thinking (*sob and long pause*), and one of the aspects that has helped me a lot has been to be thankful. We (the fire department) had a house fire 2 weeks ago and it was fully involved when we got there. I was driving the new pumper. For 3 hours—this was the night before Easter—a hard time for me—in the middle of the night I was standing on top of the pumper. On the way home, just the feeling of thankfulness that I was able to experience that. Gosh, thanks a bunch! To have that opportunity just warmed my heart. Thankfulness has been an awfully strong thing for me. I take time to sit back and pay attention and notice the accomplishments and experiences and relationships that I've been able to have.

Some patients may find themselves reading their story at the end of life in the sense of not being able to affect, and consequently write, a disease trajectory or outcome. The work of the patient, his family, and caregiver is to try to read and write this portion of the patient's life story so that the narrative at the end of life constructs the personal meaning of illness in a manner that allows the patient to feel comforted. Here, Barnard and his colleagues[10] note that "the norm is frequent oscillation between hope for cure and acceptance of decline and death." The final episode of Max's story shows how this is the case.

> Another difficult thing is that for 2 years I've been searching and there's no bone marrow donor. So the transplant specialist thinks that if there's no perfect match that's not a good option for me. That's because of my background. I'm part German and part American Indian. That minority background—no one has come forward to donate. So we're still searching, but I haven't put a lot of stock in that.

> Last year the doctor asked me if I would be interested in meeting with a specialist who was doing a new procedure. I said, "Why not? I haven't got anything to lose." The average life span for people with this disease is 42 months. I'm on my 36th. So why not?

> So I went to visit with this new doctor. He is the only doctor in the country right now doing a new procedure called cord blood transplantation with adults. He found a match for me! But after doing exams and blood work, he thought that I had progressed to the next stage. He felt that I had less than 6 months to live. He wanted to do the procedure immediately. Of course, for me, that was like going back to the beginning. My wife and I sat there. We were numb. I couldn't believe it. He did another bone marrow and decided that he was wrong. I was exhibiting symptoms of second stage, but was still back in first stage. That's God working!!

> I had several bad weeks then—some virus or something—so we put off the transplant. This decision to do the transplant—that was a family decision. There is a 70% chance it won't work. So we talked about that—and cried about it. But, we all decided to try for it. I check in at the hospital next Monday. I'm okay with this. I know this is the only chance I have. I'm back in a good relationship with God now. I'm not sure what he wants of me—to be on this earth to continue this life—or to go on to some other place. It's in his hands now.

In sharing his story, Max teaches us—his caregivers, his family, and those who carefully listen—how a life is constructed and reconstructed through dealing with illness and suffering by bringing meaning to the events through storytelling. Max's story illustrates that the process of reconstruction is importantly narrative and jointly constructed by the patient and caregivers. In the end, the cord blood transplantation failed and Max died. But it is clear from the last time we listened to his story that he and his family jointly constructed a decision based on hope but with the realization of his likely death.

Using Stories in the Education of Caregivers

In the first part of this chapter we have illustrated the importance of the patient's illness story to both suffering and healing. In addition, we have described the influence of the caregiver on the development of the illness story. Here, in the second part of the chapter, we turn directly to considerations of the education of professional caregivers and its impact on their relationships with patients. While we focus our arguments on the education of physicians, we recognize that the issues we raise are often relevant to other caregivers as well. After highlighting the process of conventional medical education, we review our experience in teaching medical students to honor the patient's story, and we conclude with thoughts on the role of the caregiver in the patient's narrative.

Traditional Medical Education

History taking and storytelling are central to the patient-physician relationship, and they should be central to the education of physicians. Traditional medical education is aimed at enabling medical students to develop considerable skill at constructing the disease narratives of their patients. Students are taught to direct the way their patients tell their disease stories so that the evidence, so presented, optimally constructs the differential diagnosis, or the list of most likely pathophysiological explanations for the patient's experience. Consequently, students are expected to move the patient's *subjective* telling to the more *objective* and generalizable theories that inform diagnostic conclusions and lead to treatment decisions. This process of transforming a patient's unique experience into something more universal, transcending the *particularness* of a given patient's suffering to the suffering of all who have experienced the same malady, is a useful strategy in the clinical development of the physician. It allows classification and codification and allows the clinician to move quickly to diagnosis and treatment. It is impersonal, scientific, and, for the most part, precise. Through this process, young physicians in training become quite facile in dealing with diseases, their pathophysiology and natural history, their most common signs and symptoms, and their most likely outcomes.

These traditional educational precepts have come increasingly under criticism when they are offered without additional training aimed at understanding the lived experience of illness particular to the individual sufferer. Lamenting our traditional approach, Donnelly[11] points out that "we urge students to write histories to transcend the particular as quickly as possible to reach some larger truth." While he admits that such an approach lends the information, so gathered, "great explanatory and predictive power," he warns that the particular patient's experience may be lost or dangerously misinterpreted in this transcendence. As trainees move further along the course of their clinical training, the tendency and pressure to objectify the patient's story becomes greater.[12] Coles,[13] describing his own residency training as a psychiatrist, observes:

> the farther one climbs the ladder of medical education, the less time one has for relaxed, storytelling reflection. And patients' health may be jeopardized because of it: patients' true concerns and complaints may be overlooked as the doctor hurries to fashion a diagnosis, a procedural plan.

Here Coles argues that as young physicians become increasingly adept at transforming the patient's medical story into a diagnostic theory, they lose sight of the person as a particular individual.

More worrisome, this progressive mastery of a highly specialized and scientific language and body of knowledge may be accompanied by a real sense of elitist power over those not so informed. The person seeking care and telling the story may be lost in the rush of such power. Coles[14] observes:

> No wonder so many medical reports sound banal; in each one the details of an individual life are buried under the professional jargon. We residents were learning to summon up such abstractions within minutes of seeing a patient; we directed our questions so neatly that the answers triggered the confirmatory conceptualization in our heads: a phobic, a depressive, an acting-out disorder. . . . Some of these labels, or categories of analysis, are psychological shortcuts and don't necessarily mean offense to patients or diminishment of the user. On the other hand, the story of

some of us who become owners of a professional power and a professional vocabulary is the familiar one of moral thoughtlessness. We brandish our authority in a ceaseless effort to reassure ourselves about our importance, and we forget to look at our own warts and blemishes, so busy are we cataloguing those in others.

Young physicians learn quickly how to translate what they hear and see in their encounters with a patient into a highly codified document. This traditional medical case history, a disease-focused storytelling vital to the initial diagnostic and therapeutic approach to a suffering person, is therefore a powerful device but is not without its deficiencies. Sobel,[15] addressing the poverty of the medical case history, writes:

> The medical history is a proven tool for approaching the question "What is wrong with this person?" Its virtues, however, can become vices, in part as a consequence of the dehumanizing flight from sensitive subjectivity to sanitized objectivity, from human interests to "science." The case history, because it is so useful and effective, is not likely to be profoundly altered in the future, but medical educators can make themselves and their students more aware of the serious flaws in this form of discourse, i.e., the erasure of the unique individual from his or her disease.

Bruner[16] postulates that stories construct two landscapes: a landscape of *action* and a landscape of *consciousness*. The action landscape (much like Mattingly's event-centered narrative) depicts the events of the story, and in the consciousness landscape (much like Mattingly's experienced-centered narrative), one comes to understand the meaning of those events in the lives of the story's characters. The former landscape is where traditional physician education has been focused. Students learn to ask, "What were the symptoms, when did they occur, how did they progress?" and so on, until the entire action landscape of the patient's disease unfolds before them. How medical educators are to focus their students' attention on the consciousness landscape and, more importantly, help them to become adept at accompanying the patient in an understanding of the meaning of that particular person's lived experience of illness is less clear. Some schools have attempted to create this balance through the addition of educational offerings that often reside in the humanities and social sciences portion of the curriculum, offerings often purposively placed at what some have described as the "margin" of the scientific disciplines.[17] Such courses have sprung up in medical schools around the country in efforts to direct students' attention to the lived experience of illness. The educational challenge is exacerbated by the tendency of young students with limited life experiences to consider these courses "softer" and more peripheral to the real science of medicine. These "touchy-feely" curricular add-ons bear little real importance, in their eyes, to the medical approach to the human condition. Further, traditionally and conservatively trained physicians often share their distaste for these "nonscience" educational experiences, and such attitudes come all too often to influence impressionable students.

In the case of Max, whose story we detailed earlier, the physician, who is unaware of Max's experience with dying leukemia patients, may dangerously underestimate the psychological trauma that Max's diagnosis presents. Unaware of Max's son's bed-wetting and his daughter's becoming more withdrawn, the caregiver is left unable to participate in the healing of Max's family. Clearly, how Max's children suffer his illness impacts directly on his own suffering. And the caregiver who comes to understand Max's motivation toward ministry and serving others is presented with a broader array of options in helping Max toward active mastery of his illness and dying.

We believe that the training of physicians must include a balanced education across both landscapes of suffering. Thus, it becomes critically important that young physicians develop skill at understanding not only disease but the meaning of that disease as it plays out in the lived life of a particular patient. This previously mentioned moral imperative—that caregivers must attend to the patient's illness story in the context of that person's broader life narrative—mandates that educators make students aware of the risks associated with a more exclusively disease-focused caregiving.

Teaching Medical Students to Practice in the Patient Narrative

Medical students at our institution become exposed to the value of operating in the patient narrative through writing exercises they experience during all 4 years. We highlight their experience as third-year students on their internal medicine clerkship rotation. More than a decade ago, under the leadership of Martin Kohn, who was then on our behavioral sciences faculty, a narrative ethics component was developed for the internal medicine clerkship, in which students would have the opportunity to examine the moral matter of medical work through narrative inquiry. Students begin this work by reading a short story by Ghassan Kanafani, "The Death of Bed Number 12." This story is used as a cautionary tale. That is, although the narrator of the story (a fellow patient of the young man who dies in bed number 12) feels morally compelled to reconstruct the dead man's life story, he discovers to his dismay that to understand another person's life is difficult, if not impossible. We use this story to emphasize to our students that while our attempts to comprehend our patient's lives may fall short, it is critically important that we nonetheless make these attempts.

After discussing the story, and influenced in part by the pioneering work of Rita Charon,[18] we then ask each student to write a story, in any genre, based upon fragmentary evidence of the lived life of that patient and in the voice of that patient. We encourage the student to identify a patient in whose care he or she has experienced some degree of moral turbulence (i.e., some discomfort over the lived experience of the patient). Such stories are intended to capture the interior monologue of the patient as he or she encounters caregivers through illness, and they are to be imagined to some extent, even fictionalized, based upon what the student knows of the patient at the time of the writing. In small group sessions of 8 to 10 students, with both a clinical faculty member and a behavioral sciences faculty member present, each student reads the story, and discussion ensues. For later sessions, each student is then asked to add a second voice and write an extended second story in the form of a dialogue between the patient and this second character. Subsequent group sessions provide a forum for reading these newly created stories and further discussion of the patient experience.

For example, a student encounters a 70-year-old British woman admitted for mental status change. She was recently diagnosed with lung cancer, supposedly known only to her daughter and granddaughter. Her family was described as belligerent and problematic, insisting that the patient not be told of her diagnosis. The family hovered in the emergency room, frantic that the word—cancer—might slip out. The student writes:

> . . . her eyes just seemed to say that she knew. Watching in the periphery, she would shake her head, as in disagreement to all of the medical talk. And she seemed to say, in her thick British accent, "Come close, doctor— no, closer yet," and she seemed to whisper to the ear, "Come hither, children, I want to tell you something. I am old and frail now and no one ever listens—no one listens to the old. I am going to die—you act as if I do not know—as if I do not know that there is a tumor eating away at my lungs. It will engulf my lungs until I cannot breathe. It will engulf my life. You are too afraid to look me in the eye and tell me.
>
> I am going to die. Where is my rum?
>
> Now listen, children—I don't want newfangled machines and devices. And I want it to say DNA in big, bold letters on the front of my chart."

Christopher, she means DNR. "I bloody well heard that—you think that I don't hear. DNR—just as I said, on the front of my chart—BIG BOLD LETTERS.

I know that you are angry, children—we are all angry or not, I am going to die. Say it children. Say it.

It is my right.

I want "administer chocolate" written on my arm. That is it—at my last moment I want nothing but chocolate.

I am tired now, children, let me rest. No one ever listens to the old.

Where is my rum?"

For a second "story," the student is moved to write a short poem.

Despair of an Angel

The wings are tethered.
It is by silver grey hair.
"Love and kisses to you, too, you old hag."
Surely this is she.
Ah, and brandishing an umbrella as well.
It is her self-proclaimed right of age.
There are fewer and fewer to whom she must defer.
She batters and pummels them.
They, in turn, batter and pummel her—with their silence.
Oh, my feather, it has fallen out.
My wings are tethered—by silver grey hair.

Guiding the students to use the patient's voice as a springboard for our ethics case conferences frequently leads to deeper questioning by the student of his or her personal beliefs and values, to less reliance on formalized response patterns, and to a diminished desire for formulaic answers. Students come to a greater appreciation of the *particularness* of their patient's experiences, and how each person's suffering is unique, despite how common his or her disease may be.

These storytelling experiences have been developed as a model to promote empathy among caregivers. Underlying the model is the idea that to a great extent, empathy is strengthened, if not ensured, by the exploration of the illness narrative for a particular patient. In addition, small group discussions of student experiences with patients, when constructed to allow open and honest dialog in nonthreatening environments, promote self-reflection and self-awareness, which are often squelched in traditional bedside clinical teaching. On the wards, students learn quickly to suppress their emotional reactions to a given patient's circumstances and to focus on the science and disease as the priorities.[19] Without some opportunity to reflect on the lived experience of the patient and the meaning of the disease in that person's life, the feeling and self-reflective humanist, who we hope resides in each of our students, is at risk of being slowly, but inevitably, extinguished as part of that student's ultimate identity as a physician.

The Role of the Caregiver in Narrative

As we noted early in this chapter, Bruner[20] makes the point that all stories have a common trajectory, beginning with some steady state that is breached by some crisis. The resultant disturbed state then undergoes some form of redress, from which results a return to the prior or to some new steady state. For example, in Max's story, the steady state of his life is breached by the earliest signs and symptoms of his leukemia and ultimately by the learning of the diagnosis. Max describes his trip for blood work as a continuation of his steady state, noting that his wife did not accompany him as they saw this as simply *a usual blood test.* Subsequent to the diagnosis being made, Max's life narrative is reconstructed as he assumes a new identity as a person with leukemia. In this reconstructed narrative, he comes to see the world differently, and he reassesses his meaning and value in the world. Frank[21] describes this process as redrawing maps and finding new destinations following a narrative wreckage. Caregivers play an important role in this narrative reconstruction process, a role that depends on the caregiver's ability to understand the meaning of the sufferer's illness in the context of the life of the sufferer—that is, in the consciousness landscape. The conscious caregiver can become a spiritual companion for the sufferer, assisting in constructing new trajectories, reconstructing relationships, and reconstituting hope. This is particularly true at the end of life, for example, where hope for a cure or hope for survival must be redirected. The caregiver can guide the dying person away from the sense that there is no hope, toward new hopes, including perhaps hopes for comfort, reconciliation, closure, or the hope that he or she will not die alone. Often at the end of life, much suffering results from "unfinished business," often between the dying person and others who have played meaningful roles in his or her life. The caregiver may discover opportunities to facilitate conversations to resolve such incompleteness in the sufferer's life, to encourage talking or letter writing or other discourse aimed at closure and reconciliation.

As the caregiver shares in the narrative of the patient's illness, operating in both the action landscape as well as the landscape of consciousness, the patient's suffering is shared as well. In such a relationship of compassion, the caregiver assists the sufferer with the earlier-mentioned process of emplotment, in an attempt to return coherence to the trajectory of the patient's illness or end-of-life story. This restoration of narrative coherence is in fact the essence of healing. Even at the end of life, perhaps most poignantly at the end of life, when the dying person is reconstructed, when closure, comfort, and reconciliation are achieved, when hope is restored, healing results on the eve of death. The sufferer, the dying person, becomes whole again.

17

Meaning-Centered Group Psychotherapy for Cancer Patients

CHRISTOPHER GIBSON, ALEXIS TOMARKEN, AND
WILLIAM BREITBART

The greatest lesson I have learned from working with patients facing death is that life continues and change is possible until the very end. Before working with these patients, I had the impression (that I feel many of us do) that a terminal diagnosis signals the beginning of the end and that life slowly dwindles down from there. I now know, from seeing the accomplishments of my patients, that this is not true. Until our last breath, we live. And since we live, our ability to find meaning, purpose, and growth continues. Although the nature and scope of such things may be reduced by the challenges of the illness, they remain viable nonetheless. I hope, when I face my own death, that this lesson is not forgotten.

Christopher Gibson

Introduction

As we continue to develop our understanding of the needs of palliative care patients, it is becoming more apparent that our present concepts of adequate care must be expanded in their focus beyond simple pain and physical symptom control to include psychiatric, psychosocial, existential, and spiritual domains at the end of life.[1] While such symptoms are indeed distressing to patients with advanced disease, it is clear that symptoms relating to psychological distress and existential concerns are even more prevalent than pain and other physical symptoms. Acknowledging the psychological as well as spiritual domains of end-of-life care has been identified as a priority by both medical professionals as well as by cancer patients themselves. A recent Gallup poll on "Spiritual beliefs and the dying process" demonstrates this. In this poll, 40% of those polled said that if they were dying, it would be "very important" to have a doctor who is spiritually attuned to them. Fifty to sixty percent said their greatest concerns when thinking of their own deaths are (1) not being forgiven by God, (2) not reconciling with others, and/or (3) dying when you are removed or cut off from God or a higher power. Clearly, patients are requiring more attention to the existential crisis of meaning that serious illness engenders. As healthcare providers, we often view patients as clusters of syndromes and rush to find symptom relief and reduction. Although this approach may be effective at a purely reductionistic level, it ignores the complexities of the existential crisis that serious illness often engenders.

With these issues in mind, our research group wished to develop a psychotherapy intervention for seriously ill cancer patients by acknowledging the importance of such existential crises through addressing the role of meaning and spiritual well-being. This endeavor led us to closely examine the work of Viktor Frankl and his concepts of logotherapy or meaning-based psychotherapy.[2] We acknowledge that Frankl's logotherapy was not designed for the treatment of cancer patients or those with life-threatening illness, but we felt that his concepts of meaning and spirituality clearly apply in doing psychotherapy with advanced cancer patients, many of whom seek guidance and help in dealing with issues of sustaining meaning and hope in the context of cancer and possibly death in their lives.

The Contributions of Viktor Frankl

One of the major voices in the study of meaning for humans is Viktor Frankl. Frankl viewed the suffering of his patients as a potential springboard for having a need for meaning, as well as for acquiring it.[3] For Frankl, the diagnosis of a terminal illness may be seen as a crisis in the fullest sense of the word—an experience of distress or even despair that may in itself offer an opportunity for growth and meaning as one learns to cope. Either one has a loss of sense of meaning and purpose in life (as many terminally ill cancer patients do, when they become demoralized and see no value in living out the remaining weeks of their lives[4]), or one has a sustained or even heightened sense of meaning, purpose, and peace that allow one to value even more intensely the time remaining and positively appraise events.

In Frankl's conceptualization, meaning, or having a sense that one's life has meaning, involves the feeling that one is fulfilling a purpose or gifted role in life; a responsibility in life to live up to one's full human potential. By doing this, one has achieved a sense of peace, contentment, or even transcendence by connecting with something greater than oneself.[5] It is through this connection that psychological and spiritual healing and growth take place. Frankl greatly contributed to psychology by raising awareness of the role of spirituality in the human experience and the importance of meaning (or the will to meaning) as a driving force or instinct within human suffering. As a psychiatrist who survived Auschwitz, Frankl is much respected and his insights have been widely shared.

Some of Frankl's basic concepts include (1) meaning of life—life has meaning and never ceases to have meaning, even up to the last moment of life, (2) will to meaning—the desire to find meaning in human existence is a primary instinct and basic motivation for human behavior, (3) freedom of will—we have the freedom to find meaning in existence and to choose our attitude toward suffering, and (4) the three main sources of meaning in life are derived from creativity (work, deeds, dedication to causes), experience (art, nature, humor, love, relationships, roles) and attitude—the attitude one takes toward suffering and existential problems.

Frankl felt that there are three inevitable existential problems that we all face, which he referred to as the "Tragic Triad": suffering, death, and guilt. The impact of this triad on an individual with cancer is demonstrated in Figure 17.1.

These issues are quite heightened for cancer patients. Obviously, fear of possible or impending death is a major concern for many cancer patients. Fear of suffering, whether from symptoms or from treatments such as chemotherapy and surgery, is also a strong concern for most cancer patients. Guilt is often overlooked by healthcare professionals but is a major concern for many individuals suffering from cancer. Did I do this to myself from smoking? Should I have taken better care of myself? How is my illness going to impact my family? These sort of guilt-driven ideations are often at the forefront of many patients' minds. As shown in Figure 17.1, the impact of this triad can result in diminished meaning for patients. The goal of our

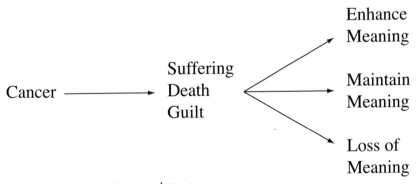

FIGURE 17.1 *Cancer and Meaning*

intervention is to at least help them maintain meaning, if not increase it during the course of their illnesses.

Understanding Meaning

We as humans have been described as "meaning-making machines." In other words, we are constantly taking appraisal of our environments and our inner states and ascribing some inherent meaning to it. Kies[6] presents an excellent example of meaning-making through the use of poetry. Read this excerpt from a poem by e.e. cummings:

> Pity this busy monster, manunkind not. Progress is a comfortable disease: your victim (death and life safely beyond) plays with the bigness of his littleness—electrons deify one razorblade into a mountain range

What does "manunkind" mean? Any computer could interpret and give the meaning and definition of any of the other words, but not "manunkind." As I was editing this piece, my computer kept catching it as being misspelled and wanted me to change it to a word it understood: "mankind." For a human, the meaning of the word is a personal search for our individual interpretation of it. When I first read it, I interpreted it as merely a play on "mankind," a use of literary license to create an interesting sounding word. On second reading, and in the context of the rest of the excerpt, I "saw" the meaning as being that of mankind as a vulnerable and feeling entity at the mercy of larger forces. Is this the "true" meaning of the word? Does a true or correct meaning exist? As with much of creative endeavor, the true meaning lies within the cognitive appraisal of the perceiver.

Such individualistic appraisals are well studied and are frequently utilized in therapeutic interventions such as cognitive-behavioral psychotherapy. For example, "cognitive distortions"[7] are often examined and modified in the treatment of depression. However, it is important to note that meaning may be viewed at both a micro and a macro level. For example, at the micro level we may make meaning of why we were able to make it to work today (we remembered to set our alarm). Micro-level appraisals of meaning involve tactical, less significant events. At the macro level, we may make meaning of why we are successful (we have studied and worked hard). Macro-level appraisals of meaning involve very significant strategic events in one's life. Serious illness, due to the serious level of threat it imposes, has its most major impact at the macro level of meaning-making. Purely cognitive-behavioral interventions are often hampered by a focus on the micro level of meaning-making. Macro-level meaning-making seems to involve more complicated issues, often at a spiritual level.

The Role of Spirituality in Meaning-Making

Meaning-making is not merely a cognitive construct. As humans, we strive to incorporate and synthesize a vast inner and outer world. For example, researchers theorize that religious beliefs may play a role in helping patients construct the meaning of suffering inherent in illness, which may in turn facilitate acceptance of their situation.[8] Importantly, recent studies have found that religion and spirituality generally play a positive role in patients' coping with illnesses such as cancer or HIV.[9] Park and Folkman[10] review the concepts of "meaning" in the context of stress and coping and describe conceptual models for meaning in relation to traumatic events and coping. They describe meaning as a general life orientation, as personal significance, as causality, as a coping mechanism, and as an outcome. Thus, positive psychological changes and an improved sense of meaning in life have been associated with cancer illness.[11] Cancer professionals have witnessed many examples of positive life change and positive reappraisals of the value and meaning of life in their work with terminally ill patients.[12]

As for a definition of spirituality, Puchalski and Romer[13] define spirituality as that which allows a person to experience transcendent meaning in life. Spirituality is a construct that involves concepts of "Faith" and/or "Meaning," according to Karasu[14] and Brady, Peterman, Fitchett, Mo, and Cella.[15] Faith is a belief in a higher transcendent power, not necessarily identified as God, and not necessarily achieved through the rituals or beliefs of an organized religion.

The importance of addressing issues of spirituality in palliative care is becoming apparent. Spiritual well-being, in general, and a sense of meaning and peace, in particular, appear to have a substantial benefit on psychological distress at the end of life. Brady and colleagues[16] found that cancer patients who reported a high degree of meaning in their lives were able to tolerate severe physical symptoms more than patients who reported lower scores on meaning and/or peace. Patients with a high sense of meaning reported high satisfaction with their quality of life, despite pain and fatigue, to a greater degree than patients with a low sense of meaning.

Our group's recent research, measuring spirituality, faith, and meaning, has helped to show the importance of these concepts in end-of-life care.[17] One of these studies examines the desire for death and the relationship and impact of treating depression in patients with terminal AIDS, and the second examines the correlates of desire for death in terminally ill cancer patients and the role of depression and the impact of treatment for depression. In the course of conducting these studies, we have collected preliminary data that sheds light on the important relationship between spiritual well-being and meaning in particular, in such critical end-of-life care issues such as depression, hopelessness, and desire for hastened death.

Spiritual well-being, in general, and a sense of meaning and peace, in particular, appear to have a substantial benefit in alleviating psychological distress at the end of life. Both spiritual well-being and meaning were strongly negatively associated with ratings on a depression severity scale. These findings suggest that psychotherapeutic interventions focusing on increasing or maintaining a sense of meaning and purpose may have substantial benefits in decreasing psychological distress at the end of life.

These data demonstrate that levels of spiritual well-being and sense of meaning are powerful predictors of both levels of hopelessness and desire for death in terminally ill cancer patients. Not only did both of these variables show a strong negative correlation with measures of hopelessness and desire for death, but these associations were independent of the effect of depression on these outcomes. These data further support the importance of developing and assessing the efficacy of interventions that focus on increasing or maintaining a sense of meaning and purpose, as such interventions may have substantial impact in reducing one's sense of hopelessness and decreasing the desire for hastened death at the end of life. From these studies, we have been able to demonstrate a significant role for spiritual well-being and meaning, particularly as a protection against depression, hopelessness, and desire for hastened death within the terminally ill cancer population.

Consequently, it became clear to us that any effective psychotherapetic intervention for meaning should include issues of spirituality. To date, use of logotherapeutic interventions with medically ill individuals has been very limited. To our knowledge, there have been no controlled studies of group psychotherapy interventions conducted with cancer patients based on a meaning-centered approach of logotherapy.

Prior Research on Psychotherapeutic Interventions for Meaning

Despite some early clinical work in transcendence and logotherapy,[18] minimal research on psychotherapy interventions for spiritual suffering or end of life has been conducted. Rousseau[19] outlined an approach for the treatment of spiritual suffering that was composed of the following steps: (1) Controlling physical symptoms; (2) Providing a supportive presence; (3) Encouraging a life review, to assist in recognizing purpose, value, and meaning; (4) Exploring guilt, remorse, forgiveness, and reconciliation; (5) Facilitating religious expression; (6) Reframing goals; and (7) Encouraging meditative practices, focusing on healing rather than cure. Rousseau has presented an interesting approach to spiritual suffering, but it is not applicable to all patients and is not necessarily an intervention that many clinicians feel comfortable providing. Rousseau's research suggests that more psychotherapeutic interventions centered on improving spiritual well-being, sense of meaning, and reducing hopelessness, demoralization, and distress are critical to develop at this time.

At this point in the development of palliative medicine and end-of-life care in the United States, meaning-centered interventions can be designed as individual or group interventions. It is clear that group psychotherapy interventions for cancer patients are time efficient, cost effective, and highly effective in improving quality of life. They also are effective in reducing psychological distress, anxiety, and depression, improving coping skills, and reducing symptoms such as pain, nausea, and vomiting.[20] Several studies have shown significant benefits in quality of life, mood, coping, and symptom control for patients with advanced metastatic cancer, including terminally ill patients.[21] Group psychotherapy is seen by some investigators as being equal to or even more effective than individual psychotherapeutic interventions.[22] Many unique benefits to group interventions are a sense of universality; sharing a common experience and identity; a feeling of helping oneself by helping others; hopefulness, fostered by seeing how others have coped successfully; and a sense of belonging to a larger group (self-transcendence, meaning, and common purpose).

The role of cancer support groups has traditionally been to provide basic information, provide support, facilitate emotional expression, and teach coping skills.[23] Very few cancer group psychotherapy intervention trials have specifically examined existential or spiritual themes or outcomes (e.g., self-transcendence, meaning, and spiritual well-being) as their main focus. A small but growing literature is developing around group psychotherapy interventions for cancer patients, which is focused on spiritually based interventions that are grounded in theoretical perspectives based on concepts and theories of self-transcendence[24] and those based on Viktor Frankl's logotherapy.[25]

The majority of this psychotherapy intervention work has utilized the related concepts of "Self-Transcendence" and "Meaning" as developed by Viktor Frankl in his logotherapy[26] and by Pamela Reed.[27] "Self-Transcendence" is only one element in Frankl's theory of man's will (instinct) to meaning; he describes self-transcendence as an inherent characteristic of humans to connect with that which is greater than one's own individual concerns and needs, and through this, in part, finding or making meaning in one's life.[28] Self-transcendence has been shown, primarily in nursing literature, to be associated with indicators of well-being and mental health in older adults, women with breast cancer, women with AIDS, gay men with AIDS, and older men with prostate cancer.[29]

It is clear that addressing spiritual issues in end-of-life care for cancer patients has become a priority in palliative care in the United States, in particular, in maintaining a sense of meaning, peace, and hope in the face of advancing cancer. As a profession, we need to develop more innovative psychotherapeutic interventions for advanced cancer patients, to help them deal with the spiritual suffering, demoralization, hopelessness, and loss of meaning that is so common (up to 17% of terminally ill cancer patients have a significant desire for a hastened death[30]. As previously noted, very few interventions have been developed, manualized, or studied for their efficacy. Our group has attempted to fill this void by designing a manualized, meaning-centered group psychotherapy intervention. We are currently involved in a randomized trial investigating the efficacy of this group by comparing it to a standard supportive psychotherapy group.

The Meaning-Centered Group Psychotherapy for Cancer Patients

The novel intervention we call "Meaning-Centered Group Psychotherapy" is based on the concepts described previously and the principles of Viktor Frankl's logotherapy. Our intervention is designed to help patients with advanced cancer sustain or enhance a sense of meaning, peace, and purpose in their lives, even as they approach the end of life. We have conducted a series of these group psychotherapy interventions using this meaning-centered approach in a cohort of advanced cancer patients in order to establish the feasibility, practicality, applicability, and acceptance of such an intervention. As a result, we have been able to manualize an 8-week (1½-hour weekly sessions) meaning-centered group psychotherapy intervention that uses a mix of didactics, discussion, and experiential exercises that are centered around particular themes related to meaning and advanced cancer. In each group, patients are assigned readings and homework that are tailored to each session's theme and then discussed in each session. Although the focus of each session is on issues of meaning/peace and purpose in life in the face of advanced cancer, elements of support and expression of emotion are inevitable in each group session (but limited by the focus on experiential exercises, didactics, and discussions related to themes focusing on meaning). The general aims of this group are to:

1. Promote an environment of communal support among cancer patients with similar challenges at an otherwise difficult time in their lives;
2. Facilitate a greater understanding of feasible sources of meaning, both before and after the diagnosis of cancer; and
3. Assist participants in their discovery of a sense of meaning in life, as well as maintenance during illness.

The ultimate goal, however, is to make the most effective use of coping through an enhanced sense of meaning and purpose and to make the most of the time that each individual group member has left, regardless of how limited that time is. It is of fundamental importance to remember that it is up to the individual group member to use the group to find the sources of meaning in his or her life. In other words, they are not to be perceived as the group leaders' passive receptors, but rather as active participants in the process. This view is essential, as we conceptualize meaning to be a creative, individual, and active process. As such, participants must be willing to help create meaning, both for themselves and the other group members.

Structure of the Group

The intention of this intervention was to help expand the breadth of possible sources of meaning, through the combination of (1) instructed teaching of the philosophy of meaning on which the intervention is based, (2) group exercises, followed by homework for each individual participant to complete, and (3) open-ended discussion, which may include interpretive comments by group leaders. The individual themes of each session are presented in Figure 17.2.

The following is a general discussion of each session. It should be noted that group leaders attempt to keep the session focused on the relevant theme. However, participant discussion and concern occasionally veers away from the theme at hand. Group leaders attempt to address these concerns while attempting to steer the conversation back to the particular theme of the given session. We have been gratified to note that these deviations are relatively infrequent, possibly indicating that the themes we have chosen are truly relevant and are in the proper progression for this population.

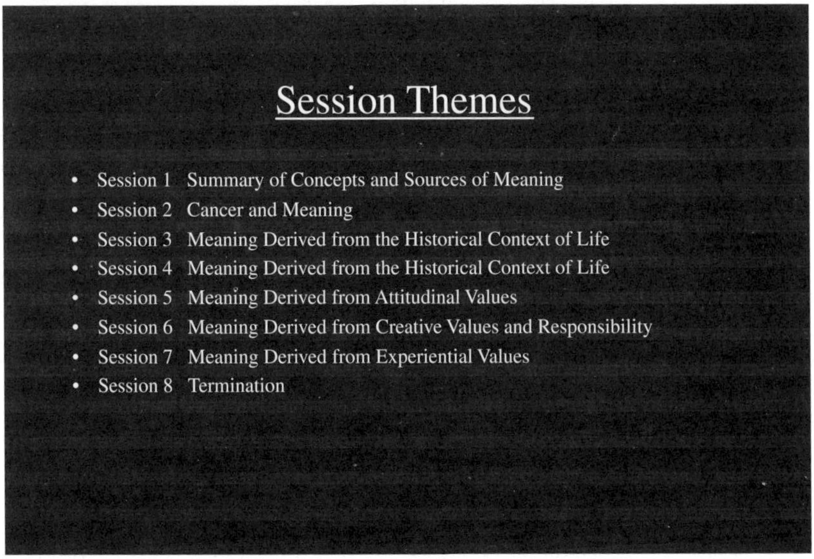

Session Themes

- Session 1 Summary of Concepts and Sources of Meaning
- Session 2 Cancer and Meaning
- Session 3 Meaning Derived from the Historical Context of Life
- Session 4 Meaning Derived from the Historical Context of Life
- Session 5 Meaning Derived from Attitudinal Values
- Session 6 Meaning Derived from Creative Values and Responsibility
- Session 7 Meaning Derived from Experiential Values
- Session 8 Termination

FIGURE 17.2 *Session Themes*

Session 1: Summary of Concepts and Sources of Meaning

The first session involves introductions of each group member and an overall explanation of the group's goals. Patient introductions include biographical/demographic
information, as well as their expectations, hopes, and questions relating to the
group. As an adjunctive to the group, all patients are given a copy of Frankl's *Man's
Search for Meaning* as a means of facilitating each patient's understanding. The session concludes with a discussion of what *meaning* means to each participant. This
discussion provides an excellent chance to more clearly define terms such as *meaning* and *purpose.* Participants are asked to list one or two moments when life had felt
particularly meaningful. These exercises help to discover how each individual finds
a sense of meaning and purpose in general, as well as specifically in relation to having been diagnosed with cancer.

Session 2: Cancer and Meaning

Session 2 is a continuation of sharing meaningful experiences, as well as a detailed
explanation of what, or who, made those experiences particularly meaningful to the
participants. In addition, each individual was asked to impart something about his
or her sense of self; this revealing process was accomplished by having each participant answer the question "who am I?" This exercise provides an opportunity to discuss how cancer has affected each participant's answers, as well as how cancer had
affected what he or she considered to be meaningful in his or her life. In addition, the
participants were asked to consider how they might have responded to these particular inquiries prior to having been diagnosed with cancer.

Sessions 3 and 4: Meaning Derived from the Historical Context
of Life

Sessions 3 and 4 focus on giving each participant a chance to share his or her life history with the group, which in turn helps participants to better appreciate past accomplishments while still elucidating future goals. This focus on future goals (no
matter how small) is continued throughout the group. This focus is intended to help
participants overcome the hopelessness that is so common among advanced cancer
patients. As a homework assignment, participants are asked to tell their life story to
the important people in their lives, highlighting proud moments or things they
wished they might have achieved. This "Life Project" is an important component of
the group and is often a theme of discussion by participants in the following ses-

sion. In session 4, participants are given an opportunity to discuss the experience of telling their stories to family members, as well as the process of recording their memoirs. Participants are asked how pleasant or unpleasant they found the experience of sharing their life story. In addition, each participant is asked if there was any moment in which he or she felt particularly moved by feelings of joy or pain while recounting his or her story.

Session 5: Meaning Derived from Attitudinal Values

This session examines each participant's views on the finiteness of life, finding meaning in his or her daily life, and moments when he or she has experienced a loss of meaning in life. This discussion is intended to allow the group to question the meaning of their existence and to contemplate ending it, particularly in the face of suffering. As a follow-up, participants are then asked to discuss what their thoughts, feelings, and fantasies are about a "good" or meaningful death. Common issues that have come up include what they expect takes place after death, funeral fantasies, family issues, the afterlife, and so on. We had designed this exercise as a way to put death and suffering in a larger context. These fantasies provide insight into ways in which people experience themselves in the larger scheme of things.

Session 6: Meaning Derived from Creative Values and Responsibility

Session 6 focuses on participants' feelings of responsibility. Each participant is asked to discuss what his or her responsibilities are, as well as for whom he or she is responsible. In addition, any unfinished business or tasks that participants may have is examined. This discussion forces participants to focus on the task at hand, as opposed to focusing only on their suffering. In addition, by focusing on their responsibility to others, meaning may be enhanced by the participants' realization that their lives transcend themselves and extend to others.

Session 7: Meaning Derived through Experiential Values

Session 7 focuses on discussing experiential values, such as art, beauty, love, and nature. Participants explore moments that felt special and discuss what exactly made that moment particularly special. Feelings concerning the group's upcoming termination are discussed at length, in preparation for the final session. In addition, individual participant's perceptions of limitations and endings are discussed.

Session 8: Termination

The final session provides an opportunity to review their life projects, as well as a review of individual and group themes. In addition, the group is asked to discuss topics such as (1) How has the group been experienced? (2) Have there been changes in attitudes toward your illness or suffering? (3) How do you envision continuing what has been started in the group? and (4) Do you have any changes to suggest for future groups? The purpose of these questions is to continue to provide a future focus for the group participants (combating hopelessness) and to help them maintain a sense of meaning through helping to elucidate what has been helpful for them from the group experience.

We have found terminations of individual groups to be quite varied. Some groups have continued meeting on their own, in coffee shops or over dinner, while other have been content to conclude with the last session. The majority of individual participant responses to the group experience have been extremely positive.

The Process of Meaning-Making within the Groups

Viktor Frankl stresses one crucial theme—that the longing to find meaning within the contents of our lives and within our existence is not just mere coincidence, but rather, it is a primary motivating force in humans. Frankl believed that life has meaning and never ceases to possess this precious meaning until we pass away. It is our hope that attaining such a sense of purpose and meaning can help to assuage the distress experienced by our group participants. However, it must be considered that what one may hold as meaningful may change over time, with the changing of circumstances. Having no control over the various facets of suffering, Frankl suggests that each individual still has the freedom to choose his or her attitude toward suffering.

This essential mutability of meaning has been very apparent in our groups. For example, some common themes noted in the early sessions include feelings of helplessness, anger, betrayal, injustice, and physical concerns, as well as interpersonal concerns such as isolation, dependency, envy, and fear of death. As the groups progress, we have noted that in later sessions themes such as the afterlife, uncertainty about the future, loss of identity, meaninglessness, and previous experiences with illnesses, or the sudden death of other family members and/or close friends come to the forefront. This progression in focus on broader, more existential themes is in keeping with Frankl's conception of human meaning-making. We feel that it is this metamorphosis of meaning that results in the positive outcomes we have noted in the groups so far.

Preliminary Efficacy of the Group

We have conducted a preliminary analysis of the efficacy of these groups in helping individuals with advanced cancers. This analysis revealed substantially stronger effects for spiritual well-being and end-of-life despair (hopelessness and desire for hastened death), while depression and anxiety were somewhat less responsive. Importantly, an analysis of the data from the 2-month follow-up assessment demonstrated that the benefits of this intervention continued to grow after treatment had concluded. The treatment effects at the follow-up assessment were substantially greater, particularly for overall spiritual well-being and meaning. Despite the small number of subjects available for analysis, these effect sizes are encouraging.

We also analyzed responses to a specific item from the Schedule of Attitudes Toward Hastened Death,[31] focusing on a sense of meaning. Responses to the item "Despite my illness, my life has meaning and purpose" increased substantially (and significantly) following this intervention (see Figure 17.3).

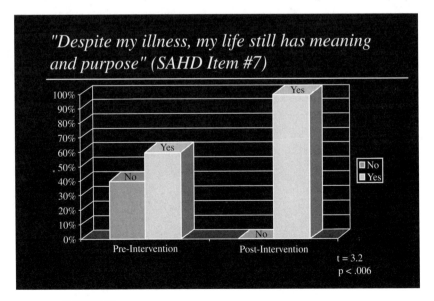

FIGURE 17.3

Prior to beginning the intervention, roughly 40% of study participants indicated that they did not perceive a sense of meaning and purpose in their lives, whereas none of the study participants perceived their life as meaningless *after* the intervention.

Conclusion

Issues of meaning and spirituality are essential components of the experience of individuals facing serious illnesses. They shape a great deal of such an individual's views of him- or herself and his or her illness and future. Unfortunately, we as healthcare providers have often overlooked them. It is heartening to note that this is changing; we are growing more aware of these issues and are exploring them scientifically. Future research should endeavor to continue to explore the complex interchange between meaning and illness. Our patients will only benefit from our expanding knowledge.

We feel that the group psychotherapy we have presented in this chapter is a step toward attempting to grapple with these issues in a therapeutic and healing manner. As we continue with our research, we hope to find better and more efficacious ways of helping patients overcome the existential challenges their illnesses present to them. We are guided by the following words: "The meaning of our existence is not invented by ourselves, but rather detected."[32] This work was supported by a grant from the National Institutes of Health, grant R21-AT01031 (to P. I. W. Breitbart, MD). We gratefully acknowledge the assistance of Haley Pessin, Brooke Myers, and Barry Rosenfeld. This work would not be possible without their tireless help and contributions. We also wish to thank the patients who participated in the groups and who have allowed us to better understand the challenges they face.

18

Reflections on Dance and Music Therapy in Palliative Care

JANET LYNN ROSEMAN

The most important lesson and gift that I have been given as a color/light therapist has been the gift of witnessing courage. When my clients tell me of their personal struggles in an often dehumanized hospital or medical environment, I am reminded of the warrior-like courage that emanates from women in their seventies and eighties. It is a profound lesson in acceptance and grace.

Janet Lynn Roseman

And the state of this soul is, there is a feeling of such utter peace and tranquility that it seems to her that her heart, and her bodily being, and all both within and without is immersed in an ocean of utmost peace, . . . and she is so full of peace that though she may press her flesh, her nerves, her bones, and other things comes forth from that peace.

St. Catherine of Genoa[1]

Dance is considered the oldest of art forms, and I am hard pressed to name a pre-Christian culture that did not dance, for dance was the predominant medium of expression to invoke the gods, to grant blessings to the community, to ensure that the crops would be plentiful, and to integrate members of the community in sacred form. Dance has always been a sacred form of self-expression and was a mystical experience when it was in pure form, uniting the body physically and devotionally. As dance evolved, the norm became the practice and training of dancers for performance, thus losing its connection to the Divine. Dance then became a form that offered self-expression from *outside* instead of *inside* the dancer. Besides the obvious religious and ritualistic aspects of movement, dance provides (through movement) the opportunity to align with the life forces of the body.[2]

According to Dr. Ross Laird, author and teacher:

> This awakeness is the essence of healing. Life stretches us thin on our bones, makes us brittle and windswept, makes us yearn for something we can't quite reach. Dance delivers us into the knowledge of the vast being that hovers over our shoulder. Dance cracks us open, makes us light as gossamer, then knits together our dry bones into a kite whose string is pulled by the invisible.[3]

The power of movement is so pure and strong that often it remains inside of us long after the movement experience has ended. I believe that the real reason that people dance (from any time period) is that it offers the human body the opportunity to become lost, to lose one's boundaries, and to experience a sacred act. That state of transcendence, or alignment with the soul embodied within, is one of the reasons that the healing aspects of dance are so powerful.

Dance therapy, as well as other therapeutic modalities, relies upon the skills and knowledge of the therapist; however, in end-of-life care, the therapist must be able to confront his or her own personal issues surrounding death if he or she is to be of service to his or her clients. By examining personal prejudices, fears, and demons about dying, then and only then, can he or she be truly present with his or her clients. We cannot place our service to someone at end of life if our minds, souls, or hearts are absorbed anywhere else. In a conversation with founding Program Director for The Wellness Community in Southeast Florida, Vicki S. Burns (January 2003) explained:

> Death is truly the last taboo in our culture. As a society, we are very uncomfortable with the dying process; talking about death, being with the dying, even grieving our loved ones. We have collectively forgotten how to be comfortable with death. The advent of the funeral industry has played a part because we have taken death out of the home. We shield our children from death and when we become adults, we are not prepared for facing death; our own or others. We have lost the wisdom that our ancestors knew; that dying is the final stage of living, that death need not be a lonely, terrifying experience for our loved ones or for ourselves. The vast majority of deaths are peaceful and the moment of death is as sacred as the moment of birth, perhaps even more so. We need many more people who are comfortable with the dying process who can be midwives to help people prepare for their crossing over to the other side.

Death is a potent teacher about living in the moment. When one faces death, emotional walls are shattered and vulnerability is ever present. Dr. Laird addresses this vulnerability poetically in the following words:

Breath and bones and blood are the instruments of the soul's expression: frail, small things prone to the many sufferings of the world. All dances are therefore devotions of vulnerability. The dancer beseeches the soul, asks to be carried into solace, into comfort, into peace. The soul's answer is movement: thumping arm, a shout emerging from the grieving heart. The sounds and movements of dance evoke all the secrets, reveal all the hidden places of refuge and sorrow.[4]

Dance Therapy in Palliative Care

Being present, although it sounds simple, is actually a difficult process. Caregivers who have worked in palliative care are aware of the enormous responsibility they have—to not only make their clients comfortable and free of suffering but to address the psychological impact of the dying process fearlessly. One of the beautiful gifts that dance therapy sessions can offer to people at the end of life is the chance to "Let go, to release the natural flow of energies inside of him- or herself. It can open up the channels of the body to clear away old emotional blockages, belief systems that no longer serve, and memories the body has held onto long after their usefulness has served."[5]

Often, in palliative care, the person who is at the end of life is reevaluating his or her life, often faced with turmoil and grief over "what should have been" and pushed into looking at unpleasant psychological realms. Dance, or movement therapy, is an ideal modality in palliative care, for it speaks its own language, a universal language. In a world overrun by a bombardment of words, the language of the body often reveals the true expression of interior emotions. Movement can also be a deeply cathartic process. Sometimes, a patient at the end of life does not want to speak, or perhaps cannot, and the gesticular language can bring him or her into the world of matter and restore him or her in the sensory world.

Dance therapy is usually indicated for people with a wide range of movement; however, it can also be utilized by clients who are not able to move. This ability (to move or not move) does not in any way diminish dance therapy's efficacy or potency. Even though the limbs of the body may be limited, dance therapy offers the person a means for soul expression, and any movement, even as simple as lifting a hand, can be infinitely significant. Even when one is unable to move the limbs, there is also a response in the body, for there is movement inside the body; muscles of the throat contract, the eyes flutter while the blood dances in the body. These silent movements can occur when both therapist and client are in the state of "what is," a reality in end of life reflecting the immediacy of life. During a session, the therapist may choose to ask his or her client to describe the pain in their bodies (perhaps in their hands or feet). Accordingly, they may also explain through movement what their life feels like or what Death looks like gesturally.

Every dance therapist works in his or her own unique manner; there are no rules to follow and no "correct response." A good therapist does not perform or teach; he or she simple guides his or her clients and follows physical and emotional cues, always aware of the client's psychological status. Being present with the client and following his or her lead, instead of vice versa, are immensely powerful acts. Most dance therapists do not employ talk therapy in liaison with their work; movement is the prime language used, and sometimes silence is all that is called for.

These encounters, in my opinion, often have a mystical quality, because the mystic is able to show things as they are and to penetrate to the heart. The mysteries of the human form are boundless, and, through dance therapy, I have witnessed transformations of a mystical quality. Often, people at the end of life are closer to these mysteries and navigate their inner and outer worlds in a manner that we would otherwise not understand unless we have had this experience personally. Furthermore, these movement sessions can be transformative for the therapist as well as the patient, and a cross-healing can occur as well. According to music scholar and musician Beverly Lomar, "Music's ability to affect the body has always been known. Since ancient times and across cultural boundaries, music has been universally associated with both worship and healing, for it enables us to both connect with the innermost core of our being and to transcend the limits of the enclosed self in mystical union with the universal other(s)."[6]

In this sense, music and dance are the ideal communicators of Truth, since the body doesn't lie. According to the dance pioneer and philosopher Isadora Duncan, "No pose, no movement in gesture is beautiful in itself. Every movement is beautiful when it is expressed truthfully and sincerely."[7]

Movement has always been revelatory. Movement reveals the soul, and what better therapy to employ in palliative care than a model that seeks to embrace the client exactly as he or she is, in the NOW, without artifice. Palliative care involves the stripping down of everything: emotions, pride, absence of body functions, and, sometimes, dependency. The nod of a head, a flex of a foot, or a tapping of a hand on a bed when one has not been able to serve themselves in bodily form can be very balancing. Dance or movement therapy can give a person who cannot move, cannot speak, or is riddled with pain a link to self-expression, which can be a divine offering. These sessions present a union with self, an elevation of self, and a union with another. The therapist's presence, the ability to be there without judgment and to offer him- or herself as facilitator, is a privilege as well as a responsibility.

The Sacred Body

Harry Rende, an artist and former physicist, described in his essay "Sadness in Art" a personal process of making art that speaks volumes about the therapeutic process. Although his essay was not intended to describe dance therapy, it is apt. He wrote:

> Sadness comes from the body, it is the body's gift. . . . That sadness be-
> longs in the physical body may at first seem strange. The sadness of the
> body is vital—it is a type of friction. . . . Hope alone has the strength to
> overcome it. Hope is without tomorrow and sadness is without yester-
> day. . . . When I try to be quiet within myself, when thought and feeling
> are the sensations of my body and [they] are not banished but seen as
> mine . . . my body reestablish[s] itself.[8]

Many caregivers, even though they are experts in palliative care, are uncomfortable with being totally present with their clients. Providing medications and fluffing up a pillow, although useful, are not the same as actually being with a patient. The possibilities can be very creative, even if the patient is limited physically. The use of rhythmic breathing or using visualization work can often foster the same therapeutic response as using movement alone. Through meditative exercises and visualizations, one can experience a sense of peace or return to a sacred place from one's memory.

The hospice movement is an important component in palliative care. In innovative hospice centers all over the world, end-of-life patients and their families are provided with the educational and psychological tools to enable their loved ones to die with dignity. Many hospice centers advocate dying at home, offering the patient support and love of their family and friends during the final stages of life. As Vicki S. Burns once said to me:

> Although, hospice encourages home deaths—something that is in the
> purview for most families—many people still opt for a Hospice Unit or
> hospital death. The motivation for that choice, I believe, is fear, and hos-
> pice has been very helpful in providing the emotional support to temper
> that fear. I worked as a Hospice Social Worker for over five years and I
> never heard a family member regret that their loved one died in their own
> home surrounded by family. I have assisted many families and patients
> as death entered and there is almost a universal experience of euphoria
> for the loved ones at the bedside of the dying. Regardless of their religious
> beliefs or lack of belief, everyone experienced the sacredness of being
> with the loved one—holding their hand, reassuring them and loving them
> as they leave—being there in the moment of death.[9]

In palliative care, certain clients, although attended to physically, do not have the support systems to express their inner worlds in a safe and inviting manner. In addition to their pain, they may experience loneliness, regret, frustration, anger, and acute depression. Dance therapy is not the answer, but *is* one of the ways that can offer a chance to feel connected, to let go of tension in the body, and to exorcise psychological states that are impeding comfort. This, of course, is contingent upon the therapist's flexibility and the ability to master his or her intuitive skills as well as his or her sense of compassion.

During one session with a client who had constant stomach pain from frequent vomiting episodes resulting from surgical complications, I sat with her and asked her to focus on her discomfort and to visualize breathing into her stomach. The vomiting caused so much tension in her stomach and impeded her breathing due to the pain. Slowly and repeatedly, she localized her breath into her belly and was able to release the pain, as well as her chronic gastric tightening. By visualizing the color blue gently floating into her body, she was able to self-medicate, to take care of herself when she felt powerless and alone.

Psychological and Spiritual Issues

Because the therapist and client interact so personally, it is essential that the therapist recognizes that he or she is working in service and that the relationship is not within a hierarchical model. One of the dangers in working in palliative care is that the therapist may believe that *he* or *she is* doing something for the client, when in truth I believe that it is the other way around. My clients have been my most valuable teachers, and I try to be mindful of that whenever I am tempted to pat myself on the back after a session.

There are no "fixes" when one is dying, and there is often not a timetable. People who have had the chance to look at their lives and reevaluate are often living in their heads or forced out of their bodies because of pain. Dance therapy is a wonderful tool for reconnecting with the body and provides the opportunity to realign with the body, mind, and spirit. The subsequent healing that dance or movement therapy can provide is not a cure, but is potent nonetheless. I know that it is not my role to decide what this healing will look like. According to Nikki Todd, a contemporary shaman and educator, "Healing does not always look like healing. Don't judge what form it is supposed to look like."[10]

When one is seriously ill, one's body image is often distorted, and the mind/body fusion can be separated. Through rhythmic movement, simple breathing, and nonconditional approval from the therapist that the client's emotions are acceptable (whatever they may be), the destructive thoughts, self-hatred, and other negative images can be "moved through." There is no verbalization or analysis needed in that moment, and the client, if working with a talented therapist, has a choice to feel acceptance. Often, clients are dependent on others for their perceptions about their body, and the information is pathologically based. The client is unable to feel his or her own body (sometimes due to medications), and he or she may have cut off his or her physical connections because of acute pain. A therapist can reflect the patients' bodies back to them, gently or strongly, depending on the physical health of the patients, to nurture and hold their lack of perceptions for them until they are able to feel themselves living inside of their bodies.

Some palliative care patients are removed from the outside world, have lost their own sense of self in body, and depend on others to reflect not only this sense of self but sense of the outside world. Through gestural movement, those abilities can be regained through therapeutic sessions. Movement offers a sanctuary to express feelings in a safe environment. For someone who has been in long-term hospital care, this opportunity to manifest rage and other toxic emotions can be very liberating.

Dance therapy is a deliberate process, not only for personal and transpersonal revelations, but because the body can serve as a direct channel for awakening the higher nature, or soul nature. During the end of life, frequently the veil between life and death is lifted, and patients reside in both worlds. What better moment to grieve, to celebrate, to explore the meaning of one's life then to use this potent art form and therapeutic model? Such soul work may not be instantly catalyzed in the dance therapy process; however, it can and should be used as an example of a spiritual practice. Healthcare practitioners who work in palliative care know that each session is a leap into the unknown. Every patient is unique and therefore has special psychological and physical needs. However, I believe that these interactions between therapist and client, when offered with an open heart, can be healing for both people, for that link to the spirit is an important and many times neglected essence of healing.

Music Therapy

Everything dances; leaves in the autumn wind, waves traversing the trackless sea, planets and stars in their languid orbits across the heavens. Those dances, ecstatic or tranquil or suffused with longing, are a way of taking a stand in the face of oblivion. In the spiraling and turning that leads ever

toward a core of aliveness, the dancer affirms the spirit, calls forth its voice,
pays attention to the patient instructions of the innermost self. Dance, and
its handmaiden music, are spontaneous and authentic prayers of the soul.[11]

Dr. Ross Laird

Music, the handmaiden of dance, has universally reflected, historically and ritualistically, the understanding between all cultures that sound is essentially a creative healing modality. The inherent medicinal powers of rhythm and harmony speak to us on both conscious and unconscious levels, beginning with our entry into the world. Mothers all over the world rock, sway back and forth, coo, and sing lullabies to their babies. Even the ancient philosophers advocated the use of music for its curative effects, although their choices for such effects were fiercely debated.

The definitions of music therapy and music thanatology differ in the sense of how music is used and received by patients. Specifically, music used in therapy is meant to engage a person in interactive experiences that support life processes. Music thanatology, on the other hand, is concerned with providing music that is simply to be received, allowing a person's "unbinding" and movement toward the completion of life.[12]

As stated by Beverly Lomar:

> Music therapists often utilize improvisation to offer patients a way of "trying out" different ways of relating, both within the self and with others. As eminent jazz musician Wynton Marsalis describes it, "Music is a way of playing life." So it is with those who seek music as a healing art— the fundamental premise on which music therapy rests is that the self is always becoming, and music, because of its intensely embodied and universally appealing nature, enables that self-discovery.[13]

Music Thanatology

Although music therapy and music thanatology both have as their goals the use of music to alleviate suffering, the training and intentions for each modality differ. Music therapy is generally practiced interactively and suggests that the patient is more attentive and responsive, whereby music thanatology is specifically rooted in palliative care and caters exclusively to the needs of that population. However, I would imagine that practitioners in both fields have worked with responsive patients at the end of life and have also used music therapy as a dying vigil. Dr. Therese Schroeder Sheker, considered to be the leader in music thanatology, created The Chalice of

Repose Project in Missoula, Montana. Her unique and visionary program of offering music with a sacred intention has offered countless patients and their families relief at the end of life. In her essay, entitled "Musical-Sacramental-Midwifery: The use of music in Death and Dying," Dr. Sheker wrote powerfully about her experiences:

> When you are peacefully present with someone whose time has come, all that matters is that they are allowed to *shine through the matrix*. I mean this implicitly and explicitly. People ask: isn't the work depressing? Are you filled with fear or sorrow? None of that exists if you are really with the dying person: *it is their time, not yours*. Any burden or sorrow, or wounds of your own disappear. You hold the person and keep vigil while they quietly, almost invisibly, shimmer an indescribably membrane of light.[14]

This practice and training in music thanatology were lovingly resurrected by Dr. Sheker, using music as a spiritual intervention based on its historical use. "Contemplative musicians tended and comforted the dying, essentially anointing the terminally ill with sound and song."[15] This privileged work calls upon the compassion, ease, and service of an individual and calls to many who consider it their life's work.

Emily Spahr, a music therapist in a large nursing home in New York, detailed her experiences working with one of the residents in the following paragraphs:

> Anna was a Russian immigrant in her late 90's. She was tiny, sweet and loved to call everyone "dahling." I visited Anna for individual music therapy sessions. Her hearing and visual losses were significant, and some days I had to write out words as big as 8 x 11 to communicate. We would go through many songs with my guitar as accompaniment and I had to practically sing into her ear so she could hear. Al Jolson was a big favorite; Jewish songs were always appreciated. After many sessions, we came across "My Bonny," which we both connected with in an indescribable manner. (I have a recording of us that speaks volumes.) Anna took that song, a song I deemed in my mind as a simple song, and ran with it. To Anna, this song she loved so, seemed to be about her many losses; her hearing, vision, husband, son. I believe that for her, singing the song was a way of expressing her sadness for those losses and simultaneously expressing her happiness. After we sang the song, she would often begin to talk about those losses.
>
> As her health deteriorated, she was placed on "comfort care." Her mental status declined, and she became agitated and paranoid, often accusing the staff and residents of attempting to poison her. Because of the strong

link we made from our sessions, I was one of the few people who could calm her. I was honored when the nurse asked me to come sing with Anna. Communication was extremely difficult, but somehow she managed to hear "My Bonny" and would listen attentively, no longer able to sing along. Possibly, it was one of the few moments at the end of her life when she knew who was in the room with her and could let her guard down and be at peace.

When Anna passed away, I had to take a lot of time processing our time together and mourning for such a wonderful soul. I made an audiotape copy of the songs and stories that we had recorded together and gave it to her daughters, who were very grateful. It's a life-altering experience to connect with someone at the end of life. There are times when the emotional burdens are heavy; however, that emotional toll is part of a beautiful connection that can happen near the end of one's life. It is hard, fulfilling, and wonderful work. I was surprised by my own feelings when I began to work with this population—I was more readily able to accept death as a natural event. I consider that a 'gift,' and feel more compelled to work with the dying because of it.[16]

Music's Healing Properties

Sound is dynamic and dramatic, and every person has a predilection for a certain sound or tone and, likewise, a negative response to many sounds or tones. We all possess our unique pitch or note when we speak, a tone that cannot be duplicated. Often, we are drawn to certain tones or types of music because it holds within it *our* particular sound. "We learn and ingest sounds with more than an auditory mechanism of our ears. The whole body responds to sound and consumes it whether we consciously hear the sound or not. Consider how the mind tunes out the ticking of a clock or the humming of a refrigerator. But even though the conscious mind can filter out the sound, the body cannot."[17]

Because our bodies, including organs, bone, muscles and tissue, are in a constant state of vibration, the use of introduced sound through music, chant, the sounding of tuning forks, crystal bowls, and other sacred instruments can produce profound healing effects. "When disease [is present], a different sound pattern is established in that part of the body which is not vibrating. . . . Therefore, it is possible through the use of externally created sound that is projected into the diseased area, to reintroduce the correct harmonic pattern and effect a curative reaction."[18]

It should be noted that a "curative reaction" does not necessarily mean survival, but certainly the offering of comfort and solace; freedom from pain and deep relaxation are all curative reactions. Sound waves, introduced by a variety of instruments, have the ability to resonate and produce sympathetic vibrations in the cells of the body. When a therapist aligns her- or himself with a patient with sound, using music or even fusing her breath rhythms with the breathing patterns of her client, she is offering a simple act that has deep responses.

Dr. John Upledger, world-renowned doctor, scholar, and the founder of Craniosacral therapy, utilizes music as a healing/creative modality, and his work promises to revitalize and revolutionize how we consider the use of music as therapy. Dr. Upledger's protocol addresses the body organs directly, and through his experienced hands, he translates the tone(s) needed from the body's consciousness and dictates the sound(s) to an accompanying cellist. His pioneering methods in music reach further than the use of music for comfort, as he speaks with the consciousness of the cells, tissues, and organs of the body guiding him to choose the appropriate note(s) he identifies.

Dr. Upledger's work is quite different than music therapy. In an interview, he explained:

> I am not interested in saying, "OK, it's your liver cell and we will play a B flat." I want to put my hand on your liver, feel the vibration and if that vibration translates to an F, a G, or A, that's what I want to hear and (the cellist will play), then the liver will respond to it and it changes its vibration. The liver is creating its own melody and it has to feel good, because I firmly believe that every tissue, every cell in your body has its own consciousness. Consciousness includes intelligence, decision making ability and it probably includes emotion and along with that, the joy of being creative. I am offering the tissues opportunity to create their own musical melody and in so doing, they get better and it helps them function better because they are happy.[19]

His work suggests a resonant response in the body that provides the cells (or tissues, or organs) a healing response and a creative outlet that can induce healing of the body's systems.

Over forty years ago, George Gershwin pondered this idea when he wrote that "Music sets up a certain vibration which unquestionably results in a physical reaction. Eventually, the proper vibration for every person will be found and utilized. I like to think of music as an emotional science."[20]

Dr. Upledger's success in using musical tones as a therapeutic means is a natural extension of Gershwin's ideas. A prominent musician in his own right, Dr. Upledger has conducted sessions with a variety of patients over the years. Although there is literature on the healing attributes of specific musical notes, Dr. Upledger extends those ideas further, taking into consideration the uniqueness of *each body*.

When Dr. Upledger worked with a client whose arm growth was stunted because of palsy, the results were astounding. The 67-year-old man's arm grew several inches after several sessions. He explained, "It's extraordinary (and not something I learned in school), but when you see it happen, what's the point of doubting? That's why the body has to dictate the music. I don't want to use music that is a healing note for all." In his sessions, as he "reads" the patient's body with his hands, the notes change while he verbally transmits the appropriate notes to the cellist, which he intuits are correct for the particular organ (or tissue, or bone). Once one note is played, the organ dictates another note, and so on.

When Dr. Upledger was asked to conduct a session with a prominent classical music conductor who had severe back pain, he discovered after playing a variety of notes that the open G note stopped his back pain. Each time the orchestra tuned up to concert A, the conductor's pain would reoccur. Dr. Upledger suggested that he stay in his dressing room during the tunings, and when in pain, he instructed him to play the note he discovered (Concert G) on a pitch pipe, alleviating the conductor's pain.

Akin to his discovery of Cranio-sacral therapy, Dr. Upledger is elevating the fields of medicine and music and expanding the parameters. His ideas for use in palliative care, although he hasn't utilized them in this population, have great potential during the death experience. He stated in our conversation, "If I had a cellist with a patient near death, and I gave them the vibration they needed (for death), they may die very peacefully. I am certainly willing to try it."

Spiritual Comforts of Sound

The frequencies of sound affect both our psychological and physiological reception, and yet many end-of-life patients are often without the benefit of healing sounds from music healers or the comforting voices of family members. Instead, many are left alone in a hospital room or nursing home with the sounds of a TV droning on and on. One can envision a different scenario, when all patients at the end of life are surrounded by healers, by family and friends who carry with them the intention of offering love to the individual. Imagine the frequencies of Gregorian chant, harp, or flute music, or even sacred silence filling their hours; then, what would their impending deaths look like?

To comfort, soothe, and offer spiritual care not only to the dying patient but to their families and friends are powerful and sacred offerings. Although the use of tuning forks, crystal bowls, and even vocal toning is often inappropriately labeled New Age;[21] these modalities can be just as practical in providing palliative care.

In our culture, music (like dance) is seen as a product; however, the sacred aspects of sound and its integral healing components are becoming more acceptable, particularly in alternative medicine. It is time to return to the ancient wisdom that music/sound can offer. Several ancient cultures recognized this potent force. "Since, the body is a bio-electrical system . . . [it makes sense] that every cell within our body is a sound resonator. It has the capability of responding to any other sound outside of the body. The various systems in the body also respond to sound vibrations as will various emotional, mental and spiritual states of consciousness."[22]

Although music therapists and music thanatologists provide a unique service in palliative care, often these services are unavailable or unaffordable. Certainly, playing taped music in the room or having a family member play an instrument of choice, especially if they are knowledgeable, can also be a potent act. I believe that the use of music and sound in an appropriate form offers a link to the spiritual world, because of the healer's intention of a loving presence. When author Sandy Boucher was undergoing chemotherapy treatments for cancer, she used music as part of her healing process. The music she listened to by singer/songwriter Jennifer Berezan was created in honor of the Goddess of compassion, Kwan Yin.

> During my cancer and the chemotherapy treatments that went on for twenty-five weeks, I listened daily to a piece of music that deeply comforted me. Entitled, *She Carries Me*, it is a chant, multi-layered and rich with voice and instrumental elements, yet simple enough to follow easily; it was composed, performed and produced by singer/songwriter Jennifer Berezan. . . . [During] those months in which I spent the first half-hour of each difficult day listening to *She Carries Me*, how it softened and strengthened me to go through the pain and loss that ruled my life at that time.[23]

Gifts of Music

Music and sound provide for a distraction from pain, offer deep relaxation, but also work on a spiritual level, offering comfort and solace. Dr. Joy Berger, Director of Hospice Institute, Hospice and Palliative Care of Louisville, Kentucky board-certified chaplain and music therapist explains:

> My training and contribution focuses on spiritual elements of life— meanings, beliefs, emotions, and transcendent moments and my methodology uses music from pivotal life-moments that holds meanings for the person, and bring past/present/future "aha" moments into the here and

now, in a "chairos" sense of time vs. a "chronos." My background in counseling/life/meaning and pastoral care and this music-meaning mode is that it is a springboard for reflection/insight/comfort for both patient and family months before death, while the patient is still alert, in the actively dying phase, and through the funeral to bereavement. It's also a wonderful method for connection with patients lost in the darkness of dementia.[24]

Many classical musicians composed their works specifically as a divine gift, and these intentions are laced through their musical offerings. Patients can be part of a cathartic release through listening to this music. For example, when my mother, Theodora Roseman, was seriously ill in the hospital, her bedmate played Vivaldi in their room day and night, and it was a comfort to each of them. In a conversation with my mother, she told me, "The music was gorgeous and helped me sleep so much better since the hospital is the worst place to try to rest. The music also distracted me from the many medical procedures I had to endure day and night."[25]

Jeri Howe, a music thanatologist and graduate of The Chalice of Repose Project, described her work with the dying:

> The vision of music-thanatology is to offer loving care to the dying through the delivery of prescriptive music, weaving together sound and silence. Because the music of the harp is not speaking to the conscious mind, it is not necessary for the patient to be awake to receive the benefits. The music is flowing soul-to-soul; connecting the visible to the invisible, the physical to the spiritual. To be at someone's deathbed is to be on holy ground. It is to be near the portal that humanity has pondered since the development of consciousness.[26]

When Howe conducted a music vigil with a friend who was dying and who lay in a coma, unresponsive, she brought her harp to his side and lovingly played for him, singing and speaking heart to heart. "Before long, tears were rolling out of his closed eyes. I knew he could hear me. I believe the music was accompanying him and helping him to let go. He died soon after I left."[27]

Such compassion is no small task. Those who are called to do such holy work know that this is not a performance and is as close to Truth as they will ever witness. Dr. Joy Berger created a prototype for musicians that she calls CORE Values: Care, Ownership, Respect, Empowerment. A brief explanation follows.

CARE: Base decisions of music from an inner core of care—over and above the standards of one's own tastes. What do you hope the music will provide? Hear, affirm, and use music from the cultural, religious, and meaning-base core of the person involved. When verbally introducing music, never assume or tell another what she or he should be experiencing, feeling, or moving toward. Be sensitive to the speed and power with which music can stir emotions. Provide an emotionally safe environment. Allow yourselves to be human with each other.

OWNERSHIP: Know, affirm, and cherish your own music—as being uniquely yours. It is your music of your soul. Hear the meanings and values it holds for you. Trace your favorite music to its deeper roots within. Likewise, honor the music of another's life story, culture, religion, experiences, and meanings. Honor and affirm these experiences as his or her own, not yours. Let yourself learn from another in the midst of your different life experiences.

RESPECT: Respect another's emotional boundaries and timetable. Emotional defenses, denial, and resistance appropriate their place in healthy mourning. In the words of Paul McCartney, let another "be." Especially in your leadership role, respect another's privacy. Respect our larger, more universal spiritual realm.

EMPOWERMENT: Seek a power and a courage for what you can do, a surrender and a serenity for what is beyond your control. With persons experiencing loss, ask not only "What do you need?" but also "What do you not need?" Seek whole truths, not mere sentimentality. This especially applies to selections and uses of musical texts, for music can move into one's core depths with speed and power. Be responsible, sensitive, and accountable. Tune into emotional wellness and health, not a pathology of pity. Know your power and your powerlessness. Refill, restore, and renew your own energies within—mentally and spiritually.[28]

Dance and music therapy and music thanatology can expand not only the patient's quality of life but the practitioner's quality of life. These modalities offer a conscious form of direct communication to the Divine and, as such, are art forms that are sacred. Difficult work, yes; however, the rewards are plentiful and abundantly rich. For too long the body, mind, and spirit have been separated, and these therapeutic models offer insights into their union. "When the whole person is recognized as a 'thou', it is no longer possible to separate the body from the soul."[29]

19

"Waking Dreams"

The Arts: A Nondenominational Tool for Reconnecting Spirituality and Medicine

BETHEANNE DELUCA-VERLEY

We hope to change the medical community's perspective of a patient's journey through illness from being impacted only by technology and scientific advances to inviting holistic questions about spirituality and creativity.

BetheAnne Deluca-Verley

Waking Dreams

It is the window of time between sleep and full consciousness. It is when I realized that there's something sacred and healing in the Self, and that creativity can release its power . . . perhaps this power is our deepest connection to God and our souls and all that we, in our busy and conscious lives, are not still enough to hear or feel.

It is for some, a creativity . . . expressed by music, sculpture, painting, photography, gardening, cooking, writing, theater, or dance.

It is a call to the true Self, to a path of growth . . . that feels full and life-giving, like the best of friendships and the greatest of loves.

It is the sparkle of the soul we feel in church or temple in the midst of our world's natural beauty . . . the beach, the mountaintops, and forests . . . the smiles of great faces . . . the giggles of children.

It is within each of us—buried, in some—amidst roles and agendas, and brilliant in others who have been graced with great intuition or forced by disease or crisis to hear the whispers of the waking dreams.

BetheAnne DeLuca-Verley

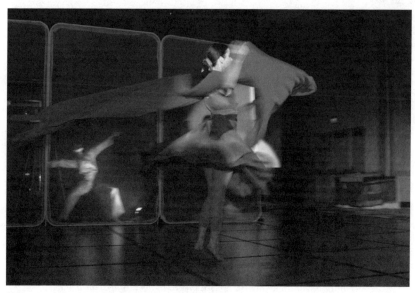

FIGURE 19.1 *"Dark Nights of Our Souls"—American Medical Women's Association 2003/Photo & Choreography WDWW.*

Introduction

Art seems to resonate with a yet undefined, fundamental energy of life that is not only timeless but also transcendent and universal. Art stirs us in a place within our bodies, tapping our dreams, our imaginations, and our prayers.

- How does art do this?
- How can art or the art process offer hope for understanding and compassion through its use of symbolism, imagination, and intention?
- Can it actually reach beyond our thoughts or cognitions to the roots of our human condition, to the core of human emotions?

Historical examples, as well as those discussed in the previous chapter, would suggest that our faith is indeed linked to art. In addition, the arts and medicine movement has recently been promoting the merits of honoring patients' spiritual journeys through dance, poetry, journaling, painting, photography, sculpture, and the collaborations between these media, as well as many others. Their work reflects an almost palpable *need* for a time and space for caring and listening to the human spirit, which is the essence of any medical care. Amidst our technologically advanced world of medicine, simple things like taking the time to look patients in their eyes, sharing their triumphs and losses, and allowing ourselves to be present to the process authentically hold value far beyond the therapies. Even when our treatments have not defeated the disease or thwarted the arrival of death, the connections or sharing lives on in our hearts. Art amplifies these connections within medicine, which cannot be bottled or quantified, but which resonate with the sublime.

Art, whether actively or passively experienced, seems to evoke emotions on both a conscious and unconscious level. This experience becomes a sacred space. The sacred space of the art experience can be used to honor the stories of those suffering from illness, crisis, or end-of-life moments, hours, days, months, or years. The art experience is a journey linking our creativity to our soul's most profound lessons.

Dancing in the Etherdome: Integrating the Arts and Medicine

The following is an excerpt from a multimedia lecture I was invited to give with the nonprofit organization Waking Dreams and Warrior Women (WDWW) at Harvard's famous Etherdome in 2002. The Waking Dreams and Warrior Women organization—as it was first known in 1998—makes the distinction between curing the mind and body and healing the spirit. We are all affected by illness and death, and we all have places to heal within ourselves. Using the arts, everyone can participate creatively in the healing process. WDWW is an organization whose mission is to explore the relationship between the arts and medicine and to discover how to integrate the two to promote spiritual or emotional healing. Their work with women living with breast cancer represents a starting point for evaluating the potential that the arts and creativity have for people facing all types of chronic illness and end-of-life issues. The Etherdome is where patients received the first form of Western anesthesia or pain control, using ether during surgery in 1846.

> As I pondered why we were graciously invited to come and share our work here at Harvard's famous Etherdome, I began to realize that Waking Dreams' desires, are not, in a sense, unlike those of Drs. Morton and Warren, "who sought to still peoples' sense of pain and bring comfort to those suffering."[1]
>
> One might view WDWW's endeavor to confront, process, and possibly transform a most elusive type of pain and suffering—the kind called emotional or spiritual pain—using the arts, as implausible! I hope tonight's multimedia experience will encourage you to wonder whether the arts

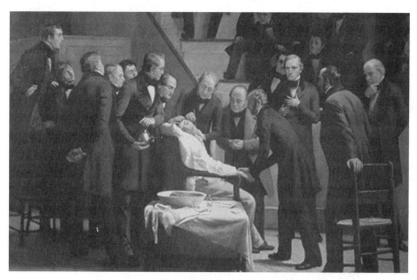

FIGURE 19.2 *Recent Multimedia Production at Harvard's Massachu-setts General Hospital.*

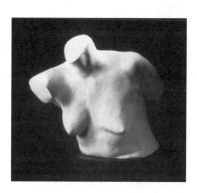

FIGURE 19.3 *"Reaching and Letting Go" Sculpture by Christiane Corbat, Sculpture and Photo Property of WDWW.*

and medicine are, indeed, related. Dr. Morton and his friends, I realized, also looked to that space between sleep and full consciousness with their pioneering use of ether. Interesting, I thought. What brought me to this point of exploration?

I was 37, still breastfeeding my third child and celebrating the opening of my solo practice in pediatric and adolescent medicine and teaching as a clinical faculty member at Brown University Medical School, when my life took a dramatic turn.

I found a lump in my breast, which proved to be malignant, along with nine lymph nodes. Due to the aggressive nature of my premenopausal cancer, I saw my colleagues' faces drop as they laid out my treatment options. Several nights later, as I struggled to find some comfort from sleep, I found myself having a "waking dream." There in the darkness of my room, with my young family asleep, an odd notion kept pressing me to rise and dance.

I recall that my medically trained mind hammered off thoughts that this was ridiculous to consider dancing . . . since I needed many surgeries, intensive chemotherapies, radiation, major luck, and prayers to beat the poor prognosis laid out before me. Nevertheless, this notion persisted, until I thought, "What do I have to lose?" Since I had not danced in nearly twenty years—I had actually stopped dancing to pursue medicine—it seemed strange that a part of me, so long forgotten, reared up as a pathway to explore my illness.

That night, I went to the other end of the house and put on some music and danced in tears. My dancing eventually gave way to an internal shift. In those hours as I danced, I met my fears and my pitiful loss of control—the control I had worked so hard to master. Within that space of awareness or some strange sense of knowing, I felt an unbelievable urge to dance and then cry and then dance and then collapse into a place within myself. It felt like I was falling into what I called deep, dark spirals, where I had the sense of falling inward. I wanted to extend apologies to those I felt I had wronged. So during those wee hours of the morning, while my family slept, I sat with a pen and paper and wrote letters of forgiveness from my heart. I felt so very much at peace, so full of compassion for myself and others who I had strained so hard to understand for so long. I recall feeling an opening through which my essential Self rose along with the rhythms of the music—feeling in unison with something far greater than myself—not alone. I felt well connected and energized for what was to be a long, intensive period of treatment for my aggressive form of breast cancer. I realized that no matter what this disease did to me, inside, my essential Self would always be there. To feel my body moving to the rhythms of the music reassured me that I was still quite whole indeed.

Then, as fate would have it, my neighbor, Christiane Corbat, an artist whose life's work has been about the arts and healing, offered me yet another interface with the art process, this time with sculpture. At her stu-

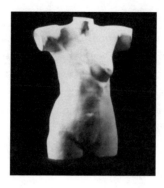

FIGURE 19.4 *"Acknowledging My Story" Sculpture by Christiane Corbat, Sculpture and Photo Property of WDWW.*

dio, with the light beaming through the vast windows, she turned the focus away from my disease and onto me and my dealing with the disease. She opened a dialogue with matters of my spirit and my emotions by using casting materials, which clinicians had long used to heal fractures, to create a series of torso castings.

She allowed me to honor all the places that somehow my frontline clinicians had overlooked or delegated to others because there was *no forum* in which to comfortably deal with this nebulous realm. From these creative experiences, I believe I was able to navigate all of my intensive treatments differently than I might have. That is not to imply that by picking up a brush one can avoid conventional treatments—this would be absolutely false. For me there was no replacing the state-of-the-art medical care I received. But did this mind-body-spirit connection, explored first here at Harvard by Herbert Benson in 1975, maximize my healing potential? Did it improve my mood and my confidence or my quality of life? Yes!

And further, was this experience unique to me? What you will see is that, in fact, I was not alone at all! There has been great interest in exploring the relationships between the arts, medicine, and spirituality. All around the world, artists, patients, and clinicians have been inquiring about the potential significance of these naturally integrative disciplines to make a difference in the "quality of the moment."

However, in my small New England town in Rhode Island, a gathering of creative yet diverse people met to ponder the possibilities. That fall night Creativity met Healing and Healing honored Spirituality. In the fall of 1998, myself, my husband, Thierry, Christiane Corbat, the artist, Donald

Acevedo, a professional dancer, Marlene Cutitar, a surgeon and the acting president of the Rhode Island Medical Women's Society (at that time), Colleen Cavanaugh, an Ob-Gyn and choreographer, a handful of patients, other physicians from the Brown University Medical School, some community members, and other health professionals sat in our living room on short notice. We mused over what might be gained in exploring the relationship of the arts and medicine. All of us shared in the excitement that this collaboration held for us in the upcoming months and years.

Our group brings people together within a shared creative process in order to awaken new ways to view and confront their illness. How do we do this? We use the transformative art experience in a process focused on improving the quality of life, one moment at a time. There are also hundreds of hospitals throughout the country with artists-in-residence programs, healing arts programs, and arts coordinators who manage hospital art collections and who organize artists to be available to work with patients. The arts are used for their own transformative power rather than for diagnosis, treatment, or interpretation, acknowledging that healing does not always mean a cure. Waking Dreams has been in the forefront of this movement, examining the meaningful collaboration of the arts within the framework of traditional medicine.

We attempt to give all those involved, on both sides of the collaborative healing relationship—patients, families, and healthcare givers—a forum or platform in which to express emotions. These emotions—pain, disappointment, anger, and sadness—reflect one's spiritual views about life, illness, judgment, death, and afterlife.

So much of the work of the last century focused upon the development of technology and mastery of the science of medicine. Then, more recently, assembly line or drive-through business models have been inappropriately applied to the sacred arena of medicine. From my unique perspective, as both patient and physician, the net result has placed corporate profits in front of the essence of healing. What exactly does this symbolize? The void that has been created within healthcare represents a call to realign our focus, to take time for listening and caring . . . whether that

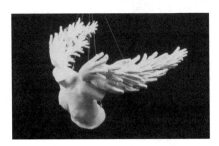

FIGURE 19.5 "WINGS OF FLIGHT": WINGS MADE FROM HANDS OF LOVED ONES DEPICTING THE TRANSFORMATIVE EXPERIENCE OF SHARING. Sculpture by Christiane Corbat, Sculpture and Photo Property of WDWW.

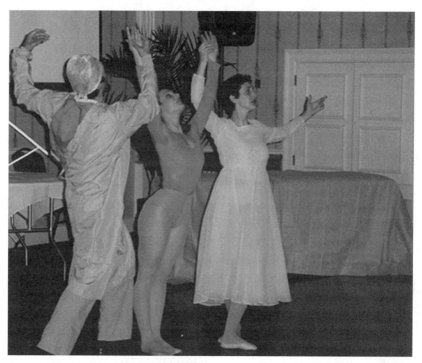

FIGURE 19.6 *"Sacred Spaces" Photo & Choreography WDWW photo WDWW choreography Bethe Anne DeLuca-Verley and Donald Acevedo.*

means being present to the patient's concerns or simply acknowledging his or her feelings. What I have heard most from people on both sides of the healing relationship is that they feel overwhelmed without the intangibles of kindness, stillness, or mutual respect. The artistic or creative experience presents us with a chance to connect on a more fundamental basis, as fellow human beings.

The Artistic Experience—Personal Dreams to Waking Reality

The artistic experience can seem nebulous or difficult to understand. However, by looking at the illness experience in three phases, one can become familiar with how simple, inexpensive, and powerful this nondenominational process we have been calling "the arts experience" actually is to create. Recall that this experience is one that moves us or elevates us to a higher sense of ourselves and others. This elevation seems to connect us with something or someone beyond our normal realm.

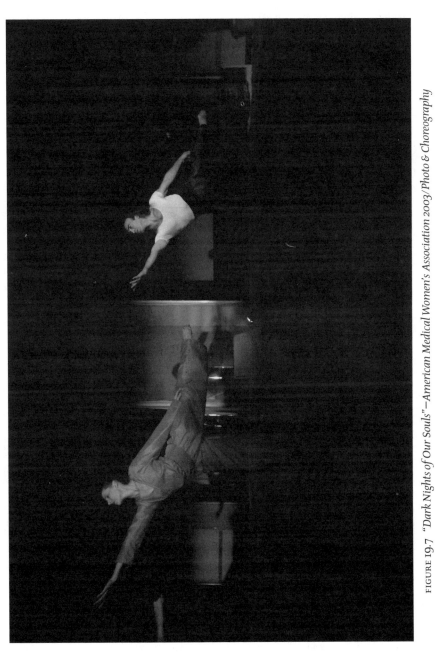

FIGURE 19.7 *"Dark Nights of Our Souls"—American Medical Women's Association 2003/Photo & Choreography WDWW.*

The Three Phases

1. Emergence of a quest
2. Acknowledgment of a personal story
3. Transformative Experience

1. Emergence of a Quest

When patients confront a diagnosis of either a chronic or fatal illness, they experience their world moving out from under them. Nothing makes sense. On a world scale it feels like September 11, 2001—when our lives were nearly severed in two—before the tragedy and after the tragedy. Our priorities seem to immediately shift. The essential issues surface to a place of great clarity while we search for solid ground. A genuine quest for meaning and often a need for closures emerge with intensity. The following small project of WDWW's will give an overview of the potential this kind of approach holds for restoring an element of dignity and compassion to the healthcare setting. This is a true story of a brave 8-year-old boy's quest.

> "Jack and the Beanstalk" was our pediatric oncology project, where Jack, a young boy with a leukemia relapse, his mother, and his sister engaged in a pilgrimage of art, spirituality, and healing through the sacred spaces of France. Here you see that loved ones can help identify a quest, which can be in the form of a pilgrimage to sacred places. Likewise, Jack and those who shared his pilgrimage were involved in a process on behalf of a cause greater than their own trials.

> "Jack and the Beanstalk" began as an idea of collectively holding the hope of recovery for young Jack. Then people offered frequent flyer miles to send his sister with him, and Air France donated two tickets for Jack and his mother. Soon there was a small group of pilgrims committed to making the trip with him, not merely in spirit, but in reality. Jack's group of eight people traveled first to Paris, to Notre Dame, then to Lisieux, to the home of Saint Thérèse of the Little Flower, and then on to Lourdes by train. On the return from Lourdes, Jack, who was in the midst of intense chemotherapy, spiked a fever and developed a unilateral rash that proved to be shingles, a varicella (or chicken pox) complication, which, if left untreated, could have become lethal in an immunosuppressed patient.

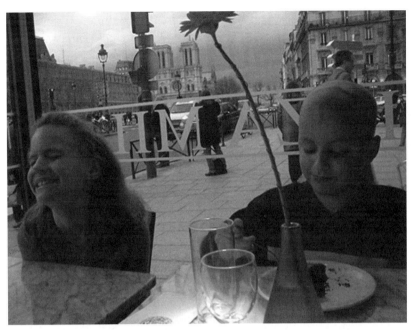

FIGURE 19.8 *Jack and Trisha in Paris with Waking Dreams during the Jack & the Beanstalk Oncology Project 2000—Photo WDWW.*

The pilgrims seamlessly and selflessly worked together to organize his medical care within a foreign country. Interestingly, before I left for Paris with Jack, I was selected to serve as his onsite physician, and I felt the need after prayer to look up the best children's oncology hospital in France. I had even made contact with staff prior to any indication of any medical problem. Between his IV therapy at Hospital Necker, Jack and his pilgrims immersed themselves in the City of Light, going to the Louvre and various other inspiring spaces. This was a celebration of life, of hope, of living in the moment as seen in this photo of Jack and his sister, Trish, eating chocolate cake against the backdrop of the spires of Notre Dame.

In this setting, the story is, in a way, physical or rhythmic, like a walking meditation. This type of creative experience is more passive in its appreciation of the arts viewed and yet active in its movement from place to place. A pilgrimage can occur either alone or in a group, such as the "Walks for a Cure," or the many popular marathons around the nation. The participants are symbolically forming a sacred circle, sharing a common intention, and honoring those suffering or lost to disease. These modern-day pilgrimages might remind us of more traditional religious journeys, which have existed throughout time and across cultures.

This search for meaning calls upon our spiritual foundation, whatever that might be. This process is truly sacred, even in its darkness and disconnects. As stated by the Carmelite author Sister Vilma Seelaus, "Something as simple as the compost heap, familiar to organic gardeners, powerfully symbolizes the reality of God's work in human life crisis. . . . The compost heap in human terms can be seen as a movement from self-possession to self-surrender. . . . Crisis tends to surface one's imperfections. These are not causes for panic. The shadow in front of the mountain is created by the nearness of God. What seems undesirable in ourselves is material for the compost heap."[2]

2. Acknowledging One's Story

How do you honor a person's story, not just the part related to his or her illness, but also the significant events of a person's life, as well as a person's connections with others? The creative process presents clues in the form similar to a collage or mosaic, with all of its conscious and unconscious meanings. The participant, whether patient or healer, has a process in which he or she leaves something behind, making a mark in the world in the form of self- expression.

Participants can use creativity to translate their pain, disappointments, and fears. They are able to highlight their triumphs and joys—some do this through writ-

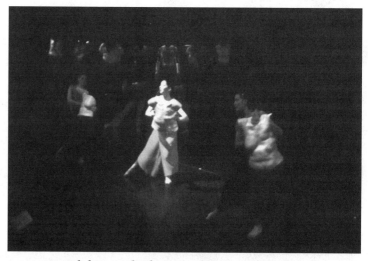

FIGURE 19.9 "Flight From Slumber"—Tour de Force, Choreography BADV, Photo WDWW—A tribal dance about breast cancer, support, and the manner in which an illness is made sacred by sharing it.

ing poems or journaling, as with Karen McLennan's WDWW workshop, "Writing for Well-Being." Karen is a writer who has inspired patients and clinicians dealing with AIDS, cancer, substance abuse, domestic violence, and depression to create narratives or stories. Karen shared a moving story about one particular woman, whom we will call Joy, living in a community home for women with HIV. Joy could not read or really even write more than her name, but who nevertheless participated in the Writing for Well-Being group.

At the second or third session Joy shared that she had an upcoming trial date in court for drug-related issues. She explained that she was very afraid that the outcome of the trial would result in her incarceration. Then she went on to say that that night she had had a strong impulse to go to the liquor store to drown her sorrows, which was how she usually dealt with problems. This time, however, Joy said, as she entered the liquor store to reach for a bottle, it struck her that she could try to write. Instead of buying alcohol that night, she bought a soda and returned to her room to write her feelings down. Note that she wrote phonetically, with many spelling and grammatical errors. Nevertheless, Joy felt some relief and pride from the creative or expressive process as she read her piece. She changed a self-destructive pattern that night and used the art of storytelling to help herself in this process. There was no mistake about her triumph and about the fact that Joy's experience illustrates that product is not the important thing; rather, it is the process. Let us dissect this story further: Joy used a pen and paper to release some of her fears and to physically put them out in the world for herself to see and to allow others to share in her experience. Karen explained that these written stories are a "means of making art of the events of our lives."[3] She elaborates further that "Writing in times of crisis puts words to fear, anger, grief, loss and a myriad of often chaotic emotions one feels."[4]

3. Transformative Experience of Connecting/Sharing

This last phase is marked by the ability of the participants to take both the *process* and the *products* of their creativity and offer them to others as a symbol of their authentic selves. There is creative freedom and clarity that emerges from this spiritual experience. There is a sense of self-acceptance, a retreat of fears, or the feeling of "Aha!"—much like the compost heap.

The differences between the process and the product—both are transformative, and yet distinct—are seen in Table 19-1.

The artistic experience can change our perspectives and give us new tools to deal with our disease or illness. This process of learning signals the transformation of frustrations, pains, and losses and the integration of new material into a more meaningful context. Who actually are the masters of this sacred ceremony? Where

TABLE 19.1

Process	Working in any type of expressive or creative medium	Writing; story-telling; dancing; playing music; poetry; sculpture; collage; gardening; sewing. cooking; traveling	Examples: Jack traveling on a pilgrimage; Joy's writing
Product	Physical or tangible item conveying underlying symbols of the journey	A journal entry, story, dance, or a piece of choreography; a painting; a sketch	Examples: A photo journal of the pilgrimage; Joy's journal entry

TABLE 19.2.
Differences between the passive versus the active transformative experience.

Passive	Viewers, audience, or anyone sharing the process or product of the creative experience
Active	Patient, clinician, family member, chaplain, or other caregiver involved in the actual creative process

do we find this sacred space within the clinical world? Can this transformative experience occur passively as well as actively (see Table 19.2)?

Masters of the Ceremony—A Circle of Participants

The key players are, of course, patients, their families and loved ones, any interested clinicians, other healthcare providers, their chosen chaplain, and anyone else viewed by the patient as capable of being present to the artistic experience or creative process. The circle of participants can be the surgical team or treatment team. For example, I recall my reconstructive surgery, when I wrote a letter of gratitude to the whole team to be read as I was undergoing anesthesia. I had had dreadful nightmares about returning to the patient role again after a period back at work in my pediatric practice. I had dreamt of ripping the mask and IVs out and scrambling for the door. While this surgery was indeed routine for these clinicians, it was not for me!

So, I drafted a letter thanking them for their skills and expertise and stated that I viewed them as participants in my healing. I asked them to join me in honoring this event by being present to this intention of healing, not only their technical prowess with the procedure. First, I had taken an active role in this sacred space, the operating room. Second, I also set the intention, inviting them to join me or share in my truth. I even drew a picture, stick-like, of a warrior with a bow and arrow shooting for the stars in hopes and with prayers of healing, both physically and spiritually.

Recall the three phases just described:

- Emergence of a quest: I found a way to cope with my fears of returning to the role of the patient.
- Acknowledging my personal story: drafting a letter to the surgical team.
- Sharing: allowing a nurse to read the letter to the team as I was put under anesthesia.

I do recall my surgeon saying, as I drifted to sleep, that I was "too much!" but, the point was that I wanted to be a part of this experience, not merely a victim or object of a disease. The surgical results startled even the surgeon, who had expected to give me multiple blood transfusions. Happily, I did not even need one. Additionally, the results were better than he had expected, needing less pain control and having fewer complications. Now perhaps this could be dismissed as coincidental, but since then I have had four surgeries, and with one I was unable to create the sacred setting with my shared intentions. That one resulted in poorer outcome, by measures of postoperative pain control, and required drainage of edema at the site for a complication of fluid accumulation.

The point here is not to dispute the merits or validity of calling forth a circle of participants, which in medicine means using randomized, double-blind studies, but rather to highlight the following points:

- The patient can be the master of the ceremony, as I described, without specific training.
- The artistic experience can be like my little drawing and thank-you letter, or photos of my loved ones, which I sometimes included.
- Setting the intention is easy, like a shared prayer.
- The ceremony does not need to be a grand display or a highly sophisticated form of artistic expression.
- The participants do not need to be trained in a special way either.
- The experience can be inexpensive, fun, and transformative!

A little letter of intention changed our perspectives that day, set a different tone, and placed us within the sacred space together.

Where Are Sacred Spaces Created?

Recognizing the three phases of the artistic experience is important to creating the sacred spaces in which an opportunity for *both* patients and clinicians can take place comfortably. This space becomes sacred by setting its intention and by creating a sense of honor for what is being shared or expressed.

The sacred space does not necessarily have to be an art studio or a formal setting. It can simply be by the bedside or in a corner of the medical ward, as in the Shands Hospital in Gainesville, Florida, under the direction of Dr. John Graham-Pole, through a medical school requirement called Arts In Medicine (AIM). It exists at hospices, such as at Brown University's community project involving creating Oral Histories, which allows patients to tell their story and have it preserved for loved ones.

The sacred space can be in clinics, such as in Intimate Expressions, where Kim Greenberg's WDWW workshop at Women and Infants Hospital, at one of Brown University's Oncology Units, involved performance art in the form of modern improvisational dance as a means to connect women who were undergoing chemotherapy with their feelings. It could be at Tufts New England's Saint Anne's Hospital, with Caryl Sickal and her meditative movement project with women at various phases of breast cancer treatment. Note that in all settings, the participants are able to sense their uniqueness, their connections to the cycle of life, and then transform their suffering.

While most of my discussion has revolved around women's issues, other venues have been exploring this nondenominational tool in work with men and children. The sculpture project of artist Joel Haas, titled "Hands of An Angel," represents an extension of our work with women's oncology to that of men during a period of affiliate development in 2001. This program stemmed from our lecture and multimedia production at the American Holistic Medical Society in Miami. It appears that artists and clinicians, especially physicians, have been drawn to the concept of using creativity as a nondenominational spiritual approach to enhance their care and connect with their patients on a more personal and more profound level.

I believe that clinicians have long feared engaging patients about their spiritual beliefs because they might not understand the specific principles underlying them. We are not a group who deals well with not having a handle on all the details. Physicians are typically control freaks—being one, I can say this! The real issues, though, are universal. These issues are the subjects of WDWW's performances. Inevitably peoples' responses to the passively shared artistic experience, such as attending concerts, exhibitions, or performances related to the arts and healing movement, touch a common chord that has not yet been fully addressed for both healers and patients in any other setting.

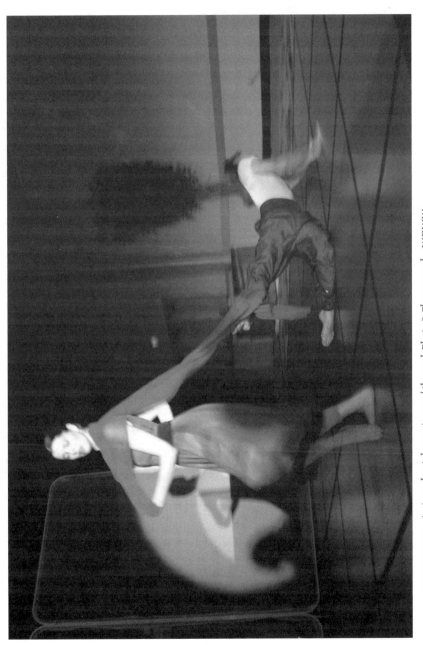

FIGURE 19.10 *A piece about depression and the soul. Photo & Choreography WDWW.*

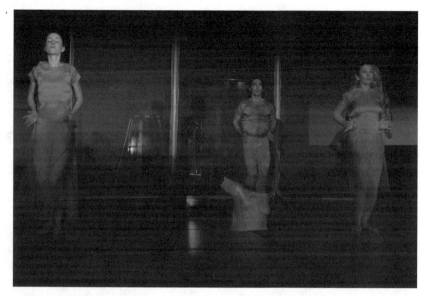

FIGURE 19.11

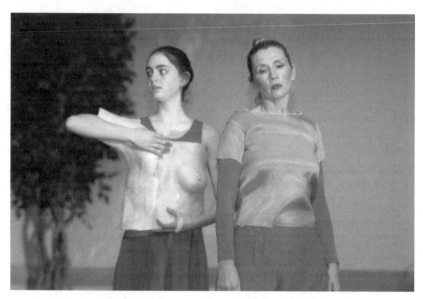

FIGURE 19.12   *"Tour de Force"—A dance piece about breast cancer, family, mothers and daughters, and community—Choreography and Photo WDWW.*

Here are some examples of the far-reaching interests of the Arts, Medicine, and Spirituality movement, which demonstrate the fact that a real desire exists to re-unite the science of medicine with the art of medicine by including compassionate care and by providing a setting for listening and reflection. The photos and brief lists below represent the broad and intense interest of various medical organizations and audiences willing to honor the sacred spaces of illness and death through both installation art exhibits and multimedia productions.

Installation Art Exhibits and Multimedia Productions in Clinical and Nonclinical Settings

- The Society for Arts In Healthcare conference with C. Everett Koop in 2000
- The American Holistic Medical conference, attended by 500 physicians in 2001
- The American Medical Women's Association's Annual meeting in 2003

Regardless of the setting, sex, race, age, religion, disease process of participants, media used, or whether it is an active or passive process, the integration of art into modern medicine has the power to be a tool for accessing people's spiritual resources.

Art is not limited to those trained in extensive study of these media but rather is a window into the soul. Art within the context of our discussion is more process related than product related. Ironically, however, the products created in this realm of illness and impending death ring so purely with the courage and strengths of the human spirit that we are often overwhelmed by the beauty of the truths and the honesty that are inevitably revealed.

20

The Role of Music at the End of Life

MICHAEL STILLWATER-KORNS AND GARY MALKIN

In bringing music to the bedside, what I have learned is an appre-
ciation for each moment, an uncompromising request for authen-
ticity, a heightened sensitivity to what is most meaningful, and a
recognition that, in the end, we simply want to love and be loved.
To enter a hospital room as a stranger and leave as a friend are only
possible because of each person's courage, generosity, and willingness
to open to the living moment once again.

Michael Stillwater-Korns

Everywhere I go, I see a real hunger for presence, for vulnerability,
and for authentic empathy. When eye contact is made, a hand is
extended in kindness, or the right music is played at the right time,
these qualities thrive. When we are willing to be real and meet
people in a human, heartfelt way, we are reminded of our inter-
connectivity as humans. We are humbled by it all: the joys, the
suffering, and the mystery of life itself.

Gary Malkin

Music is a medicine of the soul.

Plato

Music as Therapeutic Intervention

Music has played a significant role throughout time in honoring and assisting the dying process. We can imagine our ancient forebears easing a tribal member's jour-ney into the next world with the intonation of their voice, the pluck of a string, or the beat of a drum.

For people in faith traditions, hearing favorite hymns is a great source of comfort. For those in earth-based cultures, music as a part of ceremony and ritual around the dying process is essential and natural. For anyone, music that touches the heart is deeply calming, making it more possible for those surrounded by such music to embrace an attitude of compassion, acceptance, and presence.

Research has shown that music affects us physiologically, psychologically, emotionally, and spiritually. We respond to music in many more subtle and complex ways than can be proven scientifically. However, we do know that music can transport us from a waking state (Beta) to a contemplative state (Alpha) while remaining awake. New areas of research show a correlation between music and the body's release of endorphins and neuropeptides, as well as changes in the circulatory system, brain wave activity, and metabolism.[1]

That music can change our emotional state is not surprising, but new research has shown that appropriate *application-specific* music can actually reduce the need for pain medication. This is one of the reasons why music therapy is one of the fastest-growing complementary therapies in healthcare today.

As a result of this research, as well as anecdotal evidence since antiquity, singing harpists and other musicians are now being invited into hospices, clinics, and homes to provide peaceful tones to match the breathing rate of dying patients and to help unlock the soul from the body. These methods were discovered nearly a thousand years ago by the Cluny monks of France, who developed an entire body of knowledge that is now known as *musical thanatology*.

The word "thanatology" comes from the Greek word for death, *thanatos;* the term "music thanatology" was coined by Therese Shroeder-Skeker of the *Chalice of Repose Project.* As a result of her vision and dedication over the last three decades, trained musical thanatologists now provide service at the bedside of those who are dying by offering what she calls a "music vigil." Their aim is "to lovingly serve the needs of the dying and their loved ones with prescriptive music."

"In situations like these, where everyone is doing their best, the dying person may still have significant physical, emotional, or spiritual pain. A music vigil at the bedside is almost always very beneficial for both the patient and loved ones. Music can help to ease physical symptoms such as pain, restlessness, agitation, sleeplessness, and labored breathing. The vigil conveys a sense of serenity and consolation that can be profoundly soothing to those present. Difficult emotions, such as anger, fear, sadness, and grief, can find unspoken comfort as listeners rest into a musical presence of beauty, intimacy, and reverence."[2]

As medical science continually advances its practices and technologies, leaders in healthcare are becoming aware of the fact that there are many forms of suffering that elude even the most sophisticated medical breakthroughs. Healthcare professionals are beginning to recognize this and welcome these musical interventions as a complementary modality of care that provides alternatives for the alleviation of the many sources of suffering—physical, emotional, and spiritual.

Research on the benefits of music for the dying has been appearing over the years, opening the doors for more health professionals as well as lay people to start using music as a tool for creating a healing environment, as an intervention for anxiety relief for both patients and their families, and as a technique to enhance and deepen the work of the caregiver. More and more composers, musicians, music therapists, and practitioners have been exploring this field, as well as taking greater care to select the right music for its desired effect as well as for its healing characteristics.

"Music is a useful therapeutic intervention that can improve quality of life for dying patients. Physiologic mechanisms in response to carefully chosen musical selections help to alleviate pain, anxiety, nausea and induce sleep. Expression of feelings enhance mood. . . . Music, a universal language, is an important clinical adjunct that addresses individual and family needs, thereby assisting patients to achieve a peaceful death."[3]

What is it about music that has earned it such universal acceptance as a companion at the end of life? How is it that music can accelerate one's sense of connection to greater meaning, enhancing one's relationship to spirituality? How does music help to create healing environments in which there is a greater probability of engaging with one another in ways that could encourage more frequent expressions of compassion and empathy? Could it be because our sense of hearing is the first to develop in utero and the last to leave before dying, making it the most intrinsic of the human senses? Or could it be because music can be heard inside the mind, even without our external sense of hearing? Could it be because, as Leonard Bernstein once said, "music can name the unnamable and communicate the unknowable,"[4] reaffirming that we are, essentially, spiritual beings on a human journey? Or is it because music can be such an intimate companion throughout the important phases of our lives, helping us traverse life's challenges with more ease?

Music for Crossing Over

Dying is the last transition of a lifetime—some say, a passing from this world to another. Others say that it is a disappearing altogether or not going anywhere at all. Whatever a person believes, everyone agrees that something significant happens when we die—a major passage. And in the industrialized world, for every person who looks upon death with awe, wonder, and curiosity, there are at least twice as many who approach it with dread and denial.

Regardless of how we view this ultimate change, music itself is impartial. It plays on as we pass through the greatest transition of our lives.

Music inducts us into the present moment, catalyzing a direct experience with the unchartable aspects of life. It reflects back to us an invisible mystery that we never truly solve. It has been seen as a connector between worlds, with a simultaneous existence in the realm of the living as well as the realm of vibratory frequency. Music connects us to the unseen part of us, the part of us that crosses between worlds.

In the domain of the living, music resides in the heart, in the dancing feet, in the swaying body, in the songs we can't get out of our head. In the domain of vibration, music is a magnet into the mystery, a guide into the unknown. As Aldous Huxley put it, "After silence, that which comes nearest to expressing the inexpressible is music."[5]

Music can be a vessel for "crossing over," assisting us in feeling more relaxed, safe, connected, and even fearless, especially when approaching our dying time or when being with someone else approaching his or hers.

There are ancient tales of musicians or singers who used their craft to navigate to the furthest shores. The greatest of these was Orpheus, the divine singer of legend, who sang the sweetest songs on earth, "so that nothing could withstand the charm of his music."[6] He exhaled an enchanted elixir of immortality through his voice. Seeking his beloved Eurydice, he descended into the underworld, crossing the River Styx by enchanting Charon, the oarsman, as well as all the dwellers of Hades, through his irresistible song. Just as music served Orpheus, it can help us cross our own "River Styx" more peacefully.

Music has an infinite life expectancy, capable of soothing and comforting each heart that receives and treasures it. Music transcends the end of life itself, living beyond the breath-and-water dependency we mortals share. Music can pass down through generations and renew its potency, growing stronger through each repetition.

When we let music touch our hearts, the human part of us opens to be met. In the place where music meets our heart, there exists an entryway to what the world's wisdom traditions would call our *soul*. Thus, music reminds us of this ephemeral soul of ours, summoning unseen wings with which we can soar.

This is undoubtedly why Beethoven said, "Music is the one corporeal entrance into the higher worlds of knowledge which comprehends mankind—but which mankind cannot comprehend."[7]

To allow music to be our companion during our life's passages offers us practice in the art of letting go. Music can help provide a preliminary experience of meeting parts of ourselves not confined by space or time, undefined by our relational world or even by our body itself. By allowing music to be our mentor in relaxing and letting go, we nurture a relationship that will serve us throughout our lives and through our dying process as well.

Personal Journeys

(From Michael Stillwater-Korns): "I had the privilege of singing to my father before he died. After a lifetime of criticizing my choice to dedicate music to healing, he experienced me and my singing without the filter of his judgment. He opened to the love within my music, and allowed himself to feel seen and appreciated.

Inspired by the beauty and reconciling power of that encounter, I volunteered at a local AIDS hospice. I began meeting with people who were dying, to offer music and songs for their journey. Listening from a quiet place inside me to what was wanted and needed, I allowed new songs to be born in the presence of each person and family, and over time began extending this service, in private residences, nursing homes, and hospices. During this time, I created a large repertoire of songs that addressed the dying process in many ways. Some were about letting go, others about embracing love, while still others were anthems from a welcoming companion. I called the practice 'Songcare.'

With each healing encounter, I saw how the dying person was hungry for simple and authentic presence, and for music that met him or her deeply, which spoke to the soul. I witnessed how this music created a bridge between family members, giving them permission to speak the feelings in their heart. I saw firsthand how the combination of music and quiet presence was providing a key, not only for the dying person, but for family members and healthcare professionals as well.

Out of these experiences, I was inspired to explore the idea of creating a healing musical resource for all those involved with the end of life process, on a wider scale than I could personally deliver. I invited my friend, Emmy Award-winning composer Gary Malkin, to collaborate with me on this endeavor.

His own journey of opening to life's greater meaning had recently included witnessing the unexpected death of his father, and shortly thereafter, the birth of his daughter, which was endangered by complications that almost led to losing the child. The combined power of these two events led him to know, without question, that his art needed to be in service of the passages of life. His musical gift to penetrate into the core of the listener was ready to be used in a new way."

(From Gary Malkin) "For almost twenty years, I had been composing and producing music for all kinds of media projects. Looking back, the projects that were the most fulfilling to me were the ones that uplifted the spirit, awakened our conscience, or helped to better the world in some way. I knew from experience that media combined with music could produce potent 'trojan horses' of cultural influence. So when Michael Stillwater approached me to create something for those coping with life and death issues, I was intrigued. I had just experienced some major life challenges and imagined how appreciative I would have been if there had been an audio resource that could have supported me through that difficult time.

We began by recording Michael speaking a personal message to an imaginary recipient of a terminal diagnosis, while I simultaneously underscored his words with a musical soundtrack, not unlike the film scoring process. What resulted after three years of dedicated work was a unique collection of messages that were delivered by people from a variety of cultures and traditions. Compassionate teachers, speaking from an intimate immediacy of loving kindness, included death and dying pioneer Elisabeth Kübler-Ross, Mahatma Gandhi's grandson, Arun, Harvard Confucian scholar Tu Weiming, Vietnamese Buddhist monk Thich Nhat Hanh, Jewish Renewal leader Rabbi Zalman Schachter-Shalomi, and many others. The instrumental music provided both a beautiful framework and a profound enhancement to the messages, creating an alchemical listening experience, an innovation that would ultimately be described as 'a non-pharmacological audio intervention for psycho-spiritual care.' We called it Graceful Passages: A Companion for Living and Dying."[8]

Music as "Audio Medicine"

What emerged from this creative process was a result beyond what either one of us had imagined. With the creation of *Graceful Passages,* there was now a way to use both the intimacy of spoken wisdom, along with the healing power of music, to reduce fear around the dying process, helping people embrace the possibility of both acceptance and closure.

As we played the result of this work for people at various stages of dying in addition to their care providers and family members, we discovered that the alchemy of intimately spoken messages combined with a customized musical score created an experience of connection to greater meaning and a remembrance of one's spiritual essence. The music became a delivery system for a healing presence beyond words.

After the initial release of this work, we received hundreds of letters, e-mails and phone calls from people all over the world whose lives were powerfully touched by this resource. We realized there was something going on—more than met the eye. The combination of music and healing words was a whole greater than the sum of its parts, representing a new way for information to be delivered and received.

Through the numerous responses we received, we began to understand more about the effects this "audio medicine" was having on listeners. One of the most significant of these effects is the way it addressed the fear of dying itself.

The Path to Acceptance

An aversion to the subject of death and dying is understandable. It is human nature to want to focus on life and living. An ancient Hindu scripture states that the greatest wonder in the world is that while all around us people die, none of us believe it will happen to us. Denial of death and dying is universal, yet more pronounced in our Western, technological culture, where reliance upon medical science has reinforced the illusion that we are protected from death altogether—as long as we don't talk about it.

One consequence of this belief is demonstrated in the extreme measures often taken to preserve the body's life when it is naturally ending, rather than allowing nature to take its course. A focus on the psycho-spiritual aspects of the end-of-life process helps shift our attention to the quality of our relationships and the meaning of our lives.

By facing our fear of death we inevitably begin dealing with our unresolved grief. When we make peace with the significant people in our life, the quality of our relational life improves, the burden in our heart lightens, and the presence of spirit often becomes more palpable. Many who face life-threatening illnesses report feeling more grateful, more connected to their loved ones, and more aware of the preciousness of life itself as a direct result of accepting the dying process. At the same time, being fully present to a life-threatening situation, rather than in denial of it, does not in itself hasten the process of dying but rather incorporates the possibility for survival.

How do we come more easily to such acceptance? We may find it necessary to gradually ease into the awareness of a difficult predicament, such as when we are faced with a serious illness. This is where music can be a significant tool, helping people take steps toward the ultimate realization of their circumstances. Music has a way of wrapping the unspeakable with a comforting blanket. It creates a backdrop and focus of attention within which we can contemplate, reflect, and wrestle with conflicting thoughts and feelings and ultimately find a peaceful acceptance of what is before us.

As John Ortiz, in *The Tao of Music*, wrote, "Music frees souls, captures and surrenders hearts . . . and hurls the spirit into the infinite."[9]

Application in Palliative Care

When we initially released *Graceful Passages*, we included a CD of the music without the spoken messages. This music-only CD[10] allows listeners to be held in the experience of the music without needing to listen to words, particularly the words about letting go and coming to peace with dying. Through the power of music, the listener can relax, coming into a more peaceful feeling and greater receptivity to the messages. This is why Barbara Crowe, former president of the National Association for Music Therapy, says, "Music . . . can make the difference between withdrawal and awareness, between isolation and interaction, between chronic pain and comfort, between demoralization and dignity."[11]

Using music in healthcare institutions to ease the process of acceptance and to support conversations toward closure is still, unfortunately, not widespread. In spite of music's extraordinary ability to soothe anxieties during challenging times, it is rarely offered as an ongoing palliative tool. In contrast, patients and caregivers are often besieged by a constant din of noise and media static. These sounds permeate most healthcare environments and impede the healing process itself.

We have learned to live with this kind of noise pollution without questioning its effect on us or those we care for. How many times have we walked into a hospital room or an assisted living facility with an intrusive talk show filling the space? We have only begun to discover what might be possible if we used the appropriate music to help create a truly healing environment.

Still, music that appeals to one person may not appeal to another. When music is played within an environment, it knows no boundaries. Unless a personal music system is provided, the sound permeates the surroundings. For this reason, music that is created specifically for eliciting peaceful, compassionate states of mind and heart is best suited for a general listening environment.

Because our intention was to create healing environments, as well as to underscore compassionate messages, we found that when the spoken words were removed from the recording, the music itself provided an ephemeral quality that evoked compassionate communication. The environment became more conducive to healing, helping to reduce the stress and anxieties encountered there. Many healthcare practitioners reported that by lessening the fears of patients and their families, the environment became calmer and more infused with thoughtfulness, kindness, and a connection to Spirit. In such an atmosphere, practitioners felt nourished and became reminded of why they originally pursued a career in the caring professions.

While observing the relationship between practitioner self-care and optimum care for patients, we began tracking a correlation between addressing the roots of emotional and spiritual stress and strengthening practitioner resilience—not only in palliative care and hospice but systemically throughout healthcare. Our findings have been developed into *Care for the Journey,* an educational intitiative featuring music with recorded messages of innovative healthcare educators speaking directly to care professionals. By initiating the "upstream conversation" with practitioners, giving them an opportunity to reflect on their journey their feelings around mortality and the healing power of their caring presence, care professionals feel acknowledged and renewed in their practice. In the same way that a music-infused resource can serve patients, we are discovering the integrative role it can play for practitioners as well.[12]

Integrative Elements in Music

There are certain distinctions in music that are highly effective in the integration of body, mind, and spirit, thus providing an ideal resource for palliative care. These include the following elements.

Acoustic Instruments

The presence of natural acoustic instruments is one common factor. Simply the presence of the human voice, of real wood and strings, of the human touch in performance is a vital healing factor. That is why just the music of a simple Native-American flute can be so effective, or the harp and voice as messengers of Spirit. The inherent attraction to acoustic instruments, with all their natural overtones, is an innate human response, irrespective of historical age or culture.

Relaxed Tempo

Another factor we have found to be greatly effective is a slow, spacious approach to melody and harmony. A fast, dramatic piece of music that requires most of one's focused attention is generally not as conducive for healing, reflection, and letting go as

compared with those pieces that inspire contemplation while allowing the fulfillment of everyday tasks and caregiving procedures. Music set at the tempo known as
"adagio," often expressed as a distinct movement within classical music literature,
allows for this relaxed listening while engaged in activity, providing deep nourishment and a sense of spaciousness to the spirit.

Emotionally Evocative

The emotional component of a piece of music is another factor. Much of the music
that is inspired by or dedicated to Spirit will often be evocative of the kind of inner
reflection and peace appropriate to healing environments. When music can elicit
healing tears that wash away our resistance, an inner opening may be created toward
a more genuine way of being with ourselves and each other.

Because of this universality of music as a delivery system of the spirit and because of the specific properties mentioned here, music offers a way to gently approach acceptance of challenging circumstances, ultimately making it possible to
derive the most value out of difficult life transitions. Since resistance to the end-of-
life process is universal, an important role of music is also as a bridging tool, supporting communication about when it might be appropriate to discuss palliative or
hospice care as the next step.

Those in palliative care are aware of the stigma our culture associates with hospice. There is a great need to find ways to open this important discussion, in much
the same way as when patients must decide on whether they want to be kept alive
on life support long before there is any indication that it might be necessary. Appropriate music can provide a catalyst to ask the probing and vulnerable questions
that inevitably arise when in the midst of a serious health challenge. By selecting
music to help in our contemplation, we can navigate these transitions with a deeper
sense of meaning and connection and thus find ways to navigate the next steps on
our journey.

Exploring Our Relationship to Mortality

In his message on *Graceful Passages*, spiritual teacher Ram Dass conveys the idea that
"each of us contains a being that doesn't die and a being that does die." As we've mentioned before, the part of us that doesn't die is often called the *soul*. As we identify
with our soul, our relationship to life undergoes a profound change.

The sooner the inevitable is accepted, the better chance we have of being prepared for our dying, whenever that event occurs in our lives. In Tibetan culture, people are taught to begin preparing for their dying at an early age, as their religion guides them through a lifetime of practice to meet death with full consciousness. "It's not necessary to wait until death is near to begin such a practice. In fact, Tibetans bring death in an anticipatory way into life."[13]

In the West, we seem to require a different kind of preparation. For us, what seems to be most important is learning to let go. We have, as a culture, a difficult time receiving and a similar struggle around surrendering control.

Simultaneously, as we are asking our immune systems to rally against a formidable challenge, we are also learning to relax and trust in the ultimate outcome, whatever it may be. In his message on *Care for the Journey,* oncologist Jeremy Geffen, author of *The Journey Through Cancer,* defines healing as "focused action and intention wrapped in the arms of surrender."[14] While we may continue to pray for miracles, it is required of us to ongoingly let go of any expected outcomes, accepting whatever is actually happening at any given moment. When we are able to do this, a true experience of spirituality is not far away.

Music as Spiritual Practice

In describing how music can support us in both living more fully and accepting the dying process with more awareness, the following metaphor may be helpful: Imagine a river meandering toward an enormous cascade. We are each floating down the river on a raft and can hear the approaching cataract thundering in the distance. However, we assume there is plenty of time before we reach it, so we choose to ignore it.

Gently rocked by the water, we are lulled asleep and begin to dream. We imagine beautiful, haunting music causing wings to grow, sprouting from our back, to carry us over the falls as our raft falls below. It is a wonderful sensation, a sense of perfect freedom and grace.

We suddenly awaken to the roar of the waterfall, now closer than before. During our sleep we had apparently traveled further than we had supposed, and now, the falls are nearly upon us. Fear of imminent disaster grabs us. Our adrenaline begins pumping. A fragment of our dream presses at the edges of our awareness. Are we lucid enough to remember how to sprout our wings?

If the raft is our body, and the waterfall our death, then music is the breeze upon which we soar.

Music that opens the gateway to our souls offers a treasure beyond worldly value. Listen until you find such music, and then set aside special moments to truly experience it. Allow such music to hold you, to embrace you, and to give you space to breathe a different kind of oxygen. Let it come through you, so you begin to feel inseparable from it—and listen closely. Sing it through you, with a new melody all your own—and then, let your own words emerge without planning. Let the rhythm be born directly from the pattern of your breath, and let the music arise from your deepest knowing. Allow yourself to be infused and absorbed in the music of your soul.

Practice using music for "crossing over" into the unseen worlds. Activate your "wings" by listening to the most healing music you can find. Immersed in surrender, letting go into each present moment, let music lift your wings beyond the waterfalls along the way. Amidst life's inevitable challenges, let music help you come to peace, indifferent to agitation.

With this practice, you will be better prepared when the greater roar comes along. And when the thunder does grow loud, the music will seek you out. It will already be waiting, within and around you, offering you inspiration for the unfolding of your wings.

After we had invited Ram Dass to speak on *Graceful Passages*, he asked, "Who is the recording really for?" We said it was being created for people when they were dying, to give them beautiful music and messages to ease their journey. He said, "I don't think it's only for them. You want to reach people earlier, help them prepare. When someone is at the doorway, they're already beginning to listen to their own inner music. The rest of us need it even more."

It's during the end-of-life process, with the support of touch, silence, deep conversation, presence, and healing music, that we more easily identify with our souls and lean back into the arms of surrender. The quality that turns skilled healthcare technicians into healers is simply remembering the humanity we share. As more physicians, nurses, and other healthcare professionals are given opportunities to recognize the role of spirituality in the midst of their work, music can never be far behind. Music is a tool that can enhance the integration of our humanity throughout this lifetime, and whose role is particularly vital in lessening fear while supporting the end-of-life process.

As each of us face the waterfalls ahead, may our hearts sing and our wings unfold to the music, the music that reminds us of what matters most.

21

Grief

A Wall or a Door

PAUL TSCHUDI

My patients have been my most valued teachers. They have taught me that we are all living until we die, that hope does not mean cure, and that ultimately, we are all merely and magically human.

Paul Tschudi

What Is Grief?

Grief is the natural reaction to the loss of someone or something to which we have formed a strong bond or attachment. It is a universal occurrence, individually experienced and repeatedly encountered. It is an emotional, psychological, physical, and spiritual process that allows us to let go of that which was and, if we embrace it, to ready ourselves for that which is to come. Grief is part of the process of becoming more fully human. Everyone that we know has or will be touched by it.

This definition is a collaborative effort, built word by word over the course of several years with many students from diverse backgrounds. These students have been participants in several courses that I have taught on end-of-life issues, including grief and bereavement. Many lessons have been learned from these students, and it has been my honor and blessing to have had the opportunity to learn with them. For you see, no one is an expert on the subjects of grief and bereavement. The expertise lies in the experience. This aspect of human experience has been a part of our lives from the beginning of humanity. We can imagine the fear and wonderment of a tribe of ancient people who experience the death of one of their clansmen. Seeing the physical body but not understanding where the essence of the person went. A lifeless body lies before them, not breathing, not eating, not communicating. Somehow the body begins to disappear, and yet in the clansmen's dreams or memories, the person "visits" or is remembered. The deceased is "seen" or "heard" and appears in those dreams; in their childlike understanding of the world, their beloved clansman lives on somehow. The conclusion—there must be a place where people go after they die or that a part of the deceased lives on. Tears are shed, we feel sad and abandoned, someone else is forced to take up the roles of the deceased clansman, and life goes on. They are gone from our sight but are still present.

I venture to guess that we have not advanced that much since those ancient times in our understanding of loss. It is difficult to describe or feel it until it happens to us. Grief and loss are very personal experiences. There is a distinct difference among the students in my classes on end-of-life care, between those who have endured a significant loss and those who have not. So often, students will say, "I cannot imagine what it must be like to lose one of my parents," or "I couldn't continue to live if either of my parents died." But there are also those in the class who have experienced a significant loss who can tell them that "it is more difficult than you could ever imagine but you do survive." We can be there to listen, offer support, and feel a certain sense of pity or empathy for someone experiencing the loss of a loved one, but we cannot know it until it happens to us. And it does happen to each and every one of us. Once it does, we become a member of a club that we never wanted to belong to.

It is a part of life, and everyone will be or has been forced to confront the grieving process. It is a painful process—many people have described it as a ripping open of their very being, an indescribable wounding, an assault on the soul, a theft of their assumptive world, or their "own personal Armageddon."

Grief affects the way that we view life and live our lives. It is an event that is imposed upon us; it cannot be avoided and will be a recurring theme throughout our lives. Our grief is not limited to the death of a loved one but can also be experienced when we move away from home and/or a familiar place, our youth, our health, or graduate from college, leave a job, lose a pet, lose our sense of innocence or our assumptive life. But grief is not, in and of itself, a terminal condition. If it were, we would not exist, for anyone who had lived before and had experienced the loss of a loved one would have perished from the pain, but we are here. We do not die when a loved one dies. It may feel like a part of us dies, and perhaps on some level this is true, but we do continue to live, perhaps with a different worldview, perhaps with a psychic scar that will always be a reminder of a relationship that we once had. But we learn to experience our grief, live with our pain, and transform it, hopefully, into a life lesson, changing it from a wall to a door. Even though the event of grief is out of our control, the effects and direction of our grief are not. However, we need to understand this event as best we can and see the universality of it—over time, across cultures, geography, developmental stages, gender, and spiritual beliefs. We cannot know what a grieving person is feeling at any given moment. All of his or her feelings are valid for that moment—fear, anger, hostility, sadness, despair, loneliness, and even relief. It is not up to us to judge how another person is coping with his or her pain. We grieve not only for the person who has died but, to a large extent, we grieve for ourselves after the loss of someone we love. We grieve for ourselves as people who have been left behind and who must now pick up the pieces of our lives, face the pain of loss, and rebuild our future. Grief is hard work. Sometimes it may feel as though the person who has died is the lucky one: They are now free of pain, but ours has just begun.

We are, each of us, companions on the journey through life. We can provide a safe place for others to mourn, help them explore their feelings, and simply be there. Our mere and magical presence is perhaps one of the most valuable gifts that we have to offer one another.

The way we cope with and process all of these feelings is to talk about them, bring them into the light, examine them in all their rawness, and then feel them. This helps us process and absorb the reality of the loss and helps us turn from a state of victimhood of the loss into transcenders of the loss. We eventually feel somewhat more empowered and thereby better equipped to help others through their own losses—it seems to be a part of some spiritual plan—a gift that we as human beings are blessed to have. And though each loss provides us with a new lesson or experience, it does not necessarily buffer us from experiencing the same level of pain the next time. We do come away, though, with the knowledge that we have survived before and, therefore, can again—that we are resilient.

I would guess that the majority of people who have chosen to read this book are caregivers of some sort or transcenders of grief. Whether you are teachers, counselors, psychologists, medical professionals, people of the cloth, and/or parents—you are caregivers. And most of you make your choice of profession because you are caregivers not by training but by nature. This is the blessing that you have to offer to students, clients, patients, congregants, and the world; it is what makes you good at what you do—but it can also be your curse. My guess is that you are better at caring for others than you are at caring for yourselves. You're comfortable in the role of caregiver but may have problems accepting care. I would also guess that you have come to work with end-of-life care issues because you have suffered the loss of someone significant and have survived and opened another door.

How Grief Works

Theorists have attempted to describe the process of grief by using many different approaches. Some theorists describe grief in terms of a series of tasks, while others describe a set of stages, a process, or characteristics. Two of the most respected theorists on grief are J. William Worden and Kenneth J. Doka. Dr. Worden, through his

20-plus years of research and clinical work, developed the concept of grief as a series of tasks that the bereaved must accomplish before grieving can be completed. Grieving then is seen as a process, one that offers the bereft a framework within which he or she can work through the pain of the loss. In Worden's book *Grief Counseling and Grief Therapy*, he outlines the Tasks of Mourning[1] approach, which empowers the bereft to have some control and understanding of the myriad of feelings that he or she is are experiencing and to allow the person to do his or her "grief work." The following is a summary of Worden's Tasks of Mourning.

- Task I: To accept the reality of the loss. This first task of grieving is to come full face to the reality that the person is dead, that the person is gone and will not return. It is a time of shock and disbelief. It is as though the human psyche cannot process the depth of feelings and/or pain all at once that the loss of a loved one brings—just as the physical body cannot process severe pain all at once. But human beings have been given a gift, a built-in mechanism that causes us to experience shock and numbness in order to dull the pain, and acts as a transformer that reveals the pain to us in smaller doses. We exist outside our understanding. This is a wall—when we hit it, we are stunned. Part of the acceptance is the realization that the person is not coming back and that reunion is impossible, at least in this life. This is a time of yearning and searching for the missing love attachment. Accepting this reality takes time, since it involves not only an intellectual acceptance but also an emotional one.

- Task II: To work through the pain of grief. The second task of mourning involves facing the pain of the loss and working through it. This involves not only expressing the emotional pain but the physical, spiritual, emotional, and behavioral pain as well. Once the initial shock has begun to diminish, we come face to face with these powerful and painful feelings. These emotions need expression. We need to bring them out into the light, look at them in all their rawness, feel and express them before we can move on. The depth and breadth of these emotions is a tribute to our pain and to the relationship that we have lost. We become fully and painfully engaged with our broken hearts. We feel trapped behind the wall—a thick, high wall that is covered with our emotional graffiti—a wall that feels impossible to break down, climb over, or go around. But we can. For most of us, these feelings commonly involve sadness, depression, abandonment, emptiness, fear, and confusion; but there may also be emotions that seem confusing, such as anger, guilt, and even relief.

- Task III: To adjust to an environment in which the deceased is missing. This task involves learning to live life without the deceased; acquiring new roles formerly performed by the deceased, and learning to adjust to a new sense of self and how we fit into a changed world. This can be described as a period of rehabilitation—relearning to simply be in the world—we begin to learn to live life one day at a time, we have moments of feeling better and moments of terror; slipping back and retrying. We may smile at a pleasant moment and find ourselves tearing up the next. We may feel guilt because of our moments of joy. Will this mean that we will forget our loved one? But we continue to heal and to reconnect with our daily living routines, to adapt new ones, and to realize that our own life is now one that is permanently altered by our loss. But we can choose to go on, to adapt, and reclaim some control. We become engaged with life again, though tentatively. We catch glimpses of a door ahead of us.

- Task IV: To emotionally relocate the deceased and move on with life. This task can be described as learning to live fully again and form new attachments—we begin to work our way out of that which was and into that which will be. We are different; we are becoming someone new. Our level of fear has subsided, and we may choose to form new attachments, to love again, and to relocate our deceased loved one from a person who was with us on the physical plane into one who exists within us. We no longer fear forgetting our loved one but realize that he or she is now a part of our very essence. We can love again while not forgetting. The door swings open if we gently push.

Kenneth J. Doka, an ordained Lutheran minister, is currently a professor of gerontology and thanatology at the graduate school of The College of New Rochelle and Senior Consultant to The Hospice Foundation of America. In his chapter, "The Spiritual Crisis of Bereavement," from the book *Death and Spirituality*, Doka states that as counselors who work with grieving clients, we may find some value in exploring religious and spiritual themes. In a time of significant loss or in times of emotional or physical trauma, our assumptive life, or "spiritual comfort zone," is destroyed or challenged. The world no longer feels like a safe, familiar, inviting, and engaging place. "So one may also speak of a fifth task on grief,"[2] which is summarized below:

- Task V: Rebuilding faith and philosophical systems that are challenged by loss. As Doka states, "the bereaved persons may simultaneously struggle with two losses—the loss of the deceased and the loss of their own beliefs."[3] And we realize that we can and should be engaged in it. But, what about our faith? Where was God through all this? In order to explore the unknown, or matters of faith, we need to feel grounded and somewhat safe. This is a time of questioning the meaning of life and the world that we had come to accept. We have done the work, earned the badge, and now it is time for us to rebuild our faith in something outside of and perhaps bigger than ourselves. We go through the door only to find an infinite number of other doors ahead of us. We may reject or hold more tightly to our past theological and spiritual beliefs. This is a time when ritual may be of value.

Grief presents us with both a wall and a door. It is neither entirely one nor the other, but a process where we encounter both.

So, do grief and the pain of loss mean that life is over? Do we roll over and whither away? Would this be what our loved one would have wanted for us? Are we victims of grief or transformers?

In my work and in my life, I have observed and experienced that those who suffer a loss require several gifts for healing to take place:

- We need validation of our feelings.
- We need to have companions and support when we want it.
- We need to feel safe.
- We need hope (faith).
- We need time and we need rituals.

Rituals

What part do rituals play in our healing from the loss of a loved one? The obvious answer is that rituals do exist around death and grief, as in the case of the funeral service and/or memorial services. These are the major and familiar rituals around grief and loss. In many cases, especially in most Western societies, these two events or rituals are the symbolic gestures that we offer the bereft to deal with their pain and to offer support. But in Western societies, we have very little patience for things that involve a process over time. We want quick fixes for most things in life, and we tend to want to experience only one emotion—happiness. Pain is to be avoided at all costs. But where does that leave the bereft? This is where rituals can be helpful.

Rituals are social and private inventions that offer us a symbolic means of addressing life's questions. They offer us the opportunity to create concrete acts that give us answers and connections when words simply don't say enough. They create a place where the living and the dead can meet, where the forgotten are remembered, where the past and present are bound together, where our hearts, spirits, and minds can blend, and where laughter and tears feel safe and wonder is honored. They both inform and transform us. Rituals help us make sense of and comprehend our existence in a meaningful way and can be shared or solitary. They awaken us to the realms of spirituality buried within each of us and remind us of our godness. When our godness emerges, we don't stand out more—we fit in more. So, how can rituals get us through trying times and celebrate our aliveness? They provide us with doors.

Interestingly, throughout the world, rituals seem to contain a common set of tools to assist the participants in feeling attached to each other and to the presence that is being honored. The following is a listing of some of these tools:

> *Flowers*—Flowers have become a basic element in many rituals, especially rituals around death, because, although they are dead, they are still beautiful.
>
> *Prayers, Testimonials, and Readings*—These become an opportunity to personalize the relationship with the lost love and to pay tribute in a public way. They are usually familiar and comforting and may be chosen because the words or music resonate with the life of the person who is gone from us.
>
> *Music*—Music has been described as the sound of the heavens and reflects the rhythm of life and joy. Music has the ability to take us out of ourselves and to experience the divine.
>
> *Candles*—Candles create light, warmth, and a sense of hope. Fire is the gift—the element—that human beings have used since the beginning of time to bring people together to provide warmth, protection, sustenance, and wonder. It is also believed that candles light the path for the deceased to enter the afterlife.
>
> *Tokens and Mementos*—Tokens and mementos create a feeling of giving, on the one hand, and receiving, on the other. Mementos are a sacred remembrance of a shared and meaningful experience and can, in some manner, represent the lost love.
>
> *Quiet and Solitude*—Quiet and solitude give us time for reflection, peace, and appreciation of the human spirit. I am a firm believer in the courage and strength of the human spirit. We have come this far; there is no reason to believe that we will not continue, though changed, evolved, or transformed.

I have had the good fortune, or blessing, if you will, to travel around the world, spending a month or more in countries where religious beliefs were different from the ones that I inherited from my Protestant family—Hinduism, Buddhism, Islam, Judaism, and Animism. I want to insert here that I have also met some who claim to not believe in any sort of divine presence or afterlife, but in my experience this nonbelief is situational; just as there are no atheists in foxholes, I have not found any atheists in the waiting rooms of surgical suites, either. When we fear loss, we turn to a force bigger than ourselves. However, I approached each of these religions or belief systems with as much openness as I could muster, and I found several common themes:

- We live our lives the best we can.
- We connect with other people.
- We have a belief in a higher being or force.
- We often feel powerless.
- We all are confronted with life's mysteries.
- We suffer.
- We die.
- But . . . we also hope and dream, and we encounter walls and doors.

My Story

I want to share with you a story about mystery, the utility of spirituality and rituals, and my own experience with walls and doors. This is a true story and is one that recently happened to me.

In 2001, I was invited to be the speaker for an all-day workshop on "Spirituality and Health" for a group of healthcare professionals at a local university, as part of their continuing education series. I immediately agreed to accept the invitation, but then terror set in. I questioned my wisdom of agreeing to be the only speaker at an 8-hour workshop with over 100 professionals in attendance. All of the familiar old scripts that I have lived with all my life began to scream in my ears: "What if I bomb?"; "What if I have nothing to say?"; "What if I am simply not the right person for this?"; "There must be much better qualified people to do this."; "I'll be busted for being a fraud."; "How can anyone speak for 8 hours?"

I tried meditating, going for walks, cramming material in my head, and finally trying to distract myself with idiotic TV shows. I was stuck and needed something to happen to inspire me or at least push me into action. I began the futile process of pounding out an outline on my computer, only to discover that my printer had run out of paper and it was 3 AM. The spirits seemed to be working against me. Then I remembered that there was an old printer in the attic and that there might be some paper still in it. As I rummaged around, I came across a journal page that I had written sometime after my mother's death. I sat on the floor of the attic and read. Tears welled up in my eyes—I had found my inspiration. My mother had been dead for 11 years, but she was still able to get me out of a jam, as she always had. Reading the long-lost journal became a ritual for me. I would like to share that journal entry with you now.

I have always had a deep sense of spiritual energy. It filled my life with wonder and awe. But it was also my escape, and it helped me to survive living with an alcoholic and abusive father. It was my hope when I served as a medic in Vietnam; it was my strength through failed relationships, scholastic and professional challenges, and days of self-doubt and fear. Looking back, these were easy times. I have always been a fairly happy person and have been accused over the course of my life of always viewing the world through rose-colored glasses (I could never understand a preference for any other color).

My spiritual energy got me this far, and I began to have a suspicion that I was somehow immune to the negative forces out there in the world. My life had by no means been easy, but I was always able to call upon my spiritual energy to cradle me; to protect and inspire me. I was wrong to take it for granted.

I was not prepared for the devastating effect that the death of my mother would have on my life or my spirit. Rather than having the building blocks of my life occasionally disturbed, this time it was my very foundation. She had been my protector, my champion, and my living history. In January 1992 I was sitting in my office at the university when I got the call that changed my life. The aged and tearful voice of my aunt was informing me of a truth that I never wanted or believed I would hear. My mother had suffered a massive stroke and was in intensive care in Ohio. I imploded into my very core, into a speck of myself. Overcome with numbness, I somehow managed, with the help of close friends, to make the necessary arrangements for a flight to Dayton.

There I would find my mother lying peacefully in crisp white sheets with an endless web of tubes and needles piercing her soft skin. The sound of the ventilator forcing air in and out of her lifeless body caused an angry response in me. I knew that she did not want these barriers inhibiting her passage. I also knew that it would be up to me to have the machines turned off. She had given me entry into this world, now I would give her entry into the next. I sobbed unashamedly at her bedside, holding her warm but unresponsive hand in mine and whispering the secrets of my love into her ear. It was the most alone and frightened that I had ever felt in my life. I was steeped in nothingness and numbness. I wanted to hear a last word from her, a moment of clarity, but there was none. This time my spiritual energy didn't spare me. My rose-colored glasses had been brutally knocked off, and the searing reality of my mere humanness blinded me.

The days immediately following her death are now a vague blur—the funeral and cremation, the lawyers, packing up her home. A week, maybe only a day or two later, I was sitting on the floor of my mother's house alone—the house of my own childhood, emptied of everything that made it a home. A group of my childhood friends had spent the afternoon with me and had given me some comfort. Now I sat alone with my pain. I built a roaring fire in the fireplace, which flooded my mind with memories of family times. On the floor before me were strewn the photographs of my mother's life; black-and-white photos with yellowing, zigzagged edges depicting her life before my arrival. Under other circumstances, I would have found them curious and charming. Her life, her private moments, her friendships were there for me to see. It felt intrusive. These were the records of a life that had touched many people. She had been a nurse, a sister, a daughter, a wife, and a friend. Now she was gone, yet these records were left. They had meaning only to her. I carefully went through each one, gazing into it, pondering, imagining. Something came over me that caused me to begin tossing them one by one into the flames, then watching the smoke, the memories, rise in lacy swirls up the chimney. These were her memories, not mine. I didn't want anyone else to see them or to carelessly sentence them to lie unnoticed in a box at the back of my closet. No, she should have them. Hours passed, tears flowed, the smoke of the last photo was sent skyward, and sleep finally overtook me. I was awakened from my exhaustion by the harsh ring of the phone. I picked up the receiver thinking it was one of my friends calling to comfort me but I heard the unmistakable sound of my mother's voice saying, "Thank you for sending me the photographs, your Dad and I are enjoying them. We want you to know that we are happy to be together again and we are fine. Please take care of yourself."

You may interpret this call in any way that your own understanding of the world allows you to. I prefer to think that it truly was my mother. Her spirit was telling me that everything would be OK.

Four years have passed since my mother's death. My life has continued to offer me good times and good people. The road has been rocky at times, and seemingly impassable, but with each step, I am closer to becoming more fully human.

Opportunities have presented themselves to me that I never dreamed would happen—completion of advanced degrees, wonderful relationships, world travel, and the directorship of the St. Francis Center—a not-for-profit counseling and education center for grief and loss.

Today

Today, I am a professor at a major university, director of two graduate programs in end-of-life care, a private therapist specializing in grief and loss, and now making this humble attempt at putting thoughts to paper.

Initially, it took many months to begin to recover what I knew of myself. The loss of a parent is a wrenching and unreal episode in a life. I no longer have the same level of innocence or history that I once had. The arms that cradled me, the wisdom that guided me, and the history that made me no longer exist on the physical plane. I now know that I must search for meaning in life and not simply let it find me. All of the parents of the world throughout time have lost their own parents and survived, and so must we all. Spiritual energy must constantly be nurtured and not taken for granted. My mother is gone from my senses but not from my life. She lives within me and has become a part of me, of my spirit. I no longer rely on my spirit as an immunization from pain but see it as a way to better prepare me for being fully human.

My spiritual energy slowly returned and is even stronger than before, because I have survived and have been transformed by pain. I now feel more connected to everyone who has lived before and who will live after I am gone. We are all connected, and maybe that is where our spiritual energy is born. The support of those people close to me, the tie to those who have lived before me and who have influenced my life, has enriched me. I once again enjoy wearing my rose-colored glasses, but I do find that living life can cause smudges and blurs on my lenses—but you know what? I have the power to clean them occasionally, to see the world clearly, and to find my doors.

Epilogue

These things are true. That life derives from love, that love invites loss, that loss brings grief, that grief brings growth, and that growth means life—and so the circle is complete, and grief is a part of life.

The door is open, enter life.

PART IV

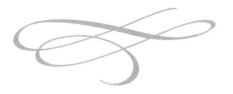

Patient Stories and Reflection

22

Transformation and Redemption through the Dark Night of the Soul

CORNELIUS BENNHOLD

I wish I could have had my cancer when I was 30. Not that my life was bad before, but it just has such a deeper and more meaningful quality to it since my cancer.

> 50-year-old woman, 5 years after she was diagnosed with
> end-stage lymphoma and given 3 months to live.

I've done all the work around my dying that I need to do. I've done all the forgiving and the healing that were needed in my life. Now it is time for the last step: the letting go of any notion that death is not okay.

> 55-year-old woman who had end-stage breast cancer,
> who passed away 3 years ago.

A couple of months ago I was asked to speak to a class of medical students about my personal experience with cancer. I began by asking them, "Assume you got up this morning and you found out that you have only 24 hours to live. Would you be sitting here in this class right now?" Of course, there were amused smiles, accompanied by answers like, "No way! This guy is crazy!"—I followed up with more questions: "Would you be here if you had, say, a week to live? Or a month? How about a year? If your answer to all those questions is no, then why are you here now? How much time would you feel you need to have, so that it would be okay for you to sit in this class today, right here, right now? What matters more to you than sitting in class today? And if it is so important, why are you not doing it, right now?"

These are some of the questions someone diagnosed with a life-threatening illness will ask: What is really important for me? What do I do with the finite amount of time I may have left? What dreams do I still want to live? How can I find out who I really am? What is my purpose here?

I used to think that the shock of being told that one has a finite amount of time left comes from having to contemplate a specific date for my death, rather than some vague time far away in the future. I now know better—the shock of being diagnosed with a life-threatening illness comes from having to actually contemplate the possibility that I may in fact die! I am convinced that, deep down, we don't really believe we are going to die. Sure, we understand it intellectually, we can think the thought, and we may say we believe it. But we don't *really* believe it at the gut level. If we would really believe it, we would live differently. Once diagnosed with a life-threatening illness, it is no longer abstract, no longer statistical, no longer someone else out there, it's real . . . it's me!

The First Round

My own journey with cancer started 11 years ago, in July 1992. My wife and I had been living in Canada and we were about to move to Washington, D.C., where I had accepted a position at The George Washington University as a professor of physics. For immigration purposes I needed to have a standard x-ray—which revealed a large, 5-inch growth in my chest. Initially, the doctors were convinced that, because of its appearance, it was a benign growth. Thoracic surgery removed the growth and the recovery went well. After 1 week we finally heard from the pathologist that it was a rare malignant tumor—synovial sarcoma—cancer! My surgeon had no trouble admitting right away that he knew very little about this kind of tumor and that he needed to do some reading and consult with experts in this field. The recommendation was to have radiation therapy as follow-up treatment. We decided to move to D.C. and begin treatment there.

There were so many questions: Why? Why me? Why now? Why this? So many questions with no answers; I was 32 years old and was just beginning my career as a university professor. I didn't need this! I didn't deserve this! I was confronted with the classic "Why do bad things happen to good people?" question. I was living a life full of expectations, with a sense of entitlement: If I work hard and play by the rules, I'm entitled to the good life! It was important for me to allow these questions to arise. Along with those questions came anger, frustration, a realization that my ideas about life were not working any more, were not valid any more. I remember talking about this with our priest, who recommended, "Allow yourself to vent this anger, but don't direct it toward yourself or your family. Direct it toward God, he can take it!" It became clear to me that my spirituality would have to be an integral part of my struggle with this challenge.

There was a key question that I had to confront myself with: What preparations had I made in my life to cope with potential challenges, to not just survive in the face of adversity but to grow and thrive with it? Rather than lamenting my predicament, how will I be able to see this test as a means for awakening, as an opportunity for growth? I had a lot of catching up to do! My starting point was books by Bernie Siegel, the cancer-surgeon-turned-holistic-medicine guru. He discusses the experiences with his patients that have lead him into the field of holistic and mind-body medicine; some patients will have exactly the same clinical condition—and therefore the same prognosis—and yet some survive and live to be cured, while others succumb to the cancer and die. He observes that many times it is their spirit, their attitude, their will to fight that appear to make the difference not only between life and death but also for the quality of life. The single most important words for me at that time was a quote from Viktor Frankl, survivor of the Nazi concentration camps, who said, "There is one last freedom that nobody can take away from us, regardless of the situation we are in, and that is the freedom to choose the way we view the situation, the freedom to choose our attitude towards the situation."[1] What does this mean? It means that I have a choice as to how I want to deal with my cancer. Do I want to give up, believe that I've received a death sentence, fold my tent and just wait for the inevitable end? Or do I want to take on the challenge, mobilize all my resources, and give it one hell of a fight? Would I let cancer run my life or would I stay in charge and incorporate cancer into my life, as a part of it—an important part, to be sure, but only a part, one part among others. This choice nothing and nobody could take away from me: no cancer, no pain, no doctor. Having a choice was empowering for me; it allowed me to take control and to assume responsibility for my life and my illness. I realized that the way I felt followed the way I thought—if I thought that there is nothing anyone can do and I am doomed, I felt deflated and depressed. If, on the other hand, I decided to think differently, to think thoughts like, "I can fight this, I can beat this!" I would feel uplifted and energized. We have all heard the line, "Life is 10% of what happens to me and 90% of how I deal with it." Using a number of tools like meditation, visualizations, and affirmations, I began changing the way I thought about my illness.

Looking back at this initial stage of dealing with my illness, today I am somewhat surprised that this process of changing my attitude toward cancer was not, in fact, harder than it turned out to be. How many times have we experienced—in our lives and in others—how hard it is to change deeply held convictions, even when it is obvious that they have outlived their usefulness? Like the same pattern of relationships that need healing or ending, but drag on and on. Like unfulfilled jobs that need to be abandoned for the dream that is yet to be realized. Like the desire to spend more time on the important things in life, yet unable to say no to new projects. How often do we find ourselves—or see others—in situations where we know some action needs to be taken, and yet we seem unable to move forward, like a deer caught in the headlights, paralyzed by some deep-seated belief that ultimately we are incapable of changing the way we think, feel, or act?

Yet, for me, the real work had barely begun. The hard lessons were yet to be learnt. I had not yet entered the Dark Night of the Soul—not yet.

One of the things I had to learn in those years was the difference between *hope* and *expectations*. We've all heard it too many times—the telling of worst-case scenarios, so that patients should not be given false hope. Let me assure you, there is no such thing as false hope! Hope is something that reflects an orientation of the soul; it comes from the heart, not from the mind. It involves a trust that needs not to be defended, needs not to be justified or argued with. Hope can never be wrong, never be false! Expectations may come with a sense of entitlement to a particular outcome, but hope allows holding the heart open to an entire range of possibilities. I use hope to focus on what is *possible*, not what is *probable*. Hope is not attached to a particular outcome; it transcends my present reality and is anchored in the faith that something has meaning regardless of how it turns out.

The Second Round

December 1995: I received a phone call from my radiation oncologist, telling me that something had shown up on my latest CAT scan. It was in the same area as before and shouldn't be there. We scheduled a small surgery in order to take a biopsy. The biopsy came back and was indeed confirmed to be a recurrence of the sarcoma. In January 1996, I had major surgery again at Georgetown Hospital. Besides the diseased area visible on the scan, there were a number of small malignant growths in the vicinity. The tumor had metastasized regionally. The surgery took 5 hours and removed a piece of chest wall, the lining of my lung (pluria), part of the diaphragm, and a few small sections of the lung.

Let me tell you a little story about my interactions with doctors at the hospital. The day after surgery I woke up in the morning with tunnel vision, seeing about ten people in white coats standing around my bed and staring at me. I was completely confused; I had no idea where I was, why I was there—even who I was! I felt extremely threatened and agitated. What had happened? During the night shift, the nurse had accidentally mixed up my pain medication; instead of the milder, prescribed drug she had given me morphine, but at the dosage of the prescribed drug that turned out to be an overdose, three times above the permitted amount. So I was on a horror trip from a drug overdose. Once they found the origin of my confusion, they took me off the morphine and pumped me full of narcane, an antidote to drug overdoses. The morning after this incident, the chief resident with the interns and medical students came by for their early morning rounds. When I realized they were all present yesterday during the incident with the overdose, I felt compelled to give them a lecture, "You jerks! You all saw me yesterday in a state of confusion, fear, and agitation. Yet none of you had the decency to reach out to me, provide some comfort, reassure me that I was safe. You all just stood there and stared at me. Your chief resident may have failed you for not modeling a compassionate physician, but all of you have failed me for not treating me with the compassion I needed as a human being!"

How did I deal with the recurrence? There were many different feelings present at the same time.

> *Disappointment:* I had made it quite far toward the infamous 5-year cancer survival mark, and now I was set back to the beginning—or even worse.
> *Failure:* I had worked so hard to make sure I would cure myself—what had I done wrong? Where had I failed? Had I not meditated long enough, visualized well enough, prayed hard enough?
> *Fear:* Has my luck finally run out? Has my time come?
> *Despair:* Oh God, please don't let me die; I don't want to die.

In March 1996, I began a chemotherapy protocol that would last about 4 months. It was the beginning of the Lenten season. My inner mental state of despair, and fear matched the season. It felt like a long, drawn-out, never-ending Good Friday. Since my spiritual tradition is Catholic, the Cross felt like a good place to linger during these weeks. This symbol of darkness and death had a comforting quality for me. When my pain was unbearable, my grief unspeakable, the Cross provided a place that could endure the emptiness and the silence without needing to hide it or fade it or fix it. Sometimes darkness is comfortable only with darkness—if the light is premature, it blinds rather than heals. If this God of mine would just be a God of the lilies in the field, he would have no credibility in this darkness. I would have abandoned him at this time in search for one that can stand in the center of the fire with me and not shrink back. Yet the God that dies on the Cross, the God that loses everything on the Cross, transcends all these simple and easy notions.

It was a time where my spirituality and my faith were stretched to their limits. In mysticism, such an experience is referred to as the "Dark Night of the Soul," a term coined by St. John of the Cross, a sixeenth-century Spanish mystic. It describes an experience that forces a reconsideration of our deepest beliefs and convictions—an experience that reveals the old mental models to be obsolete, the old ideas to be faulty; an experience that reveals what can truly sustain me from within when all else falls away. Outdated notions and concepts turn out to not work any more and must slowly burn away. It is the experience of the despairing mind, anxiously trying to maintain the illusion of control. And resistance to this process is hell. So much resentment against realizing that I must let go of this mental world that my mind has so carefully constructed all these years. An experience of such utter emptiness and loneliness, when my yearning for communion with the God I believed I could control goes unanswered and my cries seem to echo endlessly, being heard by no one but myself. This is what the Dark Night of the Soul will do; this is what it did for me. And yet, this is not *all* it does.

Hidden deep within the grief, the layers of desolation, the circles of despair, right in the center of my sorrow, there lies the potential for deeper insight into the mystery of life and death. Anguish and distress hold deep within themselves the nascent promise of a new life, radically transformed and redeemed. My own experience of the Dark Night of the Soul was a transformation that led me from the words cried out in despair from the Cross, "Father, why have you forsaken me?" to the words prayed in the Garden of Gethsemane: "Father, not my will but your will be done." The Dark Night of my soul enabled me to appreciate the difference between *giving up* and *letting go*. Giving up is accepting defeat, believing that there is nothing left for me to do, relinquishing all power and responsibility. Letting go means that even with all my healing, all my meditating, all my praying, there comes a time when I need to turn over what I have no control over. Learning to let go brings forth the gift of discernment: It allows me to distinguish that which I am responsible for—my present inner mental and emotional state—from my future physical well-being, which I cannot control. Letting go means that, while I can always promote my healing, I cannot enforce a cure. Letting go means trusting that there is a purpose to my process, even if I don't comprehend it. It means that while I may not know or understand why things happen, I trust I will be okay, no matter what.

Letting go means surrendering into the unknown with no safety net. Letting go means not just accepting that there will be no assurances, no guarantees, but it means to actually forgo the need for such assurances and guarantees. How may we ever come to such a place, you may wonder? All I know is that it cannot be comprehended by the skeptical mind but must be surrendered into with an open heart.

The Third Round

December 2001: After 5 years we had decided to change my checkup schedule from a semiannual to an annual CAT scan, since the risk of another recurrence was felt to be minimal. It had been 6 years since my initial recurrence, when in December 2001, a checkup revealed a new tumor in the vicinity of the previous growths. More surgery removed the tumor, along with a foot of chest wall, four ribs, and some parts of my lung. Since this time the tumor appeared contained, no chemotherapy was recommended.

So how did I deal with this new recurrence? Rather than disappointment and bitterness, my inner emotional response was more one of bewilderment: "I wonder what this all means. . . . I wonder what I am to do with all this." During my years of working with my cancer, I've always known that the proof lies in the pudding. Would all that I had learned hold up in the face of renewed adversity or collapse like a house of cards? Thankfully, with all the training of the previous years, the tools that I had acquired were indeed at my disposal. I managed to stay in an observer position and not get caught up in the frenzy that accompanied the weeks before surgery. It was back to the basics: What do I need to do to support my healing right now? What can I take responsibility for, and what do I need to let go of? I found myself surprisingly free from fear and more curious than anxious about my situation. The most difficult dimension for me this time around was not my own inner state—I knew how to care for myself—but the emotional welfare of our 3-year-old daughter, Catalina. Thankfully, my wife and I, along with the support of friends and family, had enough emotional resources left to face this challenge in a healthy manner.

What lessons came along with this new recurrence? To this day, not all have revealed themselves. I am still processing the emotional fallout, and much inner work remains to be done. One lesson has been with regard to time; I must admit that I was quite surprised to notice how much I had bought into the 5-year survival benchmark that cancer is usually associated with in our medical culture. Even though I was quite aware of the usual qualifiers, I had clearly assimilated the belief that after 5 years I would be home free. Now time has been released from any artificial markers; 5 years have no more meaning than 3 years or 7 years or 10 years. There was a grieving process that I had to undergo to let go of this safety marker. On the other hand, it allows me to stop wondering whether I will make the infamous 5-year mark or not—what a liberating feeling!

Another teaching came from my interactions with others who accompanied me on this journey. My being able to openly share my process and inner state in the critical weeks before and after surgery had a profound impact on family and friends around me. Some have felt moved to examine their own mortality in greater depth. This taught me that the benefits I continue to receive from my illness are not just for me to keep but are meant to be shared and passed on. This chapter you are reading right now is a consequence of this lesson. At times, people tell me how inspired they are and how much it had strengthened their faith to see me go through yet another recurrence, holding my head up high and coming out on top, beating the cancer back one more round. And yet, at times the thought coming to my mind, often left unspoken, is: "How would your faith be if I had *not* survived the last surgery? Is your faith strong enough so that you can be okay with me dying without despairing? Or will you be devastated, crushed, and lose all hope if this cancer does kill me in 6 months? How much do you need me to live for your faith to remain intact?"

It has been 18 months since my last recurrence. What will the future bring? I don't know . . . but it doesn't matter. What matters is that I am not just surviving my cancer, not just getting by in the face of adversity, but I am living a life of abundance, I am prospering, I am thriving! What matters is that I feel like I am living; my life has never been fuller, never been happier! And I am doing this not *in spite of* my cancer but *because* of my cancer. What matters is that I have been blessed beyond measure by this strange companion of mine, which has been with me for the past 11 years and will be with me for the rest of my life, may it last 5 months or 5 years or 50 years. It is my cancer that keeps me attentive, that keeps me focused, that keeps my priorities in order. It keeps reminding me that each day, each hour I have is a precious gift that I want to and can and will use wisely and deliberately, filled with intention and awareness. What matters is that I am in touch with my inner voice, which continues to lead me on this journey of exploration and transformation, one moment at a time, right here, right now.

23

Rhonda—Patient as Teacher

RHONDA OZIEL AND DENNIS OZIEL

On April 13, 1994, my sister was one of 25,000 women diagnosed with ovarian cancer each year. It was a day that would change our family's life forever. Surgery was scheduled for the next day. Not only did we have little time to learn about her illness, but we also had very few places to turn. We were all scared.

A research librarian by profession, Rhonda led the charge to find information. Our family got its strength from Rhonda as she took an active role in managing her treatment. She taught us about chemo, CT scans, CA 125 levels, and clinical trials—but most of all she taught us about hope.

Rhonda not only taught our family the importance of knowledge and advocacy, but she had the opportunity to address medical students at George Washington University Medical School as well. Because of this opportunity, given to Rhonda by Dr. Christina Puchalski, she also had the unusual opportunity to get to know many of these students. Unfortunately, shortly after her last lecture, she spent much of the next 3 months at GWU Hospital as a patient. There was a constant stream of concerned students and young doctors visiting her. Many attended her funeral on June 11, 2001. I firmly believe those students that got to hear Rhonda's lectures will become better doctors because they had the experience of knowing her.

Dennis Oziel

Rhonda Oziel

The George Washington University Medical School Presentation to the Practice of Medicine Class March 2001

This is the third year in a row that I am speaking to Dr. Puchalski's class. I am really grateful. After I gave one of my talks last year, I headed over to the Ambulatory Care building to get a dose of chemotherapy. Today, I've brought my chemotherapy along with me [shows the pump]. More about the pump later. Let me begin.

If I had asked my doctor to tell me straight out how long I'd live with ovarian cancer, and had I believed him, it's not entirely clear that I would have survived to be standing here talking to you today. I'd be dead.

The truth is, if you pay attention to the statistics, the outlook for women diagnosed with ovarian cancer is not a very pretty one. If diagnosed and treated early, when the cancer is confined to the ovary, the 5-year survival rate is about 93%.

But, due to ovarian cancer's "quiet" symptoms, only 24% of all cases are found at this early stage. Because of this, the overall 5-year survival rate for women with ovarian cancer is only between 35% and 47%, depending upon the type of tumor.

On April 13, I will celebrate 7 years of living with ovarian cancer. And thanks to my doctor, Jeffrey Lin, here at GW, my sheer will and determination, the love and support of my family, my friends, the support group at GW where I attend every week, and the other ovarian cancer survivors that I've met through the Ovarian Cancer National Alliance that I am here talking to you today.

Here's what I would like to do today.

First, I'll tell you my cancer story. Then, I'll talk about how I cope with knowing that I have a finite time on this earth. Interspersed with my personal story, I'll tell you what I've learned and how I wish that you, as doctors, would deal with your patients—how I think doctors should treat patients.

Here's my story.

About 7 years ago, just around this time, end of February, beginning of March, I put my hands on my stomach and felt some masses. Some lumps. Looking back on it, I had some of the silent symptoms—fatigue, bloating, loss of appetite. I have some information cards that tell you the symptoms of ovarian cancer that you can take away with you today [shows the cards].

I went to my gynecologist (Dr. Grossman, who was the acting Dean, right.) He did a pelvic exam. Felt masses. Arranged for me to get an ultrasound and set up an appointment with Dr. Lin. That day I think Dr. Grossman knew this was a serious situation, but he was very calm. He didn't even mention cancer.

The day I met Dr. Lin, he examined me, looked at the ultrasound again, and told me straight out that he thought there was a 90% chance that I had ovarian cancer. In the room with me were my husband and my sister-in-law.

How did Dr. Lin deliver the news? Straight. All I did was take notes and ask about the surgery and what would happen there. I did not ask any questions about the disease. It was hard enough to digest the word *cancer*.

I appreciate bluntness when it comes to things like this—giving bad news. But bad news must be tempered with hope. More on hope later.

Back to my cancer story. I had the surgery. I was diagnosed with stage IIIb ovarian cancer serous papillary cystadenocarcinoma, and Dr. Lin removed all the cancer he could see. I had cancer in both ovaries, none in my tubes or uterus. Cancer in my omentum, which I did not know I had until it was removed. And I was left with less than a centimeter of cancer on my diaphragm. There was no lymph node involvement.

Treatment was chemotherapy: six rounds taxol/cisplatin. I responded beautifully and was cancer free for almost 3 years.

How I did feel about all of this?

Scared, yes. The only thing I really knew about ovarian cancer was that Gilda Radner had died of it and that she had been very sick.

It took me about 3 months to really read anything about ovarian cancer and to read those really lousy statistics that I quoted to you. I found out that my family knew them, but no one mentioned it to me.

Seven years ago the Internet was just beginning, and I was hungry for information on my cancer. I found lots of good material from the National Cancer Institute. In the course of my research, I discovered a wonderful article on cancer and statistics written by Stephen Jay Gould. He's an evolutionary biologist who teaches at Harvard. He is the author of at least 10 popular books on evolution and science, including, among others, *The Flamingo's Smile, The Mismeasure of Man,* and *Wonderful Life.*

The essay is called the "Median Isn't the Message." Steve Dunn, creator of the CancerGuide web site, has reproduced it there. Steve says it is the wisest, most humane thing ever written about cancer and statistics. It is the antidote both to those who say that "the statistics don't matter" and to those who have the unfortunate habit of pronouncing death sentences on patients who face a difficult prognosis. Anyone who researches the medical literature will confront the statistics for their disease. Anyone who reads this will be armed with reason and with hope.

"The Median Isn't the Message": You've all studied statistics, right? So you know the definition of the word *median.* Well, in 1982 Gould was diagnosed with abdominal mesothelioma—a very rare and very serious disease. He reports how after his surgery he asked his doctors what was the best technical literature he could read about his cancer. They said there was nothing worth reading.

Gould is a scientist and intellectual. So trying to keep him away from the literature was a fruitless effort. As Gould tells it, he went to the Harvard medical library, punched in mesothelioma, and an hour later was surrounded by the literature of his cancer. It was not a pretty picture, he reports. And he knew why his doctors told him there was nothing worth reading—mesothelioma is incurable, with a median mortality of only 8 months after discovery.

Gould was stunned, but as he says, "If a little learning could ever be a dangerous thing, I had encountered a classic example. Attitude clearly matters in fighting cancer. We don't know why (from my old-style materialistic perspective, I suspect that mental states feed back upon the immune system). But match people with the same cancer for age, class, health, socioeconomic status, and, in general, those with positive attitudes, with a strong will and purpose for living, with commitment to struggle, with an active response to aiding their own treatment and not just a passive acceptance of anything doctors say, tend to live longer." I believe he's talking about me.

Gould then goes on to talk about medians and curves, which, being a scientist, he knew about. And he figured out that he could be at the tail end of the distribution. That, based on his personal characteristics—being young, with an early diagnosis, the best medical treatment, the world to live for—he would survive. He found hope in that literature.

This is probably the most important bit of patient wisdom I can impart to you today. HOPE. Each patient is a unique individual, not a number. In 1994, I was not one of 14,500 women diagnosed with ovarian cancer. And, believe me, the statistics for ovarian cancer in 1994 were grimmer than they are today. I tell every doctor that I meet that I am a statistic of one.

Treat each person that you see as a person, not as a disease. Don't think ovarian cancer. Yes, she's gonna die. Yeah, she may die. But she needs hope. And hope is a lot of things. It's being at the tail end of that distribution. Hope is reading those grim statistics and deciding that you have a 50-50 chance of surviving and that you are going to be at the tail end of those distributions.

Give your patients HOPE. Tell your patients the grim numbers if they want to know, but assure them that you will be there with them every step of the way, fighting with them. Be honest and supportive.

One of the reasons I think I have survived is the love and support I have around me. It's a security blanket for me. I'm fortunate to have a wonderful family—parents, brothers, sisters-in-law, nieces, nephews, and wonderful friends, the angels from the support group I go to every week, and the other ovarian cancer advocates that I've met.

So, maybe not everyone has such a supportive environment as I do. But I think you as physicians can provide some of that support for your patients.

Give your patients as much information as they need. Encourage them to ask questions. You can listen to your patients. Let your patients talk to you. Sometimes all a person needs is to talk to someone. Respond to your patients. Let them know you are fighting with them. And know when to stop talking. Know when your patient needs to be left alone.

A patient has to go through a lot in fighting cancer. Chemotherapy, scans, radiation, getting a port, blood draws, hair loss. These are new experiences for your patient. Tell patients what to expect. Patients are afraid of these things. Fear is paralyzing. You can help your patients learn about what will happen to them when they have chemotherapy. What it will feel like.

If your patient is going to have chemo, arrange for him or her to go to the cancer center, the hospital, or wherever they will be receiving treatment before the first day of treatment, so that he or she can see the place and meet everyone beforehand. Your patient will be scared enough that first day, and being familiar with the surroundings will lessen that fear.

If your patient has never had a CT scan or radiation, arrange for him or her to go to the place where they will get the scan or have the radiation before appointment day. Again, familiarity lessens the fear.

Encourage patients to go to a support group. Tell them it could help them survive their disease. If they do not feel comfortable in groups, perhaps you can give them the name of another patient who has gone through the same thing as they are going through.

Also, I think an information packet containing information on cancer, chemotherapy, radiation, and side effects of treatment would be helpful. If your patient does not feel comfortable reading the information right away, maybe they will read it at a later time. Or a family member might read the information.

Let me talk about the rest of my cancer story. All was well for almost 3 years since my diagnosis. And then in 1997 my cancer recurred.

We found some small tumors on my spleen. Dr. Lin advised more chemotherapy. I was still trying to absorb the fact that the cancer had come back, and I wanted to be sure of what to do. After doing some research in the library on my own, talking to other gynoncologists, and talking with a surgeon about whether or not to remove my spleen, I decided that we should do chemotherapy. Sometimes you have to let your patients decide and come to their own conclusions.

How did I cope? How did I not get depressed? I never really thought I would die. And the reason for that is the love and support I get from family, friends, and my support group, and all of the people I've met through the Ovarian Cancer National Alliance.

The Alliance is a national organization whose mission is to raise awareness about ovarian cancer. We, in the Alliance, believe that by educating physicians and women about the symptoms of ovarian cancer, we can save lives. We also believe that more research is needed to develop a tool for early detection of this horrible disease. We want a pap smear or mammogram-type test for ovarian cancer. I am energized by this work.

How else do I cope? Well, I'm Jewish, and every year on Rosh Hashanah, the New Year, I renew my name in the Book of Life. I pray that God will inscribe my name there. The first year I had cancer was very difficult for me. I was still in treatment and I stood in the synagogue and cried because I believed God had forsaken me. That God, the year before, had not inscribed my name in the Book of Life. I was truly frightened. But I survived treatment and pray every year that my name will be inscribed in the Book of Life. I believe in the power of prayer, but I'm not an active observer of my faith. My father and mother are religious and they pray for me every Saturday. There are candles being lit for me in churches, too. Every morning when I go out and walk my dog, Fred, I look up at the sky and thank God to be alive.

I've also attended spiritual support groups sponsored by the Washington Jewish Healing Network. In fact, I'll be going to group tonight. I'm convinced I've survived this disease because of all the support groups I attend and from the strength that I've found from knowing other people dealing with similar situations to mine.

Before I said that I never really thought I would die. But that doesn't mean I didn't think about it or worry about it. Whenever I would get bad news, like my CA125 tumor marker was rising and that I would need more chemotherapy, or when I found out that I would have to have a second cancer surgery, a chill would come over me. It was the deepest fear I had ever known. I was afraid that I would die and be all alone.

In the summer of 1999 my husband, Hillel, who was my biggest supporter in all of this, died from complications after coronary artery bypass surgery. It was devastating. I was the one who was supposed to die. Not him. A few months after Hillel died, my CA125 tumor marker number rose again and I had to have a CT scan. It turned out OK. But, you know, I didn't get that chill I spoke of before. Yes, I was afraid, but not like I had been before Hillel died. Now, after Hillel's death, I am not that afraid of dying. Because I know that when I die I won't be alone, I'll be with Hillel again, and that makes me content. Not that I want to die. There are still too many things to do.

Back to my cancer story: In April 1998, 5 months after completing chemo for the recurrence on my spleen, we found a tumor on the colon wall. Dr. Lin removed it, along with 6 inches of my colon. My whole family was there the day of surgery. I am lucky and grateful to have this support net. Plus my support-group friends and my colleagues in the Ovarian Cancer National Alliance were all pulling for me.

Before the surgery and afterward I was terrified, and yet I kept going. Dr. Lin was great. We agreed we would just keep trying until we got it right. No more cancer. And we're still trying. I had another recurrence on my spleen in July of 1998 and had 20 weeks of low dose carboplatin and taxol. And then at the end of May of 1999, we found something on my liver. So it was back into treatment. I had 26 weekly treatments of herceptin and taxol. I took a chemo break until last July when we discovered more tumors on my spleen and liver. We decided to remove the spleen and get rid of the tumors on my liver. All the cancer was removed, and I spent a week in the hospital surrounded by family and friends. It was a hard recovery, but I made it.

Then last December we discovered more tumors on the vaginal cuff. Back into the hospital for another surgery. This time Dr. Lin removed the tumor on the vagina but discovered that there were small seedings of ovarian cancer cells all over my peritoneum. This was the first time he could not remove all of the cancer. We started new chemotherapy. It didn't work. I wound up being hospitalized with low blood counts and then again with high fever spikes. A CT scan showed that tumors were blocking the ureters in one of my kidneys and that I had more cancer in my abdomen. Plus my stomach was bloated, which indicated that I had ascites—fluid filled with small seedings of the cancer.

In the course of almost 7 years, this was the worse news I had ever heard. Last week I started a new course of chemotherapy. A continuous infusion of chemo. Hence the pump. Or, as I call it, my new friend, Claude.

I've had a hard time adjusting to the fact that I really will die from this disease. But I'm still coping. I've made a list of dreams I'd like to live out before I die—taking trips with my family, speaking before you today. I'm preparing a power of attorney and a healthcare power of attorney in case I can't make my own decisions. These are things I haven't done in 7 years of dealing with this disease. And I'm going to a Jewish spiritual support group to gain some strength in dealing with what is happening to me. Maybe I'm getting close to the end of that distribution. But maybe I'm not. I'll be fighting every step of the way.

I am an almost 7-year survivor of ovarian cancer. Cancer is part of who I am. I am a person with ovarian cancer.

Remember that all of your patients are people. Treat them as the unique individuals they are. You will feel better and so will your patients.

Thank you very much.

24

Hope for the Future

CHRISTINA M. PUCHALSKI

*Rhonda Oziel and many of my patients who have taught in my
courses in medical school who have allowed my students into their
lives or who have allowed me to walk the final journey with them
all share something in common, beyond their illness and life struggles—these people want to make a difference, they want to know
that their stories will be heard and will somehow impact future generations of doctors. My patients want to have the hope that their
struggles and their lessons learned will improve the care of patients
in the future, so that all patients will be cared for in a compassionate system of healthcare. When Rhonda shared with me her dream
list of things she wanted to do in the final months she had left, one
of her items was teaching my course on end-of-life care. I felt that
given her frailty this might not be wise or even practical, but I supported Rhonda in her dream, because for her that item was one of
the most important on her list. With cane in hand, Rhonda showed
up for class. In spite of her frailty, Rhonda radiated as she talked to
the students, sharing and inspiring them with her story. She told me
this was one of the most meaningful things she had done, particularly knowing this would be her last class. It made her feel that her
hopes for the future had the chance of being heard and realized
through others. It made me even more aware of how important it is
for us to listen, learn, envision, and work toward a future of compassionate healthcare.*

Christina M. Puchalski

As research and development continue to expand our scientific horizons, science
holds the promise of longer life—but it also raises the question of whether this
longer life is indeed a better life. We cannot live indefinitely. But whatever time we
have can challenge us to live to the fullest, living every moment as if it were the last.

Sunrises become more radiant, flowers more fragrant, music more rhapsodic, love more passionate, and friendships more intimate if we live and appreciate the present moment rather than long for the future.

The joy of living, based on a foundation of love toward others and toward life, is immeasurable. The experiences I have as I serve others is awe inspiring. My patients have enlightened my life. The relationships that I form with my patients have enriched my life, and I hope that the lives of my patients are enriched as we work together toward healing. While I respect what science has to offer, as I grow in my clinical practice, I see that it is often the immeasurable, the mystery, or the spiritual that impacts people's lives more than the results of technological prowess. The challenge for me is to integrate science and spirituality for the good of the patient.

My patients have impacted my spiritual life immensely. The experience of being with another in the midst of suffering and woundedness opens me up to my own suffering and woundedness, as well as to questions about the very nature of what life is, who God is, and who I am in the midst of life, God, and others. St. Edith Stein wrote that "service is the effect of love and because love varies from person to person, so does the entire spiritual life."[1] My patients affect my spiritual life; my work is my spiritual practice.

As I work with my patients in a healthcare system that is increasingly becoming devoid of compassion and mercy, I find myself becoming more committed to changing the system on a larger scale. We can no longer sit by complacently as forces within society that tend away from value-centered organizations drive our healthcare system into destruction.

While technology is not a threat to be avoided, we must look at the outcomes and implications of research and scientific technology with honesty and a responsibility for the future. Are we creating technology that will bankrupt healthcare resources? Is it fair to create a future where basic healthcare is not affordable by all? Do we want to be putting our patients and loved ones through dehumanizing tests and procedures without affording them the time to be heard, to be cared for?

What is healthcare? Is it the provision of expensive technological tests and procedures, focused on cure and longevity only? Is it the success evidenced by larger, computer-sophisticated hospital systems, where the goal is financial success and technological prowess? Or is success measured by the caring that each person receives, the compassion that forms the core value of the system, and the partnerships that are formed between the patient, the patient's family, and the healthcare providers?

Spirituality is at the core of who we are as human beings. It is that part of us that helps us find meaning, especially in the midst of confusion and suffering. It is the connections we form with each other in a profound sense of community that helps all of us survive in an often isolating and dehumanizing world.

Technology does offer hope of a cure, and that is one of the strengths of research. But of what use is a cure when the attendant suffering and pain a person experiences to attain that cure is ignored, when families who cannot afford the cost of tests flounder in inequality—and when that cure is no longer possible, people become part of the "nothing more I can do" circle? Is that the type of healthcare system we want to foster and to pass on to the next generation?

We need systems of care that focus on caring as well as curing, that foster healing and creativity, that respect all people regardless of socioeconomic status, education, or stage of illness. The oft-quoted "there is nothing more I can do" response to "therapy is no longer helping" can instead be exchanged with "here are the issues we can work on together; let me walk this journey with you." At the center of all of our beings is the core of who we are—that core can be loving and giving to others. If we each make compassion and service to others the core values of our lives, then, in time, systems of care can develop that have compassion and service as their core mission. It is then that I believe there will be a time for listening and caring and a time for healing.

How can these changes occur? I don't have all the answers, but I do know that there are thousands, if not millions, of people who want the healthcare system to change, who want their spiritual values and beliefs respected, who want physicians and other healthcare providers who are caring and compassionate as well as skilled, and who want value-centered hospitals and clinics. Colleagues of mine around the country are committed to change; they, like me, feel powerless within a huge and overwhelming system. Let's turn our frustration into action by implementing a change in our own personal spiritual lives, in our interactions with other colleagues in our place of work, and with our patients. Are there changes we can make in the microcosm of our own universe? I believe that the small changes will ripple into larger ones.

Reach out to like-minded colleagues, and together we can foster a better, more caring healthcare system. Start discussion groups at your workplace, where you and your colleagues can talk about your calling and sense of mission and purpose. Think about ways to best express and nurture that sense of mission at your work. Have discussion groups around themes such as professional calling, forgiveness, service, and compassion. Learn what your colleagues are doing to handle stress, and how stress can be better handled. Form communities of caring colleagues who can together make changes to improve the work environment. Take the time to listen to your patients and your colleagues. Remember to slow down and reflect on why you are in the profession you are in and how you can make your workplace more meaningful to yourself, as well as to your colleagues and patients. Create rituals, such as memorial services for patients who died or books by patients' bedsides, where staff can write memorials for the families to keep. Perhaps a ritual honoring the work you and your colleagues do on a daily basis will help foster respect and pride in the work that is done to help others. Create a community at your workplace, changing it from just a place where work gets done.

Our patients teach us invaluable lessons. Clearly, illness has helped many experience life at a level that many of us do not attain until we are challenged by profound loss and pain. There is immense value and importance in the journeys our patients take as they navigate the rough waters of serious illness and dying. Our healthcare systems must support these journeys as much, if not more, than the treadmills of endless tests and procedures.

In this book we share our experiences and the ways we find to help meet the needs of our patients and their families and ways to help the chronically ill and dying deal with their experience in meaningful ways. We also suggest ways that caregivers might care for themselves, both in the process of caring for another and also after a loved one dies. And finally, we offer ways that we can all, in communion with each other, work together for a more compassionate and caring healthcare system.

For those of you who are caregivers, both professional and personal, we hope this will help you as you care for your patients and loved ones. And for those of you who are seriously ill, chronically ill, and/or dying, we hope that the lessons each of us have learned through our work with our patients and their families will help you on your journey. Through our patients' stories and our own, we have learned to hold sacred the most difficult moments of life—those moments for which there are no answers, no fixes, and no reasons, those moments when life seems unbearable at times and awesome at others, those moments when our struggles for answers only result in more questions: Why me? Why now? Why this? Why?

Life holds many moments of uncertainty and pain for all of us. Serious illness and loss can cause us to question the very essence of who we are and why we are alive. These experiences can make us face the fact that we are mortal beings who will die one day. It forces us to reflect and question our deepest values, beliefs, and relationships. In the midst of these questions, the uncertainty can cause deep suffering and a sense of emptiness and aloneness. While there is profound struggle in the midst of this darkness, the grace to be able to be present to that pain and to be able to accept uncertainty and confusion can help us transcend the suffering. Letting go of the need for answers and for quick fixes can help us accept our situation and open us to the possibility of finding joy and peace in the midst of seeming despair. By looking at illness or loss as a gift, one may be able to discover new meaning and new identities that enrich one's life more than was ever imaginable. These blessings, as many of my patients call their illnesses and their struggles, are the magical threads that weave our lives into wholeness.

All of us—whether patients, healthcare providers, family, or friends—are on a journey. The journey of living and dying is one we face, perhaps, in solitude, but it is not one we need to walk alone. Look for the spiritual companions in your life, in your work, in your churches, temples, or mosques, in your families and in your social communities. Healing comes out of the mysterious moments of deep connection to another person or God—the Divine in each of us. In the end, as my patients, colleagues, families, and friends faced their dying, what mattered most was their relationships with their loved ones, with God/Divine and with themselves. Perhaps that is the ultimate lesson we learn in the face of death and dying—love and service to others as the foundation of our lives. By loving and serving others and ourselves, there is the possibility and hope for change, for making a difference, and for healing.

A

Resources

NINA A. FRY

Books

The Art of Dying: The Only Book for Persons Facing Their Own Death
Patricia Weenolsen

Weenolsen is a psychologist specializing in counseling the terminally ill. Her book touches on a variety of end-of-life concerns, from the practical to the spiritual, to help the dying make the most of the remainder of their lives and find meaning in death. Coming to terms with the disease itself, managing pain, planning funerals, making peace with loved ones, deciding about terminal care, and learning what the final experience of death is like are considered in a matter-of-fact way, with a reassuring yet sensitive approach to difficult subjects.

Encyclopedia of Native American Healing
William S. Lyon

This monumental volume explores, explains, and honors the healing practices of Native Americans throughout North America, from the southwestern United States to the Arctic Circle. Designed for ease of use with maps, a detailed subject index, an extensive bibliography, and cross-references, this book is sure to fascinate anyone interested in Native American culture and heritage.

The Grace in Dying
Kathleen Dowling Singh

Dowling Singh walks readers through the final stages of death with complete honesty, yet manages to quell the ultimate fear of dying. Speaking of the "Nearing Death Experience," Singh has discovered a sequence of phases or qualities that signals when a dying person is entering the final stages of spiritual and psychological transformation. She identifies them as relaxation, withdrawal, radiance, interiority (a time of going inward), silence, sacred, transcendence, knowing, intensity, and perfection—all of which she explains in great detail.

Grace In Practice: A Clinical Application Guide from Wisdom of the World

This manual helps clinicians and caregivers integrate Graceful Passages into the daily challenges and opportunities presented in a hospital, hospice, nursing facility, counseling office, or homecare setting.

Available at http://www.wisdomoftheworld.com/products/graceful.html

Jewish Pastoral Care: A Practical Handbook from Traditional and Contemporary Sources
Edited by Rabbi Dayle Friedman

Rabbi Friedman has enlisted compassionate, experienced pastoral caregivers who are experts in their particular areas of counseling and who effectively convey the intimate details of what they provide, teach, learn, and encounter in dealing with people in need and transition. The contributors share their own wisdom, insecurities, sorrows, and joys as they accompany those whom they counsel. The reader comes to know a lot about each of the writers—getting an inside look at how it actually feels to be confronted by unexpected, awkward situations. Regardless of the pain inherent in so many of the situations addressed (terminal illness, aging, domestic violence, abuse, addiction, and family rejection of same-sex partners), the humanity of the pastoral counselor and richness of the Jewish tradition provide hope and comfort.

Jewish Paths toward Healing and Wholeness: A Personal Guide to Dealing with Suffering
Kerry M. Olitzky

Suffering is a universal experience that each of us bears in our own particular way. Whether caused by our own illness or through the pain of those we love, we all search for ways to heal from times that try our strength. In this inspiring guide, Rabbi Kerry Olitzky combines the wisdom of Jewish tradition and insight with his own personal experience and experience dealing with the illness and pain of other people—including those he loves—to show us how healing the soul is indispensable to healing the body. Each chapter helps us on our journey to wholeness, fortifying us with insights, prayers, psalms, meditations, and rituals that can help restore and strengthen our spirit. Olitzky explores: What Judaism teaches us about healing; finding the meaning of illness in Jewish tradition; how to draw on prayers, services, psalms, and other spiritual resources for healing; and how to grow by fully embracing the process of recovery.

Native American Spirituality
Speaks Lightning

Native American Spirituality, by Speaks Lightning, offers a unique glimpse into the diverse religious/spiritual beliefs and practices that are a part of everyday life among many North American nations. From ancient traditions to present-day practices, from birth to death, amidst war and peace, from fasting to feasting, this little book offers an overview for the novice. No single volume, regardless of size, could even begin to be a comprehensive and complete listing of all Native American spiritual beliefs. This book instead says "welcome" to the newcomer and promises to whet your appetite for more.

Native American Spirituality: A Critical Reader
Edited by Lee Irwin

This volume offers a multidisciplinary set of essays by noted Native and non-Native scholars that explore the problems and prospects of understanding and writing about Native American spirituality in the twenty-first century. Considerable attention is given to the appropriateness and value of different interpretative paradigms for Native religion, including both traditional religion and Native Christianity. The book also investigates the ethics of religious representation, issues of authenticity, the commodification of spirituality, and pedagogical practices. Of special interest is the role of dialogue in expressing and understanding Native American religious beliefs and practices. A final set of essays explores the power of and reactions to Native spirituality from a long-term, historical perspective.

People of the Circle, People of the Four Directions
Scott McCarthy

People of the Circle, People of the Four Directions explores the common spiritual symbols of the native people of North and South America. Drawing on poems, stories, ceremonies, and ethnological writings, McCarthy gives examples of the use of circles, the four directions, and the number four, both individually and in combination, as themes that run through all the native cultures of the Americas. The purpose of this endeavor is to encourage a sharing and understanding between cultures as they meet.

Sacred Dying: Creating Rituals for Embracing the End of Life
Megory Anderson

As the founder of the Sacred Dying Foundation in San Francisco, Anderson provides real-life examples and strong storytelling to cover all aspects of dying, including how to help someone let go of unfinished business and how to massage a dying person to help him or her let go of his or her body. Anderson lists the tools for rituals (such as holy water, incense, and markers and paper for writing final thoughts). She even devotes an entire chapter to music—a powerful tool in healing and transcendence. Anderson offers a lovely book that covers everything you need to know to help a dying person feel deeply cared for, whether you choose to read poems aloud from the final chapters or simply sit in silence, holding the hand of a loved one.

What Dying People Want
David Kuhl

In *What Dying People Want,* David Kuhl shares his education on this topic by focusing on the daily experience of patients who are learning how to broach such discussions with their caregivers and families while coming to terms with their own mortality. Personal stories are intertwined with practical suggestions, and specific instances are frequently used to illustrate techniques, processes, and the importance of telling one's story, rather than assuming your family already knows it.

Where Souls Meet: Caring for the Seriously Ill
Dillon Woods

What can you say to someone who is seriously ill or dying? How can we express our true feelings and avoid the regret of things left unsaid, acts left undone? Dillon Woods offers a tremendous number of insights in *Where Souls Meet,* an instructional book on a taboo subject. This book is relevant for friends and family of the seriously ill, as well as professional hospice workers, doctors, clergy, and those directly facing serious illness or death.

Education

Center for Palliative Care Education

The Center for Palliative Care Education is an educational resource center and training program. Its mission is to improve palliative care for people with HIV/AIDS by increasing the knowledge, skills, and comfort level of clinicians who provide this care.

    The Center develops training modules and accompanying materials on HIV/AIDS palliative care. The materials they create, although focused on HIV, are designed to be applicable to other life-threatening illnesses.

Center for Palliative Care Education
Cabrini Medical Tower

901 Boren Avenue, Suite 1100
Seattle, WA 98104-3508
Phone: (206) 685-6838
http://depts.washington.edu/pallcare/about/index.shtml

Foundations/Organizations

American Academy of Hospice and Palliative Medicine

The American Academy of Hospice and Palliative Medicine is dedicated to the advancement of hospice/palliative medicine: its practice, research, and education. AAHPM provides physicians with educational opportunities in palliative care and in the management of terminal illness, provides hospice physicians with peer support and opportunities for an interchange of information and experiences, and fosters the development of career opportunities for physicians interested in a hospice setting.

American Academy of Hospice and Palliative Medicine
11250 Roger Bacon Drive, Suite 8
Reston, VA 20190-5202
Phone: (847) 375-4712
http://www.aahpm.org

American Society on Aging

The American Society on Aging is an association of diverse individuals bound by a common goal: to support the commitment and enhance the knowledge and skills of those who seek to improve the quality of life of older adults and their families. The membership of ASA is a multidisciplinary array of professionals who are concerned with the physical, emotional, social, economic, and spiritual aspects of aging.

American Society on Aging
833 Market Street, Suite 511
San Francisco, CA 94103
Phone: (415) 974-9600
Toll Free: (800) 537-9728
http://www.asaging.org

Americans for Better Care of the Dying

Americans for Better Care of the Dying is a nonprofit charity dedicated to social, professional, and policy reform and to education aimed at improving services for patients with serious illnesses and their families.

> Americans for Better Care of the Dying
> 4200 Wisconsin Avenue NW, Fourth Floor
> Washington DC 20016
> Phone: (202) 895-2660
> Fax: (202) 966-5410
> http://www.abcd-caring.org

Center to Improve Care of the Dying

The Center to Improve Care of the Dying (CICD) was founded in the belief that life under the shadow of death can be rewarding, comfortable, and meaningful for almost all persons—but achieving that goal requires real change in the care system. CICD is a unique, interdisciplinary team of committed individuals, engaged in research, public advocacy, and education activities to improve the care of the dying and their families. Dr. Joanne Lynn, an ethicist, hospice physician, and health services researcher serves as Center Director.

> http://www.gwu.edu/-cicd

City of Hope, Pain/Palliative Care Resource Center Website

The purpose of the COHPPRC is to serve as a clearinghouse to disseminate information and resources to assist others in improving the quality of pain management and end-of-life care. The COHPPRC, established in 1995, is a central source for collecting a variety of materials, including pain assessment tools, patient education materials, quality assurance materials, end of life resources, research instruments, and other resources.

> City of Hope Pain/Palliative Care Resource Center
> 1500 East Duarte Road
> Duarte, CA 91010
> Phone: (626) 359-8111 X63829
> http://www.cityofhope.org/prc

The Compassionate Friends, Inc.

The Compassionate Friends is a self-help organization whose purpose is to offer friendship and understanding to parents and siblings following the death of a child. They have 580 chapters nationwide that provide monthly meetings, phone contacts, lending libraries, and a local newsletter. The national organization provides newsletters, distributes grief-related materials, and answers requests for referrals and information.

> The Compassionate Friends, Inc.
> PO Box 3696
> Oak Brook, IL 60522-3696
> Phone: (630) 990-0010
> Toll Free: (877) 969-0010
> http://www.compassionatefriends.org

The Dougy Center

The Dougy Center, The National Center for Grieving Children and Families, provides support groups for grieving children that are age specific (3-5, 6-12, and teens) and loss specific (parent death, sibling death, survivors of homicide/violent death, and survivors of suicide). The Center is in the process of publishing a series of guidebooks based on what they've learned from the children they have served. Titles include *Helping Children Cope With Death* and *Helping Teens Cope With Death*. Additional services include national training, consultations to schools and organizations, crisisline information, and referrals.

> The Dougy Center
> PO Box 86582
> Portland, OR 97286
> Phone: (503) 775-5683
> http://www.dougy.org

The End-of-Life Nursing Education Consortium

The End-of-Life Nursing Education Consortium (ELNEC) project is a national education initiative to improve end-of-life care in the United States. The project provides nurse educators with training in end-of-life care, so they can teach this essential information to nursing students and practicing nurses. The 3-1/2 year project, which began in February 2000, was funded by a major grant from The Robert Wood Johnson Foundation. Two new projects, funded by the National Cancer Institute (NCI), will provide education to graduate nursing faculty and to oncology nurses.

The ELNEC project is administered by the American Association of Colleges of Nursing (AACN) and the City of Hope National Medical Center of Los Angeles. The project is guided by a national advisory board that includes representatives of a variety of nursing and specialty organizations and educational institutions.

American Association of Colleges of Nursing
One Dupont Circle NW, Suite 530
Washington, DC 20036
Phone: (202) 463-6930
http://www.aacn.nche.edu/elnec

End of Life Physician Education Resource Center

The End of Life Physician Education Resource Center (EPERC) offers a number of resources online for the end-of-life care community, including a dynamic e-mail newsletter. The purpose of EPERC is to assist physician educators and others in locating high-quality, peer-reviewed training materials. This web site supports the identification and dissemination of information on EOL training materials, publications, conferences, and other opportunities

http://www.eperc.mcw.edu

Fairygodmother Foundation

The mission of Fairygodmother Foundation is to make wishes come true for loved ones facing terminal illness. The Fairygodmother Foundation strives to bring joy to the lives of individuals (18 and older) and loved ones in their time of greatest need by turning dreams into reality. Their goal is to ensure that those whose lives will be cut short by terminal illness (having a year or less to live) enjoy at least one moment of immeasurable happiness. In the process of fulfilling wishes, they create an opportunity for peace, closure, a sense of belonging, and cherished memories for everyone involved.

The Fairygodmother Foundation
2020 Lincoln Park West, Suite 37E
Chicago, Illinois 60614
Phone: (773) 388-1160
http://www.fairygodmother.org

The George Washington Institute for Spirituality and Health

The George Washington Institute for Spirituality and Health (GWish) is a university-based organization, founded by Dr. Christina Puchalski, working toward a more compassionate system of healthcare. The Institute was established in May 2001 as a leading organization on educational and clinical issues related to spirituality and health.

> The George Washington Institute for Spirituality and Health
> 2131 K Street NW, Suite 510
> Washington, DC 20037
> Phone: (202) 496-6409
> http://www.gwish.org

Growth House, Inc.

Growth House, Inc., provides an international gateway to resources for life-threatening illness and end-of-life care. Its primary mission is to improve the quality of compassionate care for people who are dying, through public education and global professional collaboration. The Growth House search engine provides access to a comprehensive collection of reviewed resources for end-of-life care. Growth House offers disease-specific guides for heart failure, end-stage renal disease, and cancer, plus overviews of key HIV/AIDS resources.

> Growth House
> San Francisco, CA
> Phone: (415) 863-3045
> http://www.growthhouse.org

Hospice Foundation of America

Hospice Foundation of America (HFA) is a nonprofit organization that promotes hospice care and works to educate professionals and the families they serve in issues relating to caregiving, terminal illness, loss, and bereavement.

> Hospice Foundation of America
> 2001 S Street NW, #300
> Washington DC 20009
> Phone: (800) 854-3402
> http://www.hospicefoundation.org

Initiative for Pediatric Palliative Care

Children with life-threatening conditions face many hurdles, and so do their families. The Initiative for Pediatric Palliative Care (IPPC—pronounced "ipsee") represents a consortium of organizations joining forces to improve the care and the quality of life of these children and their families.

The Initiative for Pediatric Palliative Care (IPPC)
Center for Applied Ethics and Professional Practice (CAEPP)
Education Development Center, Inc.
55 Chapel Street
Newton MA, 02458-1060
Phone: (617) 618-2408
http://www.ippcweb.org/index.asp

The Institute for the Study of Health and Illness

The Institute for the Study of Health and Illness (ISHI), directed by Dr. Rachel Naomi Remen, has worked with physicians for more than a decade and has seen hundreds of physicians benefit from coming together in genuine community. We have found a simple form of group process that enables us to listen deeply to one another, rediscover the joy of our work, and receive the kind of healing that only fellow colleagues can bring to one another.

ISHI/FMM
PO Box 316
[UPS/FedEx 451 Mesa Road]
Bolinas, CA 94924
Phone: (415) 868-2642
http://www.meaninginmedicine.org

Last Acts Partnership

Last Acts is a campaign to improve end-of-life care by a coalition of professional and consumer organizations. The organization believes in palliative care, focused on managing pain and making life better for individuals and families facing death. Last Acts envisions a world in which dying people and their loved ones receive excellent care and are honored and supported by their community. Last Acts and Partnership for Caring have merged to become Last Acts Partnership.

Last Acts / Partnership for Caring, Inc.
1620 Eye Street NW, Suite 202
Washington, DC 20006
Phone: (202) 296-8071
http://www.lastacts.org

The Living with Quality Foundation

The Living with Quality Foundation is committed to improving people's lives throughout the world. Their mission is to ensure that no one dies feeling alone or unloved. They are focused on making the world a better place by creating unique, forward-thinking books, tapes, and seminars that are educational and life enhancing.

> Dillon Woods
> C/O Windermere Publications
> PO Box 25109
> Los Angeles, CA 90025
> Phone: (310) 358-6043
> http://www.livingwithquality.com

National Hospice and Palliative Care Organization

The National Hospice and Palliative Care Organization (NHPCO) is the oldest and largest public benefit organization in the United States devoted exclusively to hospice care. NHPCO operates the Hospice Helpline [(800) 658-8898] to provide the general public and healthcare professionals with information about hospice care and reimbursement sources, as well as referrals to local hospice programs throughout the United States. NHPCO publishes a variety of brochures on hospice care, grief in the workplace, and bereavement.

> National Hospice and Palliative Care Organization
> 1700 Diagonal Road, Suite 625
> Alexandria, Virginia 22314
> Phone: (703) 837-1500
> Toll Free: (800) 338-8619
> http://www.nhpco.org

Positive Endings

A unique service to assist you and your loved ones at this turning point in your family's history. Positive Endings has created a safe, private, unique way to capture in words the essence of who you are and the life you have lived. Obituaries frequently fail to satisfy the needs of the family and friends left behind and do very little to tell the story of the person who lived. Positive Endings works with you to create personal obituaries and remembrance books before a person's death, to ensure the quality and meaningfulness of each, and to ease the burden of loved ones.

> http://www.rowinsky.com/resoursesondeathdyinggrief.htm

The Sacred Dying Foundation

The Sacred Dying Foundation is committed to transforming the dying experience by reintegrating spiritual and religious practices and to begin changing the way our society experiences death and dying.

Sacred Dying Foundation
PO Box 210328
San Francisco, CA 94121
Phone: (415) 585-9455
http://www.sacreddying.org

Waking Dreams & Warrior Women

Waking Dreams is a nonprofit organization, founded by BethAnne Deluca-Verley, whose mission is to explore the relationship between art, medicine, and healing.

Waking Dreams & Warrior Women
92 Governor Bradford Drive
Barrington, RI 02806
Phone: (401) 245-5449
http://wdww.tripod.com

Wellbeyond Fitness, Inc.

A wellness consulting organization committed to helping others help themselves through lifestyle change. Wellbeyond Fitness offers a number of holistic, clinical fitness programs intended to improve quality of life, diminish symptoms, and speed recovery from specific medical situations. Each program is designed with a mind/body approach and a belief that physical activity is a powerful catalyst for improving mental and spiritual states.

Wellbeyond Fitness, Inc.
PO Box 3203
Sedona, AZ 86340
Phone: (928) 282-4659
Toll Free: (866) 340-3030
http://www.wellbeyondfitness.com

Zen Hospice Project

Inspired by a 2,500-year-old Buddhist tradition, Zen Hospice Project (ZHP) is a fusion of spiritual insight and practical social action. Begun in 1987, ZHP is now nationally recognized as an innovative model in the movement to improve end-of-life care. ZHP provides a spectrum of collaborative services, including residential hospice care, volunteer programs, and educational efforts that foster wisdom and compassion in service. Each year over 100 volunteers provide an estimated 25,000 hours of practical, emotional, and spiritual support to 200 individuals and their families as they face death from cancer, AIDS, and other illnesses. Over the years, ZHP has served thousands and affected the care of thousands more through professional trainings, community caregiver workshops, and other educational efforts. Now in its second decade of service, ZHP is expanding its outreach efforts by creating an educational Institute on Dying. Continuing its commitment to local direct services, ZHP has formed this new program to develop and share its unique model with national and international audiences.

> Zen Hospice Project
> 273 Page Street
> San Francisco, CA 94102
> Phone: (415) 863-2910
> http://www.zenhospice.org

Magazines

Spirituality & Health

Spirituality & Health brings the people, the practices, and the ideas that are leading America's spiritual renaissance home to our readers in a format that combines intellectual integrity with balance and breadth. Each issue is filled with practical wisdom from best-selling authors and leading teachers, on subjects like finding new supportive relationships and deepening the ones we have, and bringing spiritual values into the workplace—living in harmony with family and neighbors.

> Spirituality & Health
> 74 Trinity Place
> New York, NY 10006-2088
> Phone: (212) 602-0705
> http://www.spiritualityhealth.com

Spiritual Life

Spiritual Life is a quarterly journal of contemporary spirituality that is published by the Discalced Carmelite Friars of the Washington Province. Spiritual Life contains articles that deal with various aspects of Christian spirituality and their application to everyday life. Carmelite spirituality is also featured, examining the meaning of the lives and writings of St. John of the Cross, St. Teresa of Avila, St. Therese of Lisieux, Blessed Elizabeth of the Trinity, and St. Edith Stein.

There are book reviews and a books and media section that highlight books and media that would be helpful to our readers on their Journey to God. Often there is a listing of spirituality resources—retreats, workshops, study programs—some following the Carmelite theme or another spiritual tradition.

Spiritual Life promises to provide its readers with intelligent and thought-provoking material that will enhance their growth in the Spirit.

Spiritual Life
2131 Lincoln Road NE
Washington, DC 20002
Toll Free: (888) 616-1713
http://www.spiritual-life.org

Music

Graceful Passages

Graceful Passages is an audio CD containing music created by Gary Remal Malkin and Michael Stillwater-Korns, with spoken passages from a variety of spiritual leaders and leaders in end-of-life care. Included are the voices of Elisabeth Kübler-Ross, Ram Dass, Thich Nhat Hanh, Arun and Sunanada Gandhi, and others. Based on an inclusive interfaith model, it includes segments inspired by Jewish, Catholic, Protestant, Confucian, Buddhist, Hindu, and American Indian traditions. Not all selections will resonate with all listeners, but there is something here for almost everyone. The moving musical score by Emmy award-winning composer Gary Remal Malkin nicely complements the spoken material.

http://www.gracefulpassages.com

Journey Songs

A CD of songs for transitions, by Michael Stillwater, Inner Harmony, 1998, Healing Music Services.

Phone: (415) 897-3801
www.innerharmony.com

Truly Loved

By Monica Perz-Waddington, this music is appropriate for miscarriage, loss of child, or any loss.

http://www.monicaperz.com

Newsletters

Science and Theology News

Science and Theology News is an independent periodical covering the field of science and religion, published monthly by Research News & Opportunities in Science and Theology, Inc. It includes editorials, recent news, feature articles, book reviews, classifieds, and a calendar of events.

> Science & Theology News
> Eastern Nazarene College
> 23 East Elm Avenue
> Quincy, MA 02170
> Phone: (919) 309-7775
> http://www.stnews.org

Online Journals

Innovations in End-of-Life Care

This international, online journal features peer-reviewed promising practices in end-of-life care, useful tools, selected bibliographies, and other resources. Previously published bimonthly, as of October 2003 the journal will no longer post new issues. All 28 past thematic issues, from January 1999 through September 2003 are now archived at this site and are available to read, download, and print for free.

> http://www2.edc.org/lastacts/

The International Journal of Healing and Caring

IJHC, an online journal, features holistic approaches, focused on the person who has the illness rather than on the illness the person has—holism addresses the growth and healing of body, emotions, mind, relationships, and spirit. IJHC is geared toward conventional and complementary healthcare providers and members of the public interested to know more about complementary/alternative therapies and integrative care.

> http://www.ijhc.org

Additional Resources

Advanced Care Directives Video for Consumers

The Center for Humane and Ethical Medical Care (CHEC) at Santa Monica-UCLA Medical Center recently completed an educational video on advanced-care planning. The video is meant chiefly for lay audiences (including young adults) as a 15-minute stimulus to further discussions about advance directives. For more information, e-mail pbhatla@mednet.ucla.edu or write: The Center for Humane and Ethical Medical Care, Santa Monica-UCLA Medical Center, 1250 16th Street, Santa Monica, CA 90404.

Approaches for Patients from Marginalized Groups

This 8-page end-of-life policy brief, sponsored by the Midwest Bioethics Center's Community-State Partnerships Program and Last Acts, reviews innovations in assessing and expanding decision-making capacity and directions for policy and research. Order free copies via e-mail: partners@midbio.org

The Bruderhof Grief Companion

This web site features writings from a variety of classic and contemporary writers that other grieving people have found helpful and comforting. Four full-length books, including the New York Times' bestseller She Said Yes (the story of Cassie Bernall, one of the Columbine victims), are fully downloadable as a public resource.

http://www.griefcompanion.org

DyingWell.org

DyingWell.org produces resources for people facing life-limiting illness, their families, and their professional caregivers. DyingWell.org works to define wellness through the end of life.

http://www.dyingwell.org

Education Development Center Creates Guide to Accompany Instructional Palliative Care Video

Last Acts' partner, The Education Development Center, Inc., recently produced a resources guide to accompany Ready or Not, a palliative care educational videotape. The film is a portrait of a small number of first-year medical students enrolled in the ground-breaking end-of-life course at Harvard Medical School, "Living with Life-Threatening Illness." The guide suggests ways medical educators might use the video, both to enhance students' comfort and skill in caring for dying patients and, more generally, to enhance their ability to forge meaningful relationships with patients, no matter where patients are in their disease trajectory.

http://www2.edc.org/Innovations/ReadyorNot

End-of-Life Web Directory

This Web directory provides annotated links to the most useful end-of-life care sites on the Web today. The Robert Wood Johnson Foundation continually reviews sites and posts the best of them here.

http://www.rwjf.org

FICA© Spiritual Assessment Tool

The FICA Spiritual Assessment Tool was developed to help healthcare professionals with structured questions to take a spiritual history. The FICA acronym stands for:

F—Faith and Belief
I—Importance/Influence
C—Community
A—Address in Care/Action

This instrument is brief and patient-centered and has been published in a peer-reviewed medical journal, and is easy to remember, meeting all five qualities needed in an assessment tool. It can also be modified for self-assessment. FICA cards are available from the George Washington Institute for Spirituality and Health (GWish).

The George Washington Institute for Spirituality and Health
2131 K Street NW, Suite 510
Washington, DC 20037
Phone: (202) 496-6409
http://www.gwish.org

Final Touches

The mission of the Minnesota Partnership to Improve End-of-Life Care is to improve end-of-life care for those we serve by (1) implementing innovative care delivery models, (2) aligning and coordinating resources, and (3) eliminating barriers. The Minnesota Partnership to Improve End-of-Life Care has created Final Touches, a CEU-certified professional education packet focusing on end-of-life symptom management and communication.

http://www.bioethics.umn.edu

Finding Meaning in Medicine

The Finding Meaning in Medicine group process was developed by The Institute for the Study of Health and Illness (ISHI), directed by Dr. Rachel Naomi Remen. It is a simple form of group process that enables physicians and other healthcare providers to listen deeply to one another, rediscover the joy of their work, and receive the kind of healing that only fellow colleagues can bring to one another. This simple approach is no cost, low effort, and high return. And it's fun! If you have 2 hours a month, a living room, or some other informal meeting place, you can make this happen in your community.

http://www.meaninginmedicine.org

Five Wishes

The Five Wishes document helps you express how you want to be treated if you are seriously ill and unable to speak for yourself. It is unique among all other living will and health agent forms because it looks to all of a person's needs: medical, personal, emotional, and spiritual. Five Wishes also encourages discussing your wishes with your family and physician. Available through Aging with Dignity.

Aging with Dignity
PO Box 1661
Tallahassee, FL 32302-1661
Phone: (850) 681-2010
Toll Free: (888) 5-WISHES
http://www.agingwithdignity.org/5wishes.html

Good Endings Program

The Good Endings program consists of recruiting and training vigil teams of volunteers to sit with the dying, implementing staff education on end-of-life issues, resource libraries, remembrance services, and bereavement counseling. To learn more about Good Endings, go to:

http://www.goodendings.bigstep.com.

Healthandage.com

This web site's end-of-life care resources include a comprehensive guide as well as information and practices regarding palliative care, cancer pain, community care reform and advocacy, and grief management.

http://www.healthandage.com

Kaiser Permanente Palliative Care Program Toolkit

Kaiser Permanente has a new online version of the Kaiser Permanente Palliative Care Program Toolkit available that gives you a step-by-step guide on how you can create an innovative outpatient palliative care program within your own healthcare institution

http://www.growthhouse.org/palliative

Palliative Care Education Resource Team

The PERT Program curriculum is designed to increase the knowledge, skills, and confidence of nursing home staff in providing end-of-life care. This section of the PERT Program web site provides information about the curriculum and how to participate.

http://www.swedishmedical.org/PERT.htm

Palliative Clinical Assessment and Research Tools

Promoting Excellence in End-of-Life Care announces its online resource: "Key Clinical Assessment and Research Tools." The primary goal of the collection is to provide an easy way for providers and researchers to access the tools.

http://www.lastacts.org/scripts/la_eln01.exe?FNC=SeeFeature4__Ala_eln _features_html___5171

Patient Education and Caring: End-of-Life (PEACE) Series

Free, downloadable pamphlets available from American College of Physicians-American Society of Internal Medicine web site for patients regarding palliative care and hospice.

http://www.acponline.org/ethics/patient_education.htm

Precepts of Palliative Care for Children/Adolescents and Their Families

Palliative Care for Children/Adolescents and Their Families is the comprehensive management of physical, psychological, social, spiritual, and existential needs. It is a suitable approach to care for children/adolescents who are born with serious medical conditions, as well as those who develop such illnesses at a later stage of childhood or adolescence. Although palliative care may be an appropriate part of the treatment of any complex or serious illness, it is vital in the care of life-limiting and incurable, progressive conditions.

http://www.lastacts.org/files/misc/lastactsprecepts2.pdf

Toolkit of Instruments to Measure End of Life (TIME)

An authoritative bibliography of instruments to measure the quality of care and quality of life for dying patients and their families. Assembled with funding from the Nathan Cummings Foundation and the Robert Wood Johnson Foundation. The Toolkit instruments are available at no charge.

http://www.chcr.brown.edu/pcoc/toolkit.htm

Web Sites

http://www.companionarts.org—Educational Programs and Resources for Transition, (415) 209-9408

http://www.nativeamericanembassy.net/—Native American Embassy

http://www.religioustolerance.org/nataspir.htm—Native American resource

http://www.wisdomoftheworld.com—Media for a Meaningful Life, (415) 209-9408

B

Religious Beliefs and Practices

CHRISTINA M. PUCHALSKI

Buddhism

General Information. Buddhism is a religion and a philosophical system of beliefs followed by 300 million people. It is based on the teachings of Siddhartha Gautama Buddha, born in Nepal in 6th century BC, who focused on living ethically in this world and achieving enlightenment. The focus on the search for awareness and attainment of unconditional compassion is encouraged. Spiritual practices such as meditation, contemplation, Yoga, and chanting provide guidance, comfort, and meaning. Relief of suffering can be achieved by following the Noble Enlightened Path.

Suffering. In Buddhism, it is believed that life is suffering, which originates in attachments and in avoiding pain. One can end suffering by letting go of attachments. Suffering results in ignorance, selfish desires, and attachments to illusions.

Diet. Different branches of Buddhism have different dietary regulations.

Death. In Buddhism, there is a belief in reincarnation, but not in immortality of both body and soul. No underlying self migrates to the next reincarnation. The dying person's state of mind is important. To help patients achieve peace of mind, family, friends, and monks read religious texts and repeat mantras to the dying person. After death, the body is washed, dressed in burial clothes, and cremated. Some Buddhists believe the dead person's conscious soul remains around or in the body for several days, so monks are invited to chant sacred texts to assist the dead person's passing to the spiritual world.

Ethical Issues. Buddhists believe that it is good to continue living, but when the mind is no longer alert or the person is in excessive pain, a natural death is preferable. Allowing a person to die a natural and peaceful death is essential.

Christianity

General Information. Christianity is a religion followed by 1.8 billion people. It is based on the life and teachings of Jesus Christ, who is God incarnate, fully divine and fully human. In Christianity, there is a belief in humanity and the need to develop selfless and unconditional love for God and other people, following God's example of his love for humankind. Christians believe in the doctrine of the Trinity, which affirms that God is three in one being (Father, Son, and Holy Spirit). Guidance and inspiration comes from the Bible. It is believed that Jesus died so that man's sins are atoned for. The Scriptures and the Ten Commandments describe the righteous life. Spiritual practices such as prayer, sacraments, rituals, meditation, and religious service offer comfort and meaning.

Suffering. Some Christians believe suffering is caused by sin; others see suffering as an unexplainable part of living or a result of alienation from God. Suffering is relieved by surrender to God's will for the person and acceptance of God's will.

Diet. In Christianity, diet varies with tradition. Some people choose to fast on particular religious days. Catholic Christians abstain from eating meat on Ash Wednesday and the Fridays of Lent (hospitalized or ill patients are excused).

Death. In Christianity, death is seen as a natural part of life. It is believed that each person has a soul that is unique and immortal. Some Christians welcome dying as a way to a full union with God and believe that in life one prepares for dying and for that union with God. Many Christians believe death results in a temporary separation of body and soul; full union will occur after Christ's second coming. Many Christians also believe that after death, the soul is judged and either remains in heaven or hell. Family, friends, priests, or ministers pray or sing at the bedside of the dying person. For Catholic Christians, the sacrament of the Anointing of the Sick (formerly known as Last Rites) or prayer ritual, called Viaticum, bring peace and comfort. Christian funeral practices vary from simple observance to elaborate rituals.

Ethical Issues. End-of-life care organ donation decisions vary. Most Christians put emphasis on respect and value of life but also view quality of life and dignity of the human person as central to decision making.

Hinduism

General Information. Hinduism is a religion of 700 million people, an amalgam of many traditions, rituals, devotions, and philosophical beliefs developed over the past 4,000 years. Polytheism (worshiping of or believing in more than one deity) is the basis of Hindu worship, although Hindus believe in the essential oneness of ultimate reality, called Brahman (God). Spiritual practices, such as Yoga, focus on developing selflessness and transforming awareness and finding meaning. Devotional prayer and Hindu scriptures provide comfort and insight.

Suffering. There are thee main causes of suffering in Hinduism:
Physical and psychosocial pain: This can be alleviated with medication.
Ignorance: This can be alleviated with education and increased insight.
Restricted sense of being: This can be alleviated by realizing that an eternal self (*Atman*) underlies the human self, which is part of the ultimate reality.

Diet. Vegetarianism is recommended.

Death. In Hinduism, death is considered natural and unavoidable, but not real. Only Brahman and Atman are ultimately real. Hindus believe in an eternal soul that transgresses from one reincarnation to another. Religious rites and ceremonies provide support to the dying person and family members. A son or relative puts water from the Ganges River in the person's mouth to bring peace. Family members and friends sing devotional prayers, read Hindu scriptures, and chant. After the death, the body is washed, anointed, and dressed in new clothes. The hair and beard of the person are trimmed. Cremation offers the best way for the soul to begin its journey.

Ethical Issues. Mercy killing, assisted suicide, and suicide are disapproved of, but letting nature take its course is acceptable. Having a living will and organ donation are both individual choices.

Islam

General Information. Islam is a religion of approximately 970 million people that is based on the teachings of the Prophet Muhammed. Muslims believe in one God who is all-powerful, compassionate, and immortal. After death, the soul is judged by God, and remains in either heaven or hell. Guidance and comfort are provided by the Koran, prayer, rituals, and fasting. Muslims believe that the Five Pillars of Islam, the Ten Commandments, and the Golden Rule describe the righteous life.

Suffering. According to Islamic belief, suffering is caused by alienation from the will of Allah and relieved by total surrender to His will, as embodied in the Koran.

Diet. Most Muslims follow rigid dietary guidelines (no pork, no alcohol) and are required to wash specific parts of the body before each of the required daily periods of prayer. Assisting with daily prayer and dietary and hygiene requirements is important for spiritual care of Muslims.

Death. In Islam, creation, death, and resurrection are linked. Life is viewed as a time of preparation for the soul to pass into life after death. To struggle against death is viewed as resisting the will of Allah. Muslims who are dying usually want to lie toward Mecca. When a Muslim person is dying, family members repeat prayers, read Islamic scripture, and encourage the patient to repeat the statement of faith. After death, the unwashed body is wrapped in a plain sheet, the feet are tied together and the face is bandaged to keep the mouth and eyes closed. At the mosque or at the person's home, the body is bathed, perfumed, wrapped in white cotton, and buried as soon as possible.

Ethical Issues. It is permissible to use life support to save and lengthen life. The purpose of oppressive medical intervention is to maintain the process of life but not to postpone death. While it is not permissible to disconnect life support, because that will cause death, it is also not permissible to cause harm to the patient with equipment and drugs when the futility of such treatment is established by the medical team. Physician-assisted suicide is prohibited.

Judaism

General Information. Judaism is a religion of 17 million people, which is based on the belief of one eternal God who is omnipotent and all-knowing. Followers rely on the Hebrew Bible, including the Ten Commandments, for spiritual authority on righteous living. Scriptures, religious rituals, family relationships, and their history as a people provide comfort, identity, and meaning.

Suffering. In Judaism, suffering results from the disobedience of God's laws as described in the Torah. Suffering is relieved by asking for God's forgiveness, living in accordance with God's divine will, and living in a righteous way for the good of the whole.

Diet. Many Jews observe a kosher diet.

Death. There is a wide range of beliefs in Judaism concerning the afterlife, from no specific belief to immortality of the soul. Death is viewed as a necessary part of God's creation, not a punishment for sin. Some Jews believe in hope for personal salvation and the coming of a Messiah. Others view salvation as an assurance of the continued existence of the whole of creation rather than eternal life for an individual. The Jewish tradition is to focus primarily on how life is lived on earth rather than on events after death. There is a belief that dying patients should be attended to constantly. Family, the rabbi, and friends read from specific religious texts and recite psalms. The dying are encouraged to pray for forgiveness. After death, the body is washed and prepared for burial, which is done within 24 hours. The Kaddish (mourner's prayer) is recited after the funeral service. A 7-day period of mourning is observed.

Ethical Issues. The importance of life is fundamental to all decision making, but the belief that dying must also be done with dignity also imparts decisions. There are many different views on removing life support. It's important to consult the family and the rabbi in each circumstance.

Native American Spirituality

General Information. Many followers of Native American spirituality regard their beliefs and practice as an integral part of their being, not so much as a religion. Because of the wide range of habitats in North America, different tribes evolved different spiritual beliefs and practices to match the lifestyle and needs of the individual tribe. Many Native Americans follow other religious traditions, such as Christianity, yet also retain their traditional beliefs and practices. Many tribes have complex forms of sacred forms of writing; others have passed on their spiritual beliefs as an oral tradition. Native Americans may believe in a Deity; some believe in a dual divinity—a Creator responsible for creation, who is recognized in ritual and prayers, and a mystical individual who teaches culture and behavior. There are also spirits who control the weather, inhabit the underworld, and interact with humans. Shamans are healers whose bodies are occupied by spirits during ceremonies.

Suffering. According to Native American beliefs, everything physical has a spiritual counterpart that is more important. Everything and everyone has an inherent purpose. A person has a spiritual definition; when that spiritual definition is not recognized in others or in oneself, suffering occurs.

Diet. Varies.

Death. In general, native religions have no precise belief about life after death. Some believe in reincarnation. Others believe that humans return as spirits, and others may believe that nothing can definitely be known about life after death. Dying at old age is a blessed event, a time to celebrate the prosperity of the community; the life of the deceased is commemorated and placed in eternity. An untimely death at a young age may be seen as a sign of trouble ahead.

Ethical Issues. Most Native Americans view death as natural. However, for specific preferences for treatment at the end-of-life, one needs to discuss that with each person, family, and/or shaman, as beliefs and values can vary.

References

Armstrong, K. (1993). *A history of God.* New York: Ballantine.

Doka, K. J., & Morgan, J. D. (1995). *Death and spirituality.* Amityville, NY: Baywood.

Hamel, R. P., & Lysaught, M. T. (1994). Choosing palliative care: Do religious beliefs make a difference. *Journal of Palliative Care, 10,* 61-66.

Interfaith Committee of the Department of Chaplaincy Services and Pastoral Education. (1999). *Religious beliefs and practices affecting healthcare.* Charlottesville, VA: University of Virginia Health System.

Kramer, K. P. (1988). *The sacred art of dying: How world religions understand death.* New York: Paulist.

Markham, I. (1996). *A world religions reader.* Boston: Blackwell.

Muck, T. C. (1993, April). *Coping with a hospital experience: It matters where you are from.* Paper presented at the Texas Society of Patient Representatives Conference, Austin, Texas.

Native American Spirituality. Accessed at www.religioustolerance.org/nataspir.htm.

Neuberger, J. A. (1993). Cultural issues in palliative care. In D. Doyle, G. W. C. Hanks, & N. MacDonald (Eds.), *Oxford textbook of palliative medicine* (pp. 507-513). New York: Oxford University Press.

Parrinder, G. (1984). (Ed.). *World religions: From ancient history to the present.* New York: Facts on File.

Reflections on Native American Spirituality. Accessed at www.augsburg.edu/ppages/-lindelan/NAReflections.htm.

Smith, H. (1991). *The world religions: Our great wisdom traditions.* New York: HarperCollins.

Storey, P., & Knight, C. F. (2003). *Alleviating psychological and spiritual pain in the terminally ill.* New Rochelle, NY: Mary Ann Liebert.

C

Protestant Advance Directives

The following were compiled by Dr. Denise Reeves, physician and member of the Vestry of Grace Episcopal Church, Muncie, Indiana, which was one of my parishes. The documents are examples only. It is necessary to check what is important in your state or province.

Document 1

LIVING WILL DECLARATION

Declaration made this _____day of_____, 200____.

I, _____, being at least eighteen (18) years of age and of sound mind, willfully and voluntarily make known my desire that my dying shall not be artificially prolonged under the circumstances set forth below, and I declare:

If at any time my attending physician certifies in writing that:

(1) I have an incurable injury, disease, or illness;

(2) my death will occur within a short time; and

(3) the use of life-prolonging procedures would serve only to artificially prolong the dying process, I direct that they be withheld or withdrawn and that I be permitted to die naturally, with only the performance or provision of any medical procedure or medication necessary to provide me with comfort, care or to alleviate pain, and, if I have so indicated below, the provision of artificially supplied nutrition and hydration. *(Indicate your choice by initialing or making your mark before signing this declaration)*:

I wish to receive artificially supplied nutrition and hydration, even if the effort to sustain life is futile or excessively burdensome to me.

I do not wish to receive artificially supplied nutrition and hydration, if the effort to sustain life is futile or excessively burdensome to me.

I intentionally make no decision concerning artificially supplied nutrition and hydration, leaving the decision to my healthcare representative, appointed under IC16-36-1-7, or my attorney in fact with healthcare providers, under IC 30-5-5.

_____

WITNESS:

_____

Date:

_____

Document 2

GENERAL DURABLE POWER OF ATTORNEY

I, _____, now residing at _____, by this instrument, do hereby make, constitute, and appoint the person or persons hereinafter named as my true and lawful Attorney-in-fact, for me and in my name, place and stead to do any lawful act for me as provided in this instrument.

THIS Power of Attorney SHALL NOT BE AFFECTED BY MY SUBSEQUENT INCOMPETENCY, DISABILITY, OR INCAPACITY, OR BY LAPSE OF TIME.

I HEREBY REVOKE all other general powers of attorney that I may have executed, if any.

1. WHEN EFFECTIVE.

My Attorney-in-fact shall not exercise this Power of Attorney until a physician familiar with my condition states in writing to my Attorney-in-fact that I am unable to manage my affairs. My Agent shall be free from any liability for any action taken under this Power of Attorney in reliance upon the physician's statement. My Attorney-in-fact shall stop using this Power of Attorney when a physician familiar with my condition states in writing to my Attorney-in-fact that I am unable to manage my affairs.

2. ATTORNEY(S)-IN-FACT.

As my Attorney-in-fact, I name _____, whose address is _____.

(A) **Limited Liability.** My Attorney-in-fact shall be liable only for willful default, gross misconduct, or fraud, and not for errors of judgment. My Attorney-in-fact shall have the power to bind me or my property without binding my Attorney-in-fact personally. A Successor Attorney-in-fact shall have no duty to inquire into the acts of any prior Attorney-in-fact and shall not be liable for any act or omission of any prior Attorney-in-fact.

(B) **Resignation.** Any person serving as my Attorney-in-fact may resign by delivering a written resignation in such person or persons remaining as my Attorney-in-fact, or, if none, to me.

(C) **Successor.** If my original Attorney-in-fact fails, or ceases to act as my Attorney-in-fact, I appoint as my Successor Attorney-in-fact, _____, whose address is _____.

3. **ACCOUNTING.** Upon termination of this Power of Attorney, or if my Attorney-in-fact fails or ceases to act, my Attorney-in-fact, or the legal representative for my Attorney-in-fact, or his/her estate, or my Attorney-in-fact's beneficiaries or heirs, shall account, within thirty (30) days after termination of the date when my Attorney-in-fact fails or ceases to act, to me, to my immediate Successor Attorney-in-fact, to my legal representative, to my estate or to the beneficiaries or heirs of my estate, for all money and property that come into the possession of my Attorney-in-fact.

4. **POWERS.** I give to my Attorney-in-fact, or any Successor Attorney-in-fact, the powers and authority as follows:

(A) **Real Property.** General authority with respect to real property transactions pursuant to I.C. 30-5-5-2, including the power with respect to any interests in property that I may own in joint tenancy with right of survivorship to sever the joint tenancy, or remove the property from joint ownership, and retitle my interest therein in my individual name.

(B) **Tangible Personal Property.** General authority with respect to tangible personal property pursuant to I.C. 30-5-5-3, including the power with respect to any interests in property that I may own in joint tenancy with right of survivorship to sever the joint tenancy, or remove the property from joint ownership, and retitle my interest therein in my individual name.

(C) **Bond, Share, and Commodity.** General authority with respect to bond, share, and commodity transactions pursuant to I.C. 30-5-5-4, including the power to purchase U.S. Bonds, redeemable at par for the payment of U.S. Estate Taxes, and to borrow money to make such purchases.

(D) **Banking.** General authority with respect to banking transactions pursuant to I.C. 30-5-5-5.

(E) **Business.** General authority with respect to banking transactions pursuant to I.C. 30-5-5-6.

(F) **Insurance.** General authority with respect to business transactions pursuant to I.C. 30-5-5-7 provided that references in I.C. 30-5-5-7(a) 2) and (3) to "section 8" are changed to "section 9."

(G) **Beneficiary.** General authority with respect to beneficiary transactions pursuant to I.C. 30-5-5-8.

(H) **Gifts.** General authority with respect to gift transactions pursuant to I.C. 30-5-5-9.

(I) **Fiduciary.** General authority with respect to fiduciary transactions pursuant to I.C. 30-5-5-10.

(J) **Claims and Litigation.** General authority with respect to claims and litigation pursuant to I.C. 30-5-5-11.

(K) **Family Maintenance.** General authority with respect to family maintenance pursuant to I.C. 30-5-5-12.

(L) **Military Service.** General authority with respect to benefits from military service pursuant to I.C. 30-5-5-13.

(M) **Records, Reports, and Statements.** General authority with respect to records, reports, and statements pursuant to I.C. 30-5-5-14, including the power to execute on my behalf any specific Power of Attorney required by any taxing authority to allow my Attorney-in-fact to act on my behalf before that taxing authority on any return on issue.

(N) **Estate Transactions.** General authority with respect to estate transactions pursuant to I.C. 30-5-5-15.

(O) **Healthcare.** General authority with respect to healthcare pursuant to I.C. 30-5-5-16, including authority to act as my Healthcare Representative for me in all matters of healthcare in accordance with my Appointment of a Healthcare Representative as provided in I.C. 16-8-12 and I.C. 30-5-5-17.

(P) **Living Will.** I have executed a Living Will Declaration.

(Q) **Delegate.** General authority with respect to delegating authority pursuant to I.C. 30-5-5-18.

(R) **All Other Matters.** General authority with respect to all other matters pursuant to I.C. 30-5-5-19.

PROVIDED, however, my Attorney-in-fact shall not have any power or authority which would cause my Attorney-in-fact to be treated as the owner of any interest in my property and which would cause that property to be taxed as owned by my Attorney-in-fact.

5. **THIRD PARTY RELIANCE.** Each person, partnership, corporation, or other legal entity relying or acting upon this Power of Attorney shall be entitled to presume conclusively that this Power of Attorney is in full force and effect unless written notice is given by me or my legal representatives that this power is no longer effective, revoked, or terminated. If this power is effective only upon a certificate by a physician stating that I am unable to manage my affairs, those relying upon this instrument shall be fully protected in assuming that such a certificate has been delivered to my Attorney-in-fact.

(A) **Copy.** I have only executed a limited number of original powers. Any person, partnership, corporation, or other legal entity may rely on a photocopy of this power, if the photocopy is accompanied by a timely affidavit of the Attorney-in-fact stating that the photocopy is a true and accurate copy of the power and that the power has not been terminated as to the date of the affidavit.

(B) **Application of Proceeds.** No person, partnership, corporation, or other legal entity relying on this Power of Attorney shall be required to see the application and disposition of any property either paid to or delivered to my Attorney-in-fact, or distributed in accordance with the instructions of my Attorney-in-fact.

6. **APPOINTMENT OF GUARDIAN.** In the event that a court of competent jurisdiction should determine that I am an incapacitated person, and that it is necessary to appoint a conservator, or guardian of my person or estate, or both, then, and in such event, I nominate and appoint _____, as such conservator, or guardian of my person or estate, or both, as the case may be.

7. **TERMINATION.** This Power of Attorney shall continue in effect until terminated as provided below, regardless of my physical or mental condition.

(A) **Revocation.** I may revoke this Power of Attorney by delivering a written revocation to my Attorney-in-fact, executed in the same manner as the original Power of Attorney. This written revocation shall not be effective until actually received by my Attorney-in-fact, who shall not be liable for any action taken prior to the receipt of the written revocation. My Attorney-in-fact may, in good faith, challenge the revocation in court if there is reason to believe that I am an incapacitated person. If my Attorney-in-fact challenges the revocation, then this Power of Attorney shall be ineffective until the court orders that my attempted revocation does not legally revoke the Power of Attorney.

8. **APPLICABLE LAW.** This instrument shall be governed in all respects by the laws of the State of Indiana.

EXECUTED THIS _____ DAY OF _____, 200____.

_____

_____

Taxpayer Identification Number

STATE OF INDIANA

SS:

DELAWARE COUNTY

Before me, a Notary Public in and for said County and State, personally appeared, _____, who acknowledged the execution of the foregoing General Durable Power of Attorney, and who, having been duly sworn, stated that any representations therein contained are true.

WITNESS my hand and Notarial Seal this _____ day of _____, 200____.

_____.

My Commission Expires:

Document 3

APPOINTMENT OF HEALTHCARE REPRESENTATIVE

I, _____, now residing at _____, by this instrument do hereby constitute, appoint, and designate _____, whose address is _____, as my Healthcare Representative. In the even _____ fails or refuses for any reason to act as my Healthcare Representative, then, and in such event, I constitute, appoint, and designate _____, whose address is

_____, as my Successor Healthcare Representative.

My Healthcare Representative, whether the original, a delegate, or successor, shall have full power and authority to make all healthcare decisions for me relating to my personal healthcare. By way of illustration, and not intending any limitation, I specifically grant my representative the following powers:

(A) **Employment.** The power to employ servants, companions, nurses, or doctors to care for me.

(B) **Admission.** The power to admit me to, or release me from, any hospital or healthcare facility.

(C) **Consent.** The power to consent, on my behalf, to any treatment, physical or psychiatric, or surgical procedure for any injury or disease from which I may be suffering.

(D) **Access Records.** The power to have access to any records, including medical records, concerning my condition.

(E) **Release.** The power to execute any releases, or other documents, which may be required in order to obtain medical information.

(F) **Disclosure.** The power to disclose such of my medical information as may be deemed necessary by my Healthcare Representative.

(G) **Waiver.** The power to execute such waiver or release from liability as may be required by a healthcare provider.

(H) **Healthcare Consent.** The power, as my Healthcare Representative, to act for me in matters of healthcare in accordance with I.C. 16-36-1-7, including the authorization to delegate all or part of this authority to any eligible individual who has not been disqualified as provided in said statute.

(I) **Stop Healthcare.** I authorize my Healthcare Representative to make decisions in my best interest concerning withdrawal or withholding of healthcare. If at any time, based on my previously expressed preferences and the diagnosis and prognosis, my Healthcare Representative is satisfied that certain healthcare is not or would not be beneficial, or that such healthcare is or would be excessively burdensome, then my Healthcare Representative may express my will that such healthcare be withheld or withdrawn and may consent on my behalf that any or all healthcare be discontinued or so instituted, even if death may result.

(J) **Consultations.** My Healthcare Representative must try to discuss this decision with me. However, if I am unable to communicate, my Healthcare Representative may make such a decision for me, after consultation with my physician or physicians and other relevant healthcare givers. To the extent appropriate, my Healthcare Representative may also discuss this decision with my family and others, to the extent they are available.

Prior Appointments. I hereby revoke any prior appointment or designation of a Healthcare Representative to act in matters of my healthcare.

Reliance. For the purposes of inducing any individual, organization, or entity to act in accordance with instructions of my Healthcare Representative who is authorized in this document, I hereby represent, warrant, and agree that:

(A) No person who relies in good faith upon the authority of my Healthcare Representative under this document shall incur any liability to me, my estate, my heirs, successors, or assigns.

(B) If this document is revoked or amended for any reason, I, my estate, my heirs, successors, and assigns will hold any person harmless for any loss suffered, or liability incurred as a result of such person acting in good faith upon the instructions of my Healthcare Representative prior to the receipt by such person of actual notice of revocation or amendment.

(C) Reimbursement of costs. My Healthcare Representative shall be entitled to reimbursement for all reasonable costs and expenses actually incurred and paid by my Healthcare Representative on my behalf under any provision of this document but will not be entitled to compensation for services rendered hereunder.

DATED THIS _____ DAY of _____, 200____.

_____

is personally known to me and I believe her or him to be of sound mind. I am not a Healthcare Representative appointed by this document. I am competent and at least eighteen (18) years of age.

DATED THIS _____ DAY OF _____, 200___,

_____

Witness

STATE OF INDIANA

SS:

DELAWARE COUNTY

Before me, a Notary Public in and for said County and State, personally appeared _____, who acknowledged the execution of the foregoing Appointment of Healthcare Representative, and who, having been duly sworn, stated that any representations therein contained are true.

EXECUTED at Muncie, Indiana, this ____ day of _____, 200___.

_____

Document 4

Funeral Preplanning Checklist

To be used as a guide and aid for my family upon my death. Please notify the church as soon as possible after death.

FULL NAME

_____

ADDRESS

_____

_____

I have a Last Will, and Testament and it has been filed with:

_____

_____

1. Disposition of the Body

___ Whole Body Burial

___ Cremation

___ Donation of body to medical research. Forms have been filed with:

_____

2. Pre-Funeral Preferences

My funeral wishes are on file with:

___ Grace Episcopal Church

___ Funeral Home _____

and they are: ___ Prepaid ___ Not Prepaid

___ Family Member

___ Other:

_____

Mortician

___ Body to lie in state at the funeral home

___ Casket open

___ Casket open to family, then closed

___ Casket closed

Casket

___ Wood

___ Cloth-covered wood

___ Metal

Participation in Organ Donor Program

___ My signed Uniform Donor Card can be found at:

_____

___ None

Autopsy

___ If it is helpful for research or needs of my survivors

___ Decision to be made by:

_____

___ None, unless vital to medical research or required by law

3. Funeral Preferences

Location of service:

___ Grace Episcopal Church

___ Other: _____

Type of Resurrection Liturgy

___ Burial Office with Eucharist using:

___ Rite I

___ Rite II

___ Burial Office only

___ Rite I

___ Rite II

Music

___ Organ and Hymn singing

___Hymns to be sung

___Other hymns of praise and faith

Hymn numbers from 1982 Hymnal:

_____

_____

___ Organ only

___ Other instruments, soloists, duet, etc.

Scripture Readings (See *Book of Common Prayer* p. 470, 475, 480 or 494-495)

Old Testament (Name of Reader optional)

_____

Psalm (Name of Reader optional)

_____

Epistle (Name of Reader optional)

_____

Gospel

_____

Homily (Name of Priest optional)

_____

Personal Tribute (Name optional)

_____

Additional Ceremonies

_____ Incense

_____ Asperges (Holy Water)

Suggested Pallbearers (minimum of 6: you may have honorary pallbearers)

_____ My family will arrange for pallbearers.

The following should be included:

Other:

Ushers:

The Parish Hall is available for fellowship and/or reception following the service.

4. Interment

Burial Location:

_____

_____ Cremation

Committal Liturgy

For whole body burial

___ At graveside, with family and friends, if possible

___ Lowering of casket into ground at the words of committal

For interment after cremation

___ Place to be arranged between family and priest

5. Additional Requests

If there is a choice and depending on circumstances, I would prefer to die:

___ At home or present residence

___ In the hospital or nursing home

I request that no extraordinary means be used to keep me alive

___ If family, priest, and doctor agree, please remove my support equipment

I understand that I may change these requests at any time, by notifying those who are holding copies.

I authorize the person(s) named here to make any necessary changes in the above requests, in accordance with their best judgment and the circumstances which exist at the time of my death:

_____

_____

_____

Other requests or instructions:

SIGNED:

_____

Date:

_____

WITNESS:

_____

Date:

_____

D

ADVANCE DIRECTIVE FOR

HEALTH CARE

A Catholic Perspective

*Approved by the Catholic Bishops
of New Jersey - 12/98*

ADVANCE DIRECTIVE FOR HEALTH CARE:
A CATHOLIC PERSPECTIVE

EXPLANATION

The Catholic Bishops of New Jersey have prepared the following Advance Directive for Health Care. The naming of a health care representative (proxy) and instruction directive are combined into one form. The New Jersey Advance Directives for Health Care Act went into effect January 7, 1992. This act allows adults to complete an advance directive. You can either choose a health care representative (proxy) or give directions about your health choices and wishes, or both. It is not a law that you must have an advance directive. You can not be refused admission to a health care facility because you do not have an advance directive.

Before completing an advance directive, it is important to think about the following:

- You should talk about your choices with your entire family. Your family may include your spouse, adult children, parents, brothers, and sisters.

- You should talk to your doctor about your health care choices.

- Your health care representative (proxy) should know you and your wishes about medical treatment. Your health care representative has the legal right to make health care decisions based on your advance directive when you cannot make decisions.

- You do not need a lawyer to complete an advance directive. You may talk to one if you wish.

- You need to review your advance directive from time to time to make sure that your wishes are still the same.

- You can decide to change your advance directive at any time.

- If you want to cancel your advance directive, put it in writing or talk to your health care representative, doctor, or family.

- You have the right to make decisions about your medical treatment.

- Medical care will not be withheld just because you become unable to make your own treatment decisions.

STEPS FOR COMPLETING YOUR ADVANCE DIRECTIVE

PART ONE:

- Choose a person whom you trust to act as your health care representative (proxy).

- Direct your health care representative (proxy) to make your health care choices in accordance with your health care instructions or wishes when you cannot make these choices for yourself.

PART TWO:

- Give directions about your health care choices and wishes to those who will be responsible for your care.

- Tell your health care representative (proxy), family member or friend to bring a copy of this form to the hospital when you are admitted.

PART THREE:

- Sign the advance directive form in the presence of two witnesses 18 years of age or older (but your health care representative, alternate health care representative or doctor cannot serve as witnesses).

- Have those two witnesses sign and date the form.

- Give copies of the advance directive to your health care representative (proxy), your doctor, and appropriate family members or friend.

- Keep the original copy of this form for yourself.

- Bring a copy of this form to the hospital when seeking medical treatment.

This document is approved by the Catholic Bishops of New Jersey.

COMBINED ADVANCE DIRECTIVE FOR HEALTH CARE
(Combined Proxy and Instruction Directive)

STATEMENT OF BELIEF

Catholics believe that life is a gift of a loving God. Life is a holy gift for which we are responsible, but do not own. We believe that assisted death and suicide destroy human life and are never allowed.

As an adult, I have the right to make decisions about my health care. As a Catholic, I may never choose my own death as an end or a means. There may come a time when I am unable to express my own health care decisions. By writing an advance directive, I give instructions and wishes for my future health care decisions. This advance directive for health care shall take effect when I am not able to express my own health care decisions, as determined by my attending doctor. I direct that those responsible for my care make health care decisions according to my stated wishes. I direct that this advance directive be included in my permanent medical record.

PART ONE: NAMING MY HEALTH CARE REPRESENTATIVE

A) I have chosen the following person to be my Health Care Representative.

Name _____

Address _____

City _____ State _____ Zip _____

Telephone Number _____

He or she will be my health care representative to make my health care decisions when I am not able to speak for myself. If my wishes are not clear or events take place that I have not talked about, I ask that my health care representative make the decisions based upon what he or she knows of my wishes.

I have talked with my health care representative about this responsibility. He or she has willingly agreed to accept this role.

B) I have chosen the following person(s) as my Alternate Health Care Representative, if the person I have chosen above is not able, not willing or not available to act as my health care representative:

1.   Name _____

    Address _____ City _____ State _____

    Zip _____ Telephone Number _____

OR

2.   Name _____

    Address _____ City _____ State _____

    Zip _____ Telephone Number _____

He or she will be my health care representative to make my health care decisions when I am not able to speak for myself. If my wishes are not clear or events take place that I have not talked about, I ask that my health care representative make the decisions based upon what he or she knows of my wishes.

I have talked with my alternate health care representative about this responsibility. He or she has willingly agreed to accept this role.

PART TWO: TREATMENT CHOICE INSTRUCTIONS

In Part Two, you are asked to give directions about your future health care. This will mean making important and difficult choices. You need to think about and write down different situations when different types of medical treatments, including life-sustaining actions, should be given or should not be given. Before finishing this part, you should talk this over with your health care representative, doctor, priest, deacon, spouse, family members or those who may be responsible for your care. It is suggested that from time to time you look over these instructions with these same people to make sure that your wishes are still the same.

Please take time to look over all of Part Two before completing the form.

GENERAL INSTRUCTIONS: I direct the people who are responsible for my care to carry out the following:

• Initial one of the following statements - either A or B.

_____ A. I direct that all medically indicated treatments and food and water (through tubes if necessary) be given to maintain my life, no matter what my physical or mental condition. (Skip B & C)

OR

_____ B. If a serious health condition occurs and my primary doctor and at least one other doctor who has personally examined me, decide that the irreversible process of dying has begun and death is very near, I direct **not** to have treatments that would only prolong my dying. If these treatments have been started, they should be stopped. I also want to be given all necessary medical care appropriate to stop pain and to make me comfortable. (Go to C)

C. If I have been diagnosed as being in a permanent coma or in a persistent vegetative state after being examined by my primary doctor and at least one other doctor who is qualified to make this decision, **choose either 1 or 2.**

_____ 1. I direct that **extraordinary*** medical care, as understood in the teachings of the Catholic Church, including food and water (through tubes if needed) shall be used no matter what my physical or mental health.

OR

_____ 2. I direct that **extraordinary*** medical care, as understood in the teachings of the Catholic Church, shall not be used. I direct that food and water (through tubes if needed) be continued unless or until the benefits of this food and water are clearly outweighed by a definite danger or burden, or are useless.

---

*extraordinary medical care is understood as those medicines, treatments or operations which may be very expensive, may cause excessive pain or other extreme difficulties or which may offer no reasonable hope of benefit.

Examples of extraordinary measures that I would want are as follows:

_____

_____

_____

_____

D. If I am **pregnant** and I am diagnosed as being in a permanent coma, in a persistent vegetative state or that the process of dying has begun and death is near, I direct that all medically indicated measures and food and water (through tubes if necessary) be given to maintain my life, regardless of my physical or mental condition, if this could maintain the life of my unborn child until birth.

E. The State of New Jersey recognizes the irreversible cessation of all functions of the entire brain, including the brain stem (also known as whole brain death), as a legal standard for the declaration of death. Generally, physicians will follow this standard. However, if you cannot accept this standard because of your personal religious beliefs, you may request that it not be applied in determining your death by initialing the following statement:

_____   To declare my death on the basis of the irreversible cessation of all functions of the entire brain, including the brain stem, would violate my personal religious beliefs. I therefore direct that my death be declared solely on the basis of the traditional criteria of irreversible cessation of cardiopulmonary (heartbeat and breathing) function.

F. Please initial one:

_____ Upon my death, I am willing to donate any parts of my body that may be beneficial to others.

_____ Upon my death, I am **not** willing to donate any parts of my body that may be beneficial to others.

PART THREE: SIGNATURE, WITNESSES AND COPIES

A. Signature: By writing this advance directive, I ask that my wishes, as stated, be put into effect by those people indicated to make health care decisions for me when I can no longer make them for myself. I have talked about the terms of this agreement with my health care representative. He or she has willingly agreed to accept the responsibility for making decisions for me according to this advance directive. I understand the purpose and effect of this document. I am signing it willfully, voluntarily and after careful consideration.

Signed today on (month, day, year) _____

Signature _____

Name (print name)_____

Address _____City _____ State _____ Zip _____

B. Witnesses: I state that the person who signed this document above did so in my presence, and appears to be of sound mind and free of duress or undue influence to complete this advance directive. I am 18 years of age or older, and am not designated by this or any other document as this person's health care representative.

1. Witness signature_____ Date _____

   Print witness name_____

   Address _____ City _____State _____ Zip _____

2. Witness signature_____ Date _____

   Print witness name_____

   Address _____ City _____State _____ Zip _____

C. COPIES: A copy of this advance directive has been given to the following people: **(It is important to provide your doctor, your health care representative, and appropriate family members or friends with a copy of this document. You keep the original.)**

1. Name_____

   Address _____ City _____ State_____ Zip _____

   Telephone number _____

2. Name_____

   Address _____ City _____ State_____ Zip _____

   Telephone number _____

COPY OF THIS DIRECTIVE SHOULD BE GIVEN TO YOUR HEALTH CARE REPRESENTATIVE, YOUR DOCTOR, AND APPROPRIATE FAMILY MEMBERS OR FRIENDS.

*Developed by the Health Literacy Committee
of Saint Peter's University Hospital.*

E

Jewish Advance Directives

Jewish Medical Directives for Health Care

The Committee on Jewish Law and Standards
The Rabbinical Assembly

This Medical Directive has been approved by The Committee on Jewish Law and Standards of The Rabbinical Assembly which serves as halakhic guide for the Conservative Movement.

Rabbi Aaron L. Mackler, Chairman of the Law Committee's Subcommittee on Biomedical Ethics, served as editor of this document which is based upon papers authored by Rabbi Avram I. Reisner, Beth Tikvah-New Milford Jewish Center and Rabbi Elliot Dorff, University of Judaism.

INSTRUCTION DIRECTIVE TO GUIDE HEALTH CARE DECISIONS

NAME _____

I am a Jew. I express that affiliation in a variety of ways in my life, and I want Jewish teachings and values to guide and inform the way in which I live through all times in my life, including times when I may be temporarily unable to communicate, am seriously ill, or in the final stages of my life. I know that at some point I may not be able to make decisions about my health care, and so I have completed this form to help make my wishes known.

Judaism values life and demands that we seek medical care. I share Judaism's respect for my body, the creation and possession of God, and I consequently wish that all prudent medical treatment be extended to me with the aim of effecting my recovery. Nothing in this directive should be construed as a wish to die, but rather as a wish to live in accordance with the traditions of Judaism and God's desires. In accordance with the Jewish tradition's respect for the life God has given us and its consequent bans on murder and suicide, I unequivocally reject any form of active euthanasia ("mercy killing") or assisted suicide.

I ask that my health care agent, and anyone else participating in the making of medical decisions on my behalf, consider carefully my wishes as reflected in this document or otherwise ascertainable. This document should not be understood as a rejection of care, but as an indication of my preferences about medical care, including desires to have specific types of treatments administered. I understand that my wishes as expressed in this document, or as articulated by my health care agent or another surrogate deciding on my behalf, will not have greater power to compel treatment than would be the case if I could contemporaneously state my views.

I intend this document to help guide my medical care in a variety of situations, including the last period of my life. Let me say in advance that I fully appreciate the loving care given to me by my family and friends and by members of the health care professions. If I cannot thank you personally at that time, I wish to do so now from the depths of my heart. You are performing a true act of "hesed," an act of devotion and love. If the pain I suffer at that time makes me cranky and hard to tolerate, please forgive me. Please understand that I may not be in control of my reactions at that time and that, no matter what I say or do, I deeply appreciate the many kindnesses you have bestowed upon me throughout life and especially at that critical stage. In the tradition of our people, I ask that the spirit, strength and comfort of God abide with us always.

PROXY DIRECTIVE
Durable Power of Attorney for Health Care

1.   I, _____, hereby appoint:

name _____

address _____

phone number(s) _____

as my health care agent to make health care decisions for me. This proxy shall take effect when and if I become unable to make or communicate my own health care decisions, due to physical or mental incapacity, and shall remain effective during the period of incapacity.

My agent should make decisions in accord with my wishes. If my wishes are not known and cannot with reasonable diligence be ascertained, my agent should decide in accord with my best interests. In either case, decisions should to the extent reasonably possible reflect my beliefs and values, including my commitment to Jewish teachings as understood within Conservative Judaism.

My agent should consult with one or more health care professionals before making health care decisions for me. I want my agent to be able to receive all medical information and records necessary to make informed decisions regarding my health care.

2. Instructions for agent: *(Please mark one statement)*

☐   In an associated *instruction directive* I have expressed some of my preferences concerning health care decisions that may arise. I want my agent strictly to follow that document, and only to rely on other sources of knowledge about my wishes and values in situations not covered therein.

☐   In an associated *instruction directive* I have expressed some of my preferences concerning health care decisions that may arise. I realize, however, that I cannot fully anticipate what will happen to me in years to come, future developments in medical practice, or the particular health care decisions which will have to be made on my behalf. I want my agent to be able to draw on all sources of knowledge about my wishes and values, and to have ultimate authority to make decisions for me if I cannot do so for myself.

☐   I have not completed any document expressing preferences with regard to health care decisions. My agent should consider all sources of knowledge about my wishes and values.

Other instructions: _____

_____

A. GENERAL VIEWS

1. Goals of treatment: *(Please mark one statement)*

Approved by All:*

Inconsistent with Rabbi Reisner's opinion:*

☐   It is my wish that all prudent medical treatment should be extended to me with the aim of effecting my recovery. Should that be deemed impossible, all nutrition, hydration, medication and necessary surgical procedures should be continued where these are understood to be effective measures for extending my life. Medical knowledge, however, may find itself at a loss as to which form of treatment is best for me, or whether a given treatment will be helpful or harmful. In such circumstances I would want a course of action that protects me from unnecessary pain and degradation while pursuing the goal of life.

☐   *It is my wish that all prudent medical treatment should be extended to me with the aim of effecting my recovery. Should that be deemed impossible, I want those caring for me to act for my benefit, interpreting that value in light of the choices I have made below and any other knowledge you have of me. In some cases in which I am terminally ill or permanently unconscious, choices to withhold or stop life-sustaining treatment may be consistent with my wishes and my understanding of Jewish teachings.*

Comments:_____

_____

2. Knowledge of my condition: *(Please mark one statement)*

☐   I wish to know all relevant facts of my condition. I can cope better with a known threat than with the unknown.

☐   I do not wish to know all the details of my condition, especially if the news is bad. I fear that such knowledge will diminish my will to live and will cast a shadow over the time left to me.

Comments:_____

_____

3. Health care agent: *(Please mark one statement)*

☐   In an associated proxy directive I have appointed _____ as my health care agent to make decisions on my behalf. I want my agent strictly to follow this document, and only to rely on other sources of knowledge about my wishes and values in situations not covered by this document.

☐   In an associated proxy directive I have appointed _____ as my health care agent to make decisions on my behalf. I cannot fully anticipate what will happen to me in years to come, future developments in medical practice, or the particular health care decisions which will have to be made on my behalf. While I am filling out this document to educate myself and give my agent some idea of my attitudes in these matters, my agent should draw on all sources of knowledge about my wishes and values. It is not this document, but my agent, who has ultimate authority to make decisions for me if I cannot do so for myself.

☐   I have not appointed a health care agent. I would want those making decisions on my behalf to rely on this document in determining my wishes and values.

Comments:_____

_____

*See introduction for explanation.

The Rabbinical Assembly

4. Rabbinic consultation: *(Please mark one statement)*

☐   If I can make my own decisions about my health care when critical decisions must be made, I intend to consult my rabbi for further advice about the specific issues which arise in the medical situation in which I actually find myself. If I cannot make my own decisions regarding my care, I would ask that those making decisions for me likewise review them with my rabbi:

name _____

address _____

phone number(s) _____

Should he or she be unavailable, it is my wish that some other Conservative rabbi be consulted. If no Conservative rabbi is readily available, The Rabbinical Assembly (3080 Broadway, New York, NY 10027; (212) 280-6000) should be contacted for an appropriate referral.

☐   I would leave the decision about rabbinic consultation to the discretion of those deciding on my behalf.

Comments:_____

B. IRREVERSIBLE, TERMINAL ILLNESS:

If I am diagnosed with an irreversible terminal illness, such that death is expected within six months no matter what treatment is provided, and if that diagnosis is confirmed by more than one physician, the following statements should assist my agent or other decision maker in deciding on my behalf.

1. Diagnostic tests if I am terminally ill: *(Please mark one statement)*

☐   I wish to have available all possible information concerning my condition. Should I be unable to understand such information at the time, I wish my agent, family members, and physicians to have such information available. Even if my condition is medically hopeless, further analysis of my disease may someday help doctors help someone else, including members of my own family who may be prone to the same disease.

☐   I do not wish to have diagnostic tests performed on me unless they are clearly related to the effort to make me well.

Comments:_____

---

2. Surgery if I am terminally ill: *(Please mark one statement)*

Approved by All:

☐   I would consent to reasonable surgery as proposed by my physicians.

☐   All surgery carries an implicit risk through anesthesia, the increased possibility of infection, and trauma to the body. I do not consent to such risk except if it is required to extend my life, to restore me to health, or to free me from unbearable pain.

Comments:_____

Inconsistent with Rabbi Reisner's opinion:

☐   *All surgery carries an implicit risk through anesthesia, the increased possibility of infection, and trauma to the body. I do not consent to such risk except if it is required to restore me to health or to free me from unbearable pain. I would not accept such risk if it would merely prolong my life.*

The Rabbinical Assembly

3. Amputation if I am terminally ill: *(Please mark one statement)*

☐   I desire above all to live. I am prepared to lose a limb if, in the best medical judgment of my physicians, this is necessary in order to prolong my life.

☐   There may come a time when my physicians feel that my life is threatened by infection, and that the most effective defense lies in amputation of the affected limb. I find the notion of amputation unbearable, and the risk of such an operation intolerable. I prefer all other treatments to fight the infection, even if they are significantly less likely to prolong my life.

Comments:_____

_____

4. Modes of feeding if I am terminally ill: If I am not able to feed myself or to eat and drink through the mouth even with the help of others, the following would represent my wishes: *(Please mark one statement)*

Approved by All:

☐   I would want to receive artificial nutrition and hydration (food and water delivered through a tube) when this would help to strengthen my body, improve my well-being or prolong my life. I understand that this procedure may at some point require restraint so that I do not dislodge the tubes (in the case of naso-gastric tubes), or require surgery to place a tube in my stomach or intestine.

☐   I would not want to be fed through feeding tubes at all. I fear the risks that such procedures entail. Whatever nourishment can be provided intravenously should be provided.

Inconsistent with Rabbi Reisner's opinion:

☐   *I would want to receive artificial nutrition and hydration on a trial basis. A decision about continuing treatment should depend on its effectiveness in helping to strengthen my body, improve my well-being or prolong my life; and on the degree of pain or severe discomfort that the treatment appears to impose.*

☐   *I would not want to be fed by artificial means at all. I fear the risks that such procedures entail. I prefer to eat normally for as long as I can, and when I can no longer do that, to let nature take its course.*

Comments:_____

_____

5. Aggressive medical or surgical procedures if I am terminally ill: *(Please mark one statement)*

☐   I wish above all to live. To that end I would undertake any regimen, however difficult, which stands a reasonable chance of helping me.

☐   Aggressive medical or surgical procedures, such as aggressive radiation and chemotherapy, can be most debilitating and destructive. While I desire to fight my disease with all effective tools at my command, I do not wish to undertake treatments which have not been shown to offer meaningful, measurable results. If my physician determines that a given mode of therapy will probably not produce remission or recovery, I prefer to engage in hospice care, accepting the inevitability of my impending death, curbing pain as much as possible, and living out the remainder of my life to the fullest.

Comments:_____

_____

The Rabbinical Assembly

6. Mechanical life support if I am terminally ill: *(Please mark one statement)*

☐   I consider that as long as my brain is still active, even if I must breathe with the aid of life support equipment, my God-given life has not yet been called back. These technologies should therefore be maintained. I recognize, however, that if the total absence of brain activity can be verified, I will be considered dead despite mechanically induced respiration and heartbeat.

☐   If mechanical means of life support cannot contribute to my recovery, I consider them to be impediments to my death at God's behest, even though they may prolong biological function. Therefore, I wish that they be forgone or withdrawn when my agent or designated representative, in conjunction with my physicians, conclude that they offer me no reasonable chance of return to unaided functioning.

Comments:_____

_____

7. Cardiopulmonary resuscitation if I am terminally ill: *(Please mark one statement)*

☐   Should my cardiopulmonary system fail for any reason, in every case I would like the utmost done in my behalf.

☐   If my heart has stopped beating and my condition is such that there is no reasonable expectation of my recovery, I would consider cardiopulmonary resuscitation, by whatever means, to be contrary to God's will, and therefore ask that my body not be subjected to such handling. In such a case I would consider a Do Not Resuscitate order to be appropriate.

Comments:_____

_____

8. Pain relief and risk if I am terminally ill: *(Please mark one statement)*

Approved by All: *Inconsistent with Rabbi Reisner's opinion:*

☐   If I am in pain or significant dis-   ☐   *If I am in pain or significant discomfort, I*
comfort, I desire that I be given appropriate   *desire that I be given appropriate medication and*
medication and other care to relieve my pain   *other care to relieve my pain and make me as*
and make me as comfortable as possible.   *comfortable as possible. In the unlikely event that*
However, I do not want any treatment which   *no alternative measures could adequately reduce*
would impose a risk of greater than 50% of   *my symptoms, I would want sufficiently large*
hastening my death.   *dosages of medication to avoid pain even if such*
                                                 dosages may entail great risk of the side effect of
                                                 indirectly shortening my life.

Comments:_____

_____

9. Pain relief and sedation if I am terminally ill: *(Please mark one statement)*

☐   I will accept considerable periods of sedation to avoid pain.

☐   If I remain alert, I am prepared to accept a reasonable amount of pain in order to maintain my awareness.

Comments:_____

_____

10. Hospital or home care if I am terminally ill: *(Please mark one statement)*

☐   I prefer to be supported by the best medical technology. To that end, if my death is not sudden, I wish that it occur in the confines of a hospital.

☐   To the extent that it is practicable and not an undue hardship upon my family, I would prefer to die at home or in a congenial supportive care facility such as a hospice rather than in a hospital. When hospital care is no longer able with confidence to effect my recovery, I would prefer such comfort-oriented care, with the clear understanding that all essential medical care that would accord with my wishes will be continued.

Comments:_____

_____

C. PERMANENT LOSS OF CONSCIOUSNESS:

If I am diagnosed to be permanently unconscious, a diagnosis tested over a reasonable period of time and confirmed by more than one physician with appropriate training and expertise, but I am not terminally ill, the following statements should assist my agent or other decision maker in deciding on my behalf.

1. Cardiopulmonary resuscitation if I am permanently unconscious: *(Please mark one statement)*

☐   Should my cardiopulmonary system fail for any reason, and there is a reasonable likelihood that cardiopulmonary resuscitation would be effective in extending my life, I would like the utmost done in my behalf.

☐   If my heart has stopped beating and my condition is such that there is no reasonable expectation of my recovery of consciousness, I would consider cardiopulmonary resuscitation, by whatever means, to be contrary to God's will, and therefore ask that my body not be subjected to such handling. In such a case I would consider a Do Not Resuscitate order to be appropriate.

Comments:_____

_____

The Rabbinical Assembly

2. Other treatments if I am permanently unconscious: *(Please mark one statement)*

Approved by All:

☐   I would want to receive all treatments that would be effective in extending my life, including mechanical interventions such as respirators, even if there is no reasonable hope of my regaining consciousness.

☐   All nutrition, hydration, medication, and necessary surgical procedures should be continued where these are understood to be effective measures for extending my life, even if there is no reasonable hope of my regaining consciousness. I would consider mechanical means of life support to be an impediment to my death, and would want them withheld or withdrawn.

Inconsistent with Rabbi Reisner's opinion:

☐   *All means of nutrition and hydration should be continued where these are understood to be effective measures for extending my life, even if there is no reasonable hope of my regaining consciousness. I would want any machines or medications (including antibiotics) used to keep me alive to be withheld or withdrawn.*

☐   *If there is no reasonable hope of my regaining consciousness, I would want to forgo all treatments and interventions extending my life, including artificial provision of nutrition and hydration, which I consider to be medications. If artificial means of providing nutrition and hydration were used during the period in which my diagnosis was being formed and tested, I hereby ask that the feeding tubes (wherever they are attached to my body) be removed once the diagnosis is confirmed, just as other medications and machines which have proven to be ineffective in effecting my cure may be removed.*

Comments:_____

_____

D. WISHES IN CASE OF DEATH:

1. Organ donation: *(Please mark one statement)*

☐   I am aware that Jewish law permits and commends the donation of organs and other body parts for transplantation. Accordingly, I desire that when I die any or all of my vital organs and other body parts be donated for the purpose of transplantation. The rest of my remains should then be buried in a Jewish cemetery in accordance with Jewish law and custom.

☐   I would want my organs and other body parts to be donated for transplantation only if there is someone who needs them at, or shortly after, the time of my death. The rest of my remains should then be buried in a Jewish cemetery in accord with Jewish law and custom.

☐   I would want the following body parts to be donated for purposes of transplantation:

_____ Kidneys   _____ Heart   _____ Skin   _____ Corneas

_____ Liver   _____ Pancreas   Other _____

The rest of my remains should then be buried in a Jewish cemetery in accord with Jewish law and custom.

☐   I do not wish that any part of my body be used for purpose of transplantation.

Comments:_____

_____

The Rabbinical Assembly

2. Autopsy: *(Please mark one statement)*

Approved by All:

□   I do not want an autopsy performed unless it is absolutely required by government authorities. If such an autopsy is performed, I ask that it be conducted with all possible respect and that all of my body parts subsequently be buried in a Jewish cemetery in accordance with Jewish law and custom.

□   I would allow an autopsy to be performed if necessary to provide information that would help save the life of a family member or other identifiable individual. If any autopsy is performed, I ask that it be conducted with all possible respect and that all of my body parts subsequently be buried in a Jewish cemetery in accordance with Jewish law and custom.

Inconsistent with Rabbi Reisner's opinion:

□   *I would allow an autopsy to be performed either to help save the life of an individual or if it would enable physicians to learn more about my disease because my case is not routine. If any autopsy is performed, I ask that it be conducted with all possible respect and that all of my body parts subsequently be buried in a Jewish cemetery in accordance with Jewish law and custom.*

Comments:_____

_____

As God is my rock and my fortress and my deliverer, so may God be my refuge, my shield and my salvation, forever.

Signature: _____
Name: _____
Date: _____
Address: _____
City: _____

I declare that the person who signed this document, or asked another to sign this document on his or her behalf, did so in my presence, that I know him or her to be the person named as the subject of this document, and that he or she appears to be of sound mind and acting of his or her free will, free of duress or undue influence. I am eighteen years of age or older, and I am not designated by this or any other document as the person's health care agent or alternate health care agent.

Witness 1:   Witness 2:
Signature _____   Signature _____
Name _____   Name _____
Date _____   Date _____
Address _____   Address _____
City _____   City _____

Notarization is not necessary unless required by your state law.

The Rabbinical Assembly

F

Muslim Advance Directives

Chapter 4

III. Advance Medical Directives

A. About *Resuscitation / Life Support*

1. Life. Life is a gift from our Maker provided in the form of a physical body, soul, a manual for its proper daily use (obey the commands of its Creator described in the Qur'an) and a purpose (worship the Master, The Creator, in the manner He ordered). The Creator also produced a role model for us to follow certain pathway and avoid other distractions. During this life there are rough times (illnesses) and the solutions (treatments, and not against beliefs) until come to a dead end (death) for a transfer to another destination (Barzukh). Afterwards we will be resurrected for an eventual eternity. We can not change our life span nor commit a suicide (unless plan to be in hell). Every life is sacred regardless of their religious beliefs or lack of; we must respect and appreciate it.

In today's material world we walk about do our daily life affairs half sleep and in some degree of euphoria. As soon as death occurs we suddenly become fully alert and wake up to reality of the (inescapable) and;

You will see with absolute certainty with your own eyes (the Real Truth). Then you will be asked on that day about every blessing that you had received (from Allah (SWT) while living). (Surah Takathur 102: 7-8)

ثُمَّ لَتَرَوُنَّهَا عَيْنَ الْيَقِينِ ﴿٧﴾ ثُمَّ لَتُسْـَٔلُنَّ يَوْمَئِذٍ عَنِ النَّعِيمِ ﴿٨﴾

2. Illness. When an illness is terminal or so seems to be, for this one must think ahead and be prepared to face the ultimate truth. Ask the following questions with the help of medical experts and scholars. Is this treatment likely to succeed or merely prolonging the time on artificial ventilation, other machines or other treatments 'which if withdrawn will result in death. *"End of the life"* may not be easily visible to the family members but the medical team familiar and working with the given patient may give some insight about odds ratio or the likelihood from their experiences, but only Allah (SWT) knows the actual Truth of the final time. Discuss and educate yourself ahead of time. It is not un-Islamic.

3. A Decision. When some one is critically ill and is hooked to life support equipment, a decision needs to be made as to what point the *futile* forms of the medical procedures to sustain organ functions should be terminated when the actual existence of the soul in the body is extremely doubtful. A brain dead person is in deep coma and no sign or chance of recovery. So if the treatment is not a treatment (change in outcome) but is an attempt to keep the patient "alive" then one (who has the power of attorney or such decision making authority) must make a realistic and perhaps a tough decision to let the departing soul go and stop the agony of dying. Everyone involved in this process needs to understand this. In reality we must think ahead, should one come to such a cross road and a decision is required. What would you decide then, if you were able to and under these circumstances you wouldn't be?

A person capable of making sound decisions should learn, and discuss in advance the possible medical issues and that after a preferred and or alternative choices of a treatment plan is/are selected are made, when enough is enough ? Those who help or actually make such decisions should also consider patient's *values, intensity of illness, preferences of the patient, available treatment options, and real likelihood of success (not just a delay)* based upon a honest information from the involved medical provider/s. Express these concerns or decisions ahead of time during health, with your family and also in your documents of the Will. These are called *Advance Medical Directives* in relation to any possible heroic treatment measures at the end of life situation. *Table 4:1* outlines some of these considerations for you to express in your Living Will and the Durable Power of Attorney.

My Advance Medical Directives;

In the event a medical emergency arises and I am unable to voice my choices for my health care, the following guidelines should be observed and added to my Living Will and the Durable Power of Attorney.

My name _____ social security # _____

	Yes-(Full)	Yes-(Reasonable trial)	No
1. CPR (cardio-pulmonary Resuscitation)___			
2. Intubations, Ventilation___			
3. Intravenous Lines, Medications, all___			
4. Feeding Tubes, (stomach, intravenous) ___			
5. Dialysis___			
6. Pace Maker, Intra-Aortic Balloon Pump___			
7. Maintain Life Support (all the way)___			
8. Placement issue;			
Intensive Care___			
Nursing Home/Rehab Unit___			
9. Other___			

10. My desire for Organ/s Donation is _____ No _____Yes (which one/s) _____

_____

_____

In case I am unable to make my own decision/s about my health care then this power of decision making will be given to _____

Whose social security # is _____

Address _____

_____

My relationship is _____

My signature _____ Date _____

Witness _____ Witness_____

4. CPR. Ordinarily, Cardio-Pulmonary-Resuscitation is done in many situations when a person suddenly collapses and resuscitated by providing simple basic thump on the chest and blowing air into his/her mouth and sequentially compressing the chest to restart or maintain the life. When CPR is done by the medical personnel after few cardiac shocks, often more patients recover provided no pre-existing or new irreparable damage has occurred to the heart or brain that cannot be recovered. CPR is not against Islamic beliefs. Every one should learn CPR to help some one else, some day help may be returned to you too, unexpectedly. **DNR,** *do not resuscitate* orders written in the medical records imply that when a patient suffers a cardiac arrest no CPR is to be performed. It is requested by the authorized guardian or "agent" of the patient with Durable Power of Attorney or from prior Living Will of the patient.

5. Death. Upon death, the soul departs from the dimension of the human body in which it lived in, leaving behind a lifeless and helpless heap of flesh, the body. Death is defined in various different ways by the religious (spiritual) and medical (physical) experts in their fields. In a given situation some times there may be confusion in defining it.
If this definition is given:
- By Islamic Scholars (Ulamaa); it is when the soul leaves the body.
- By the medical doctors; when heart (circulatory system)and lungs (respiratory system) stop working without recovery or when all functions of the brain (including the brain stem) stop working and no brain activity is present without any recovery (brain dead).

These determinations are made by appropriate specialists. These medical findings of the brain death with no recovery suggest that the person is in deepest form of coma. Does that mean the soul has now departed with no return (has death occurred)? Mechanical ventilation by artificial means can continue the heart, kidney, and lung functions for a long time. The heart and kidneys can function for a short while in a *brain dead* person. Soon the heart will stop beating too, once the ventilator is turned off.

B. Living Will and Durable Power of Attorney
There are some differences in these forms of the representations and are briefly described.
The Living Will. This represents patient's autonomy and the preferences and is used only to refuse the life prolonging measures in the usual settings of terminal illness. It is invoked under the presumption that the patient has adequate knowledge as what will be withheld after refusing of the life prolonging interventions.
The Durable Power of Attorney. This is to be exercised by the patient's designated "agent" who is supposed to know which alternatives are available to manage the patient's health condition, besides patient's preferences and values. Loss of decision making capacity of the patient is the only requirement to enact this permit of conveyance to another person so authorized, to make health care decisions.

C. About Autopsy
This is not be done unless it is required for medico-legal reasons to determine cause of death or required by coroner in case of murder, (poisoning, etc.) or in the cause of

scientific research for the advancement of medical knowledge for helping humanity. Body desecration is un-Islamic.

D. About Organ Donation

This issue needs serious reflections by every Muslim because we may be sometime confronted with the situation. There are no clear directions or rules in the Qur'an and Sunnah. The Islamic scholars of Fiqh have expressed opinions both against organ removal, transplantation during life or other after death, or in agreement for transplantation, in given situations.

1. Mutilation of Body

If the organs are removed from the dead body with the intention to insult, degrade transgression or damage or the *mutilation* of any parts of the body it will be a grave sin and injustice and is strictly prohibited in Islam. Any form of disrespect to the corpse is forbidden. The body is created by Allah (SWT) and He owns all of the rights without exceptions, and is not subject to inheritance either. There can be no monetary values attached to it. We must honor it because Allah (SWT) has given the honor (Surah 17:70)

2. Organ Removal

The removal of organs for the sole purpose of helping someone else to improve quality or extend the lifespan by the Will of Allah (SWT) should be considered, not a mutilation, but an extension of a helping hand. This is true in both the living donor for kidney transplant or cornea/heart, etc. posthumously. As long as the donated organ is functioning in the new body who is enjoying its living benefits, it should be viewed conceptually as better than its decay, destruction and eventual disappearance in the dead body. By doing this, organ donation can be considered for receiving an ongoing reward for the deceased for helping someone live, either longer life or give better quality of life? Sadaqa-e-Jariyah! Therefore the loss to the deceased for not having an organ in the body physically is far less than the gains and honoring of the life of the living without intention of disrespect to the dead. This is why most of the contemporary Islamic scholars have given their approval in support of organ donation. NOT a befitting example but:

The *mo'min* prioritize others over their own needs (   ), whenever a situation arises as exemplified by the Sahabah in the battlefield. When those who were badly injured and were in need of water and upon hearing someone else's voice for water, they would refuse to drink and pass it on first for other/s (to drink) who in turn will repeat the same act, despite the desperate need of their own to the point of losing life.

3. Those who are against it

They cite the following reasons:

    a. Verses from Surah *Nisa* 4:29 and Surah *Baqara* 2:195. Don't kill yourself or contribute to your own destruction.

    b. Hadith; breaking up the bone of a dead person is a sin equal to the sin and aggression of doing the same to him or her when the person is alive.

    c. Body and its parts are as Amanah and we are to take good care of them until we meet our Creator (from Hadith), just as we take care of the body and its parts during life.

d. When in doubt, don't do it. Good and bad are clearly evident. It's the in-between we must be even more careful lest we stray into the forbidden (from Hadith).

4. Supporters of organ donation

They reason the following;

a. Breast-feeding of the baby by the nanny is the transfer of one part (milk) of a body into another, is already well-known and permissible in Islam.

b. One companion of the prophet (S) who had his nose cut off in a battle implanted an artificial cover over it, made of gold (sort of a metallic prosthesis). Prophet (S) permitted it.

c. Blood transfusion is fluid shaped but an organ of the body transferred to another.

d. Needs of the necessity of saving or improving quality of a life of a living person are to be given preference over the needs of the dead by transplanting organ from the dead into the living.

e. Fatwas are issued in favor of organ transplant by scholars from Makkah, Jeddah, and India, when such a necessity arises and benefits are clearly defined, trained experts are able and available to perform the procedure and the suitable donors are available willingly, except corneal (eye) and the heart transplants, which can be taken only from the already deceased donor. These opinions are issued by:

    1. *Council of Islamic Fiqh Academy of the Muslim World League*, Makkah (1985)

    2. *Council of Islamic Fiqh Academy of the Organization of Islamic Conference* Jeddah, Saudi Arabia (1988)

    3. *Islamic Fiqh Academy* – New Delhi, India (1989)

5. Pre-requisites/Conditions for Organ Donation

A. Adult, sane, alert, legally competent and fully beware of the situation as what is about to happen. Such consent must be in writing, notarized and be specific about such willingness and about which organs to be donated. If there are any changes down the road, they should also be documented in writing either for or against it, about such change of mind.

B. Consenting donor should have it written on a card to be kept in the wallet, should a situation arise unexpectedly it can then be acted upon expediously.

C. If an organ is donated by the living (one out of the two kidneys, part of the liver, bone marrow) then no harm should come to the donor's life.

D. It must be only voluntary without any coercion

E. No monetary gains to the recipient exist; otherwise it can create wrong precedents.

F. This must meet very strict criteria of the established need, urgency, lack of alternative methods, proven benefits exceeding risk, consent of both parties (recipient and donor or all of his /her heirs or documented in the Will) and practical feasibility.

G. Timing. The organ/s especially the most vital ones, must be removed in most desirable timely manner and transported for immediate implantation other wise delays will result less chances for its success. Less vital organs i.e. bones, cartilage, skin and even cornea can stand the delay up to 12-24 hours if the body is immediately preserved in the cooler. Both the donor's family and the medical workers need to be aware of the urgency.

The organ transplantation can be performed;
1. From the same body, removing one part of it to put it in another location, i.e. skin graft. (Auto Transplant)
1. From one human to another human, i.e. heart, liver, kidney. (Homo Transplant)
2. From animal tissue to humans, i.e. pig heart value into human heart.   (Hetero Transplant)
3. Prosthetic or artificial devices, implantation. Artificial knee or hip joints   replacements, pace maker, artificial heart, or valves, Dacron-fabricated artery, etc.   (Device Implantation)
4. Artificial bone or limbs.

E. A Necessity.
There is growing recognition of the *necessity* and the resulting benefits of organ donation to the mankind in help saving a life or to improve the quality of the living. Giving to or taking an organ from non Muslim is acceptable according to the same scholars although first preference should be given to and from a Muslim whenever it is possible and is available.

Thus one must consider seriously about possible organ donation to be permitted or not permitted on self. During life, organ donation is frequently done and it is both ethically and socially correct and not against Islamic Shariah. Examples; blood transfusion and bone marrow transplantation, kidney, liver, lung transplantation between the close relatives and the life goes on for both donor and the recipient. If this is considered or decided about one way or another, then describe it in the Will, as how do you feel about it, although some scholars disagree its inclusion in the Will. Then how the surviving heirs ought to know what did you want at the given time decision will have to be made? This is in addition to your views or instructions about the *advanced medical directives about life support* during the terminal illness. Discuss with the physicians and Islamic scholars ahead of time for more insight.

Notes

Chapter I

1. Institute of Medicine. (1997). *Approaching death: Improving care at the end of life*. Washington, DC: National Academy Press.

2. Lo, B., Quill, T., & Tulsky, J. (1999). Discussing palliative care with patients. ACP-ASIM End-of-Life Care Consensus Panel. *Annals of Internal Medicine, 130*, 744-749. See also Karlawish, J., Quill, T., & Meier, D. (1999). A consensus-based approach to providing palliative care to patients who lack decision-making capacity. ACP-ASIM End-of-Life Care Consensus Panel. *Annals of Internal Medicine, 130*, 835-840.

3. Remen, R. (1997). *Kitchen table wisdom: Stories that heal*. New York: Riverhead Books.

4. Doyle, D., Hanks, G. W., & MacDonald, N. (Eds.). (1993). The interface between oncology and palliative medicine. In *Oxford textbook of palliative medicine* (pp. 11-17). Oxford: Oxford University Press.

5. SUPPORT Principal Investigators. (1995). A controlled trial to improve care for seriously ill hospitalized patients: The study to understand prognosis and preferences for outcomes and risks of treatment (SUPPORT). *Journal of the American Medical Association, 274*, 1591-1598.

6. Puchalski, C. M. (1999). Touching the spirit: The essence of healing. *Spiritual Life, 45*, 154-159.

7. Wald, F. S. (1986). *In search of the spiritual component of hospice care*. New Haven, CT: Yale University Press.

8. The Hospice Consult. (2002). The hospice consult: A plan to bring palliative care into patients' lives earlier. *State Initiatives in End-of-Life Care, 17*, 7.

9. Ita, D. (1994). Predictors of patient and primary caregiver ability to sustain a planned program of home hospice care. (UMI No. 9526600)

10. Sontag, M., Kerwin, M., & Richason, G. (1994, October). *The UW-EC Hospice Research Project: A national profile of hospice programs and professionals*. Paper presented at the National Hospice Organization, Washington, DC.

11. Ibid.

12. Berube, M. (Ed). (2001). *Webster's II: New College Dictionary*. Boston: Houghton Mifflin.

13. Hardwig, J. (2000, March-April). *Spiritual issues at the end of life: A call for discussion*. (Hastings Center Report, p. 28). New York: Hastings Center.

14. Koetzsch, R. (1996). *Conference on dying and the inner life*. Kalamazoo, MI: The Fetzer Institute.

15. Ellor, J. (1997). Spiritual well-being defined. *Aging and Spirituality, xi*, 1.

16. Ibid.

17. Association of American Medical Colleges. (1999). *Report III—Contemporary issues in medicine: Communication in medicine, Medical School Objectives Project (MSOP III)*. Washington, DC: Association of American Medical Colleges.

18. Frankl, V. (1984). *Man's search for meaning*. New York: Simon & Schuster.

19. Reese, D. J., & Brown, D. R. (1997). Psychosocial and spiritual care in hospice: Difference between nursing, social work and clergy. *The Hospice Journal, 12*, 29-41.

20. Larson, D. B., & Larson, S. S. (Eds.). (1994). *The forgotten factor in physical and mental health: What does the research show?* Rockville, MD: National Institute for Healthcare.

21. Ibid.

22. Puchalski, M. P., Kilpatrick, S. D., McCullough, M. E., & Larson, D. B. (2003). A systematic review of religious variables in palliative medicine. *Palliative and Supportive Care, 1*, 7-13.

23. Puchalski, C. M. (2001). Reconnecting the science and art of medicine. *Academic Medicine, 76*, 1224-1225.

24. Boston, P., Mount, B. M., Orenstein, S., & Freedman, O. (2001). Spirituality, religion, and health: The need for qualitative research. *Annals, CRMCC, 34*, 368-374.

25. Gallup, G. (1990). *Religion in America*. Princeton, NJ: Princeton Religion and Research Center.

26. The Gallup Organization for CNN/USA Today. (1999). Survey of 1,037 adults 18 years and older. *USA Today*, December 9-12, 1999.

27. Reed, P. G. (1987). Spirituality and well-being in terminally ill hospitalized adults. *Research in Nursing and Health, 10*, 335-344.

28. Reed, P. G. (1986). Religiousness in terminally ill and healthy adults. *Research in Nursing & Health, 9*, 35-41.

29. Thomas, J. M., Jr., & Weiner, E. A. (1974). Psychological differences among groups of critically ill hospitalized patients, noncritically ill hospitalized patients, and well controls. *Journal of Consulting and Clinical Psychology, 42*, 274-279.

30. Roberts, J. A. et al. (1997). Factors influencing views of patients with gynecological cancer about end-of-life decisions. *American Journal of Obstetrics and Gynecology, 176*, 166-172.

31. Conrad, N. L. (1985). Spiritual support for the dying. *Nursing Clinics of North America, 20*, 415-26. Moberg, D. O. (1982). Spiritual well-being of the dying. In G. Lesnoff-Caravaglia (Ed.), *Aging in the human condition* (pp. 139-155). New York: Human Sciences Press.

32. The George H. Gallup International Institute. (1997). *Spiritual beliefs and the dying process: A report on a national survey*. Conducted for the Nathan Cummings Foundation and the Fetzer Institute 2, 31-43. Available at www.ncf.org. New York: Nathan Cummings Foundation.

33. Ibid.

34. Ibid.

35. Gallup, G. (1990). *Religion in America*. Princeton, NJ: Princeton Religion and Research Center.

36. McNichol, T. (1996). The new faith in medicine. *USA Weekend*, April 5-7:4-5. Survey conducted of 1,000 U.S. adults for *USA Weekend* Feb. 16-20, 1996, by ICR Research Group.

37. Ehman, J. W. et al. (1999). Do patients want physicians to inquire about their spiritual or religious beliefs if they become gravely ill? *Archives of Internal Medicine, 159*, 1803-1806.

38. King, D. E., & Bushwick, B. (1994). Beliefs and attitudes of hospital inpatients about faith, healing, and prayer. *Journal of Family Practice, 39*, 349-352.

39. Yankelovich Partners, Inc., for TIME/CNN, June 12-13, 1996.

40. McNichol, T. (1996). The new faith in medicine, *USA Weekend*, April 5-7:4-5. Survey conducted of 1,000 U.S. adults for *USA Weekend* Feb. 16-20, 1996, by ICR Research Group.

41. Levin, J. S., & Schiller, P. L. (1987). Is there a religious factor in health? *Journal of Religion and Health, 25*, 9-36. Levin, J. S., Larson, D. B., & Puchalski, C. M. (1997). Religion and spiri-

tuality in medicine: Research and education. *Journal of the American Medical Association, 278*, 792-793.

42. Larson, D. B., & Larson, S. S. (Eds.). (1994). *The forgotten factor in physical and mental health: What does the research show?* Rockville, MD: National Institute for Healthcare. Craigie, F. C., Jr., Liu, I. Y., Larson, D. B., & Lyons, J. S. (1988). A systematic analysis of research on religious variables. *Journal of Family Practice, 27*, 509-513. Larson, D. B. et al. (1986). Systematic analysis of research on religious variables in four major psychiatric journals. *American Journal of Psychiatry, 143*, 329-334.

43. Oxman, T. E., Freeman, D. H., & Manheimer, E. D. (1995). Lack of social participation of religious strength and comfort as risk factors for death after cardiac surgery in the elderly. *Psychosomatic Medicine, 57*, 5-15.

44. Cook, J. A., & Wimberly, D. W. (1983). If I should die before I wake: Religious commitment and adjustment to death of a child. *Journal for the Scientific Study of Religion, 22*, 222-238.

45. Roberts, J. A. et al. (1997). Factors influencing views of patients with gynecological cancer about end-of-life decisions. *American Journal of Obstetrics and Gynecology, 176*, 166-172.

46. Yates, J. W. et al. (1981). Religion in patients with advanced cancer. *Medical and Pediatric Oncology, 9*, 121-128.

47. McNeill, J. A., Sherwood, G. D., Starck, P. L., et al. (1998). Assessing clinical outcomes: Patient satisfaction with pain management. *Journal of Pain and Symptom Management, 16*(1), 29-40

48. Kaldijian, L. C. et al. End of life decisions in HIV patients: The role of spiritual beliefs. *AIDS, 12*, 103-107.

49. Tsevat, J., Puchalski, C. M., Sherman, S. N., et al. (2003). Spirituality and religion in patients with HIV/AIDS. *JGIM, 18*(suppl 1), 234.

50. Cohen, S. R., Mount, B. M., Strobel, M. G., et al. (1995). The McGill Quality of Life Questionnaire: A measure of quality of life appropriate for people with advanced disease. *Palliative Med, 9*, 207-219.

51. Alcoholics Anonymous. (1976). *Alcoholics Anonymous.* New York: World Services.

52. Puchalski, C. M. (2003). *Caregiver stress: The role of spirituality in the lives of family/friends and professional caregivers.* Americus, GA: Caregiving Book Series.

53. Doyle, D. (1992). Have we looked beyond the physical and psychosocial? *Journal of Pain Symptom Management, 7*, 302-311.

54. Folkman, S., Chesney, M., Cooke, M., Coccellari, A., & Collette, L. (1994). Caregiving burden in HIV-positive and HIV-negative partners of men with AIDS. *Journal of Consulting and Clinical Psychology, 62*, 746-756. Reed, P. G. (1987). Spirituality and well being in terminally ill hospitalized adults. *Residential Nursing Health, 10*, 335-344.

55. Cupertino, A. P., Aldwin, C., & Schultz, R. (1998). *Religiosity, emotional strain, and health: The caregiver health effects study.* San Francisco: American Psychiatric Association.

56. Jivanjee, P. (1994). Enhancing the well-being of family caregivers to patients with Alzheimer's disease. *Journal of Gerontological Social Work, 23*, 31-48.

57. Wyatt, G., Friedman, L., Given, C., & Given, B. (1999). A profile of bereaved caregivers following provision of terminal care. *Journal of Palliative Care, 15*, 13-25.

58. Kaye, J., & Robinson, K. (1993). Spirituality among caregivers. *Image: Journal of Nursing Scholarship, 26*, 218-221.

59. Chang, B. H., Noonan, A., & Tennstedt, S. (1998). The role of religion/spirituality in coping with caregiving for disabled elders. *The Gerontologist, 38*, 463-470.

60. Doka, K. J., & Morgan, J. D. (Eds.). (1993). *Death and spirituality.* Amityville, NY: Baywood. Puchalski, C. M. (2002). Spirituality and end-of-life care: A time for listening and caring. *Journal of Palliative Medicine, 5*, 289-294.

61. Foglio, J. P., & Brody, R. (1988). Religion, faith and family medicine. *Journal of Family Practice, 27,* 473-474.

62. Roberts, J. A. et al. (1997). Factors influencing views of patients with gynecologic cancer about end-of-life decisions. *American Journal of Obstetrics and Gynecology, 176,* 166-172.

63. Cook, J. A., & Wimberly, D. W. (1983). If I should die before I wake: Religious commitment and adjustment to death of a child. *Journal for the Scientific Study of Religion, 22,* 222-238.

64. Bearon, L. B., & Koenig, R. G. (1990). Religious cognitions and use of prayer in health and illness. *Gerontologist, 30,* 249-253.

65. Benson, R. (1996). *Timeless healing: The power and biology of belief.* New York: Simon & Schuster.

66. Koenig, H. G. et al. (1997). Attendance at religious services, Interleukin-6, and other biological parameters of immune function in older adults. *International Journal of Psychiatry and Medicine, 27,* 233-350.

67. Stuart, E., Caudeill, M., Leserman, J., Dorrington, C., Friedman, R., & Benson, R. (1987). Nonpharmacologic treatment of hypertension: A multi-risk-factor approach. *Journal of Cardiovascular Nursing, 1,* 1-14.

68. Benson, H., Alexander., S., & Felman, C. L. (1975). Decreased premature ventricular contractions through use of the relaxation response in patients with stable ischemic heart-disease. *Lancet, 2,* 380-382.

69. Caudill, M., Schnable, R., Zuttermeister, P., Benson, H., & Frieman, R. (1991). Decreased clinic use by chronic pain patients: Response to behavioral medicine interventions. *Clinical Journal of Pain, 7,* 305-310.

70. Jacobs, G. D., Benson, H., & Friedman, R. (1996). Perceived benefits in a behavioral-medicine insomnia program: A clinical report. *American Journal of Medicine, 100,* 212-216. Jacobs, G. D., Rosenberg, P. A., Friedman, R., Matheson, J., Peavy, G. M., Domar, A. D., & Benson, H. (1993). Multifactor behavioral treatment of chronic sleep-onset insomnia using stimulus control and the relaxation response: A preliminary study. *Behavior Modification, 17,* 498-509.

71. Benson, H. et al. (1978). Treatment of anxiety: A comparison of the usefulness of self-hypnosis and a meditational relaxation technique. *Psychotherapy and Psychosomatics, 30,* 229-242.

72. Selye, H. (1978). *The stress of life.* New York: McGraw-Hill. Benson, H. (1996). *Timeless healing.* New York: Scribner.

73. Stefano, G. B., Fricchione, G. L., Slingsby, C. T., & Benson, H. (2001). The placebo effect and relaxation response: Neural processes and their coupling to constitutive nitric oxide. *Brain Research Review, 35,* 1-19.

74. Pargament, K. I. et al. (1990). God help me: Religious coping efforts as predictors of the outcomes to significant negative life events. *American Journal of Community Psychology, 18,* 793-824.

75. Pargament, K. I. et al. (1998). Patterns of positive and negative religious coping with major life stresses. *Journal of the Scientific Study of Religion, 37,* 710-724.

76. Rutherford, R. (1980). *The death of a Christian: The rite of funeral.* New York: Pueblo.

77. Klass, D. (1993). Spirituality, protestantism and death. In K. J. Doka & J. D. Morgan (Eds.), *Death and spirituality* (p. 61). Amityville, NY: Baywood.

78. Ryan, D. (1993). Death: Eastern perspectives. In K. J. Doka & J. D. Morgan (Eds.), *Death and spirituality* (p. 81). Amityville, NY: Baywood.

79. Grollman, E. A. (1993). Death in Jewish thought. In K. J. Doka & J. D. Morgan (Eds.), *Death and spirituality* (pp. 25-27). Amityville, NY: Baywood.

80. Vandecreek, L., & Nye, C. (1994). Trying to live forever: Correlates to the belief in life after death. *Journal of Pastoral Care, 48.*

81. Irion, P. E. (1993). Spiritual issues in death and dying for those who do not have conventional religious beliefs. In K. J. Doka & J. D. Morgan (Eds.), *Death and spirituality*. Amityville, NY: Baywood.

82. Meagher, D., & Bell, C. (1993). Perspectives on death in the African American community. In K. J. Doka & J. D. Morgan (Eds.), *Death and spirituality* (pp. 113-119). Amityville, NY: Baywood.

83. Alcoholics Anonymous. (1952). *44 questions: Questions and answers about Alcoholics Anonymous*. New York: AA World Services.

84. Larson, D. B., Larson, S. S., Puchalski, C. M., & Koenig, H. G. (2000). Patient spirituality in clinical care: Clinical assessment and research findings—Part I. *Primary Care Reports, 6*, 165-172. Strachan, J. G. (1982). *Alcoholism: Treatable illness: An honorable approach to man's alcoholism problem*. Center City, MN: The Hazelden Foundation. Koenig, H. G. (1997). Use of religion by patients with severe medical illness. *Mind/Body Medicine, 2*, 31-37.

85. Puchalski, C. M. (2002). Spirituality and end of life care. In A. M. Berger, R. K. Portenoy, & D. E. Weissman (Eds.), *Principles and practice of palliative care and supportive oncology* (2nd ed., pp. 799-812). Philadelphia: Lippincott, Williams & Wilkins. Sulmasy, D. P. (2002). A biopsychosocial-spiritual model for the care of patients at the end of life. *The Gerontologist, 42*, Special issues III, 24-22.

86. Cassel, E. (1982). The nature of suffering and the goals of medicine. *New England Journal of Medicine, 11*, 639.

87. Ibid.

88. Cassel, E. (1991). The importance of understanding suffering for clinical ethics. *Journal of Clinical Ethics, 2*, 81-82.

89. Nouwen, H. J. M. (1972). *The wounded healer: Ministry in contemporary society*. New York: Doubleday.

90. Remen, R. (1997). *Kitchen table wisdom: Stories that heal*. New York: Riverhead.

91. Frankl, V. (2000). *Man's search for meaning*. New York: Perseus.

92. Robert, S. (1996). *Theological perspectives in suffering*. Betty Rolling Ferrell (Ed.). Sudbury, MA: Jones & Bartlett. P. 166.

93. Lo, B., & Tulsky, J. (1999). Discussing palliative care with patients. ACP-ASIM End-of-Life Care Consensus Panel. *Annals of Internal Medicine, 130*, 744-749. Lo, B., Ruston, D., Kates, L. W., Arnold, R., Faber-Langendoen, K., Puchalski, C. M., et al. (2002). Discussing religious and spiritual issues at the end of life: A practical guide for physicians. *Journal of the American Medical Association, 287*, 749-754.

94. Joint Commission on Accreditation of Healthcare Organizations (JCAHO). (1999). *Comprehensive accreditation manual for hospitals (CAMH): The official handbook, patient rights and organization ethics. Update 3, RI-15*. Oakbrook Terrace, IL: CAMH.

95. Puchalski, C. M., & Larson, D. B. (1998). Developing curricula in spirituality and medicine. *Academic Medicine, 73*, 970-974.

96. Association of American Medical Colleges. (1998). *Learning objectives for medical student education: Guidelines for medical schools*. Medical School Objectives Project (MSOP). Washington, DC: American Association of Medical Colleges.

97. Association of American Medical Colleges. (1999). *Report III—Contemporary issues in medicine: Communication in medicine*. Medical School Objectives Project (MSOP III). Washington, DC: Association of American Medical Colleges. P. 25.

98. Ibid.

99. Sulmasy, D. P. (1999). Is medicine a spiritual practice? *Academic Medicine, 74*, 1002-1005.

Chapter 2

1. Walter, T. (2002). Spirituality in palliative care: Opportunity or burden. *Palliative Medicine, 16*, 133-139.

2. Ibid., p. 133.

3. Ibid., p. 138.

4. Ibid., p. 138.

5. Ibid., p. 133.

6. Ibid., p. 138.

7. Shea, J. (2000). *Spirituality and healthcare: Reaching toward a holistic future.* Chicago: The Park Ridge Center. P. 15.

8. Ibid., p. 6.

9. Ibid., p. 24.

10. Ibid., p. 38.

11. Koenig, H. G. (2002). *Spirituality in patient care: Why, how, when, and what.* Radnor, Pennsylvania: Templeton Foundation. P. 2.

12. Ibid., p. 56.

13. Ibid., p. 66.

14. Koenig, H. G. (2002). *Spirituality in patient care: Why, how, when, and what.* Radnor, Pennsylvania: Templeton Foundation. P. 2.

15. Ibid., p. 66.

Chapter 3

1. HH The Dalai Lama. (1999). *Ethics for the new millennium.* New York: Riverhead.

2. Berube, M. (Ed). (2001). *Webster's II: New college dictionary.* Boston: Houghton Mifflin.

3. HH The Dalai Lama & Cutler, H. (1998). *The art of happiness.* New York: Riverhead. P. 114.

4. O'Donnell, E. (2003). Editorial. *Spiritual Life, 49,* 1.

5. Remen, R. N. (1997). *Kitchen table wisdom: Stories that heal.* New York: Riverhead.

6. Post, S. (2002, June). "Unlimited love," Why this choice of words? Available at http://www.unlimitedloveinstitute.org/publications/pdf/research_news/June2002.PDF

7. HH The Dalai Lama. (1999). *Ethics for the new millennium.* New York: Riverhead. P. 131.

8. Puchalski, C. M., & Larson, D. B. (1998). Developing curricula in spirituality and medicine. *Academic Medicine, 73,* 970. Sulmasy, D. P. (1999). Is medicine a spiritual practice? *Academic Medicine, 74,* 1002-1005.

9. HH The Dalai Lama, & Cutler, H. (1999). *Ethics for the new millennium.* New York: Riverhead. P. 126.

10. Post, S. Definition of unlimited love. Available at http://www.unlimitedloveinstitute .org/welcome/index.html. Post, S. G., Puchalski, C. M., & Larson, D. B. (2000). Physicians and patient spirituality: Professional boundaries, competency, and ethics. *Annals of Internal Medicine, 132*(7), 578-583.

11. St. John of the Cross. (1991). The spiritual canticle. In *The collected works of St. John of the Cross.* Washington, DC: ICS Publications.

12. Post, S. G. http://www.unlimitedloveinstitute.org/welcome/index.html.

13. Association of American Medical Colleges. (1999). *Report III—Contemporary issues in medicine: Communication in medicine, Medical School Objectives Project (MSOP III)*. Washington, DC: Association of American Medical Colleges. P. 25.

14. Quill, T. (2001). *Caring for patients at the end-of-life: Facing an uncertain future together*. New York: Oxford University Press. Pp. 41-42.

15. Remen, R. N. (1997). *Kitchen table wisdom: Stories that heal*. New York: Riverhead.

16. HH Dalai Lama, & Cutler, H. (1998). *The art of happiness*. New York: Riverhead. P. 18.

17. Leighton, S. When mortality calls—don't hang up. *Spiritual Life, 22*, 150-157.

18. DiBlasi, Z., Harkness, E., Ernest, E., Georgiou, A., & Kleinjnen, J. (1997). Influence of context effects on health outomes: A systematic review. Conducted for the Nathan Cummings Foundation and the Fetzer Institute. Available at http://www.ncf.org/reports/rpt_fetzer_contents.html. Bensing, J. (1991). Doctor-patient communication and quality of care. *Soc Sci Medicine, 32*, 1301-1310. Backmeyer, J. (1981). Doctor-patient relationships: The heart of the matter. *Alumni Bulletin School of Dentistry* [Indiana University], 34-36. Inui, T. S., Carter, W. B., Kukull, W. A., & Haigh, V. H. (1982). Outcome-based doctor-patient interaction analysis: I. *Medical Care, 20*, 535-549. Carter, W. B., Inui, T. S., Kukull, W. A., & Haigh, V. H. (1982). Outcome-based doctor-patient interaction analysis: II. Identifying effective patient behavior. *Medical Care, 20*, 550-566.

19. Inui, T. S. (1998). Establishing the doctor-patient relationship: Science, art, or competence? *Schweizerische Medizinische Wochenschrift, 128*, 225-230.

20. Bond, B. R. (1994). Doctor-patient relationships. *New Zealand Medical Journal, 107*, 253-254.

21. Peabody, F. W. (1927). *The care of the patient*. Cambridge, MA: Harvard University Press.

22. Poulton, D. C. (1996). Use of the Consultation Satisfaction Questionnaire to examine patients' satisfaction with general practitioners and community nurses. *British Journal of General Practitioners, 46*, 26-31. Carter, W. B., Inui, T. S., Kukull, W. A., & Haigh, V. H. (1982). Outcome-based doctor-patient interaction analysis: II. Identifying effective patient behavior. *Medical Care, 20*, 550-566. Inui, T. S. Establishing the doctor-patient relationship: Science, art, or competence? *Schweizerische Medizinische Wochenschrift, 128*, 225-230. Robertson, W. H. (1985). The problem of patient compliance. *American Journal of Obstetrics and Gynocology, 152*, 948-952. DiBlasi, Z., Harkness, E., Ernest, E., Georgiou, A., & Kleinjnen, J. (2001). Influence of context effects on health outcomes: A systematic review. *Lancet, 10*, 757-762. Mira, J. L., & Aranas, J. (2000). Patient satisfaction as an outcome measure in healthcare. *Medical Clinics of North America, 13*, 26-33. Vaillot, M. (1970). An invitation for life. *American Journal of Nursing*, 268-275. Kushner, L. (1994). *Honey from the rock: An easy introduction to Jewish mysticism*. Woodstock, VT: Jewish Lights. P. 32.

23. Puchalski, C. M. (2003). *Caregiver stress: The role of spirituality in the lives of family/ friends and professional caregivers*. Americus, GA: Caregiving Book Series. Kloosterhouse, V., & Ames, B. (2002). Families use of religion/spirituality as a psychosocial resource. *Holistic Nursing, 16*, 61-76. Melynk, B., & Alpert-Gillis, L. (1998). The COPE program: A strategy to improve outcomes of critically ill young children and their parents. *Pediatric Nursing, 24*, 521-527.

24. Burton, L. (1998). The spiritual dimension of palliative care. *Seminars in Oncology Nursing, 14*, 121-128.

25. Henry, L. G., & Henry, J. D. (1999). *Reclaiming soul in healthcare*. Chicago: Health Forum. P. 9.

26. Begley, S., & Underwood, A. (2001, May 7). God and the brain: how we're wired for spirituality. *Newsweek*.

27. Weissman, D., & Abrahm, J. (2002). Education and training in palliative care. In A. M. Berger, R. J. Portenoy, & D. Weissman (Eds.), *Principles and practices: Palliative care and supportive oncology* (2nd ed., pp. 819-830). Philadelphia: Lippincott Williams & Wilkins.

28. What is Real Peace [Web site]. (2003). www.hanefesh.com/Real_Peace_print.htm, National Assembly of Hebrew Students: Stimulating Torah on Real Peace.

29. Niebuhr, R. (1933). The serenity prayer. In H. C. Robbins (Ed.), *Way of light: A manual of praise, prayer and meditation*. New York.

30. Kavanaugh, K. (Ed.). (1980). The Interior castle. In *The collected works of St. Teresa of Avila* (Vol. 2.). (O. Rodrigeuz, Trans.). Washington, DC: ICS Publications.

31. Nouwen, H. J. M. (1972). *The wounded healer: Ministry in contemporary society*. New York: Doubleday.

Chapter 4

1. St. John of the Cross. (1991). The Spiritual Canticle. In *The collected works of St. John of the Cross*. Washington, DC: ICS Publications.

2. Foglio, J., & Brody, H. (1988). Religion, faith, and family medicine. *Journal of Family Practice, 27*, 473-474.

3. Chandler, E. (1999). Spirituality. *The Hospice Journal, 14*, 63-74.

4. Brown, R. M. (1986). Niebuhr, R: His theology in the 1980s. *Christian Century*, p. 66.

5. Ibid.

6. O'Donnell, E. (2003). Editorial. *Spiritual Life, 49*, 1.

7. Doka, K. J., & Morgan, J. D. (Eds.). (1993). *Death and spirituality*. Amityville, NY: Baywood. P. 79.

8. Ibid., p. 147.

9. Ibid., p. 139.

10. Kubler-Ross, E. (1997). *On death and dying*. New York: Scribner's.

11. Dowling, Singh K. (1998). *The grace in dying: How we are transformed spiritually as we die*. San Francisco: Harper.

12. Fieser, J. (Ed.). (2001). Eckhart Meister. In *The internet encyclopedia of philosophy*. Retrieved October 15, 2003, at http://www.utm.edu/research/iep/e/eckhart.htm.

13. St. John of the Cross. (1991). The ascent of Mt. Carmel. In *The collected works of St. John of the Cross* (p. 176). (K. Kavanaugh & O. Rodrigeuz Trans.). Washington, DC: ICS Publications.

14. Morello, S. A. (1995). *Lectio Divina and the practice of Teresian prayer*. Washington, DC: ICS Publications. P. 9.

15. St. John of the Cross. (1991). Saying of light and love. In *The collected works of St. John of the Cross* (p. 97). (K. Kavanaugh & O. Rodrigeuz Trans.). Washington, DC: ICS Publications.

16. St. Teresa of Avila. (1980). The interior castle. In *The collected works of St. Teresa of Avila*. (Vol. 2, pp. 1-7). (K. Kavanaugh & O. Rodrigeuz Trans.). Washington, DC: ICS Publications.

17. St. John of the Cross. (1991). The dark night/The ascent of Mt. Carmel. In *The collected works of St. John of the Cross*. Washington, DC: ICS Publications.

18. Campbell, J. (1968). *The hero with a thousand faces* (2nd ed.). Princeton, NJ: Princeton University Press.

19. Lawrence, R. J. (2002).The witches' brew of spirituality and medicine. *The Annals of Behavioral Medicine, 24*, 74-76. Retrieved October 18, 2003, from http://www.pastoralreport.com/articles/archives/000051.html.

20. Butler, R. (1963). Life review: An interpretation of reminiscence in the aged. *Psychiatry, 24*, 65-76.

21. Campbell, J. (1968). *The hero with a thousand faces* (2nd ed.). Princeton, NJ: Princeton University Press.

22. Puchalski, C. M. (2002). Forgiveness: Spiritual and medical implications. *The Yale Journal for Humanities in Medicine*. Retrieved October 18, 2003, from http://info.med.yale.edu/intmed/hummed/yjhm/spirit/forgiveness/cpuchalski.htm.

23. Worthington, E. L. (1998). *In dimensions of forgiveness*. West Conshohocken, PA: Templeton Foundation. P. 107. Freedman, S. R., & Enright, R. D. (1996). Forgiveness as an intervention goal with incest survivors. *Journal of Counseling and Clinical Psychology, 64*, 983-992. Al-Mabuk, R. H., Enright, R. D., & Cardis, P. A. (1995). Forgiveness education with parentally love-deprved late adolescents. *Journal of Moral Education, 24*, 427-444.

24. St. John of the Cross. (1991). The dark night/The ascent of Mt. Carmel. In *The collected works of St. John of the Cross*. Washingon, DC: ICS Publications.

25. Puchalski, C. M. (2002). Forgiveness: Spiritual and medical implications. *The Yale Journal for Humanities in Medicine*. Retrieved October 18, 2003, from http://info.med.yale.edu/intmed/hummed/yjhm/spirit/forgiveness/cpuchalski.htm.

Chapter 6

1. Haas, J. A. (2001). Physician discontent: A barometer of change and need for intervention. *Journal of General Internal Medicine, 16*, 496. Hadley, J., Mitchell, J. M., Sulmasy, D. P., & Bloche, M. G. (1999). Financial incentives, HMO market penetration, and physicians' practice styles and satisfaction. *Health Services Research, 34*, 307-321. Murray, A., Murray, J. E., Chang, H., Rogers, W. H., Inui, T., & Safran, D. G. (2001). Doctor discontent: A comparison of physician satisfaction in different delivery system settings, 1986 and 1997. *Journal of General Internal Medicine, 16*, 452-459.

2. Sulmasy, D. P. (1997). *The healer's calling: A spirituality for physicians and other healthcare professionals*. New York: Paulist. Pp. 10-12. Astrow, A. B., Puchalski, C. M., & Sulmasy, D. P. (2001). Religion, spirituality, and healthcare: Social, ethical, and practical considerations. *American Journal of Medicine, 110*, 283-287.

3. Heschel, A. J. (1966). *The insecurity of freedom*. New York: Noonday Press/Farrar, Strauss, Giroux. Pp. 24-38.

4. Sulmasy, D. P. (1999). Is medicine a spiritual practice? *Academic Medicine, 74*, 1002-1005.

5. Sulmasy, D. P. (2002). A biopsychosocial-spiritual model for the care of patients at the end of life. *The Gerontologist, 42*(Suppl. 3), 24-33.

6. Remen, R. N. (1997). *Kitchen table wisdom*. New York: Riverhead. Pp. 63-65.

7. Osler, W. (1906). "Aequanimitas." In *Aequanimitas, with other addresses to medical students, nurses, and practitioners of medicine* (3rd ed., p. 5). New York: McGraw-Hill.

8. Ibid., p. 6.

9. Ibid., pp. 7-8.

10. Nicholl, D. (1987). *Holiness*. New York: Paulist. Pp. 145-146.

11. Camus, A. (1991). *The plague*. (S. Gilbert, Trans.). New York: Vintage. P. 219.

12. Bernanos, G. (1965). *The diary of a country priest*. (P. Morris, Trans.). New York: Carroll & Graf. P. 298.

13. Kash, K. M., & Holland, J. C. (1990). Reducing stress in medical oncology house officers: A preliminary report of a prospective intervention study. In H. C. Hendrie & C. Lloyd, (Eds.), *Educating competent and humane physicians* (pp. 83-195). Bloomington, IN: Indiana University Press. Kash, K. M., Holland, J. C., Breitbart, W., Berenson, S., Dougherty, J., Ouellette-Kobasa, S., & Lesko, L. M. (2000). Stress and burnout in oncology. *Oncology, 14,* 1621-1633.

14. Sulmasy, D. P. (1997). *The healer's calling: A spirituality for physicians and other health-care professionals.* New York: Paulist. Pp. 68-70.

15. Short versions of these presentations can be found in the *Yale Journal for Humanities in Medicine* at: http://info.med.yale.edu/intmed/hummed/yjhm/spirit2003/spiritintro2003.htm.

Chapter 8

1. Gyatso, T., & HH The Dalai Lama. (1985). *Kindness, clarity, and insight.* Ithaca, NY: Snow Lion.

2. Rinpochay, L., & Hopkins, J. (1979). *Death, intermediate state and rebirth in Tibetan Buddhism.* London: Rider.

3. Thurman, R. A. F. (1989). *The Tibetan book of the dead.* London: Aquarian.

4. Rinpoche, S. (1992). *The Tibetan book of living and dying.* London: Rider.

5. Carr, C. (1993). Death and near-death: A comparison of Tibetan and Euro-American experiences. *Journal of Transpersonal Psychology, 25.*

6. Kapleau, P. (1987). *The wheel of life and death.* New York: Doubleday.

7. Rinpochay, L., & Hopkins, J. (1979). *Death, intermediate state and rebirth in Tibetan Buddhism.* London: Rider.

8. Gyatso, T., HH The Dalai Lama, et al. (1991). *MindScience: An east-west dialogue.* Boston: Wisdom.

9. Thurman, R. A. F. (1989). *The Tibetan book of the dead.* London: Aquarian.

10. Kapleau, P. (1987). *The wheel of life and death.* New York: Doubleday.

11. Rinpochay, L., & Hopkins, L. (1979). *Death, intermediate state and rebirth in Tibetan Buddhism.* London: Rider.

12. Rinpoche, S. (1992). *The Tibetan book of living and dying.* London: Rider.

13. Kapleau, P. (1987). *The wheel of life and death.* New York: Doubleday.

14. Mullin, G. H. (1986). *Death and dying: The Tibetan tradition.* Ithaca, NY: Snow Lion.

Chapter 9

1. Field, M. J., & Cassel, C. K. (Eds.). (1997). *Approaching death: Improving care at the end of life.* Washington, DC: National Academy Press. P. 4.

2. Sumner, C. H. (1998). Recognizing and responding to spiritual distress. *American Journal of Nursing, 98,* 26-31.

3. O'Gorman, M. L. (2002). Spiritual care at the end-of-life. *Critical Care Nursing in North America, 14,* 171-176.

4. Ibid.

5. Ibid.

6. Byock, I. R. (1996). The nature of suffering and the nature of opportunity at the end-of-life. *Clinics in Geriatric Medicine, 12,* 237-252.

7. Cassell, E. J. (1982). The nature of suffering and the goals of medicine. *New England Journal of Medicine, 306,* 639-645.

8. Frankl, V. E. (1963). *Man's search for meaning.* New York: Washington Square Press/ Simon & Schuster. P. 104.

9. Swigart, V., et al. (1996). Letting go: Family willingness to forgo life support. *Heart & Lung, 25,* 483-494.

10. Ibid.

11. O'Gorman, M. L. (2002). Spiritual care at the end-of-life. *Critical Care Nursing in North America, 14,* 171-176.

12. Dickinson, E. (1978). *Complete poems of Emily Dickinson.* Boston: Little, Brown & Company.

13. Heschel, A. J. (1966). *The insecurity of freedom.* New York: Noonday Press/Farrar, Strauss, Giroux.

14. John Paul II. Address at the Rennweg Hospice in Vienna, Austria, June 21, 1998. Retrieved March 10, 2003, from http://www.macathconf.org/message_to_the_sick_and_sufferin.htm.

15. National Council of Catholic Bishops. (2001). *Ethical and religious directives for Catholic healthcare services.* Washington, DC: United States Catholic Conference Directive 61. P. 23.

16. Ibid.

17. Ibid. Directive 32, p. 15.

18. Ibid. Directive 58, p. 23.

19. Baltimore Plenary Council Staff: The Baltimore catechism: Catechism of Christian Doctrine. (1994). Rockford, IL: TAN Books & Publishers. No. 3, Chapter 13, question 136.

20. Flannery, A. (Ed.). (1996). Constitution on the Sacred Liturgy. In A. Flannery (Ed.), *Documents of the Vatican Council.* Northport, NY: Costello.

21. Glen, G. (2002). Going forth in the spirit. In *Recovering the Riches Of Anointing: A Study of the Sacrament of the Sick: An International Symposium.* Collegeville, MN: National Association of Catholic Chaplains, International Symposium Staff, Liturgical Press. P. 117.

22. Huels, J. M. (1983). Ministers and rites for the sick and dying. In *Recovering the Riches of Anointing* (p. 103).

23. International Commission on English in the Liturgy, A Joint Commission of Catholic Bishop's Conferences. (1983). *Pastoral care of the sick: Rites of Anointing and Viaticum.* New York, NY: Catholic Book Publishing Company. Section 117. P. 100.

24. Ibid., sections 104-107, pp. 93-94.

25. Ibid., section 193, pp. 167-168.

26. The Gallup Organization of Princeton, New Jersey. (1996). Survey to Measure Knowledge and Attitudes Related to Hospice Care and Other End-of-Life Issues. Survey conducted for National Hospice Organization.

Chapter 10

1. Enriching Our Worship 2: Ministry with the Sick and Dying. (2000, December). *Burial of a child.* New York: Church Publishing. P. 127.

2. Frank, A. Quote found on the walls of a cave where Jews were known to have been hiding.

3. Church of England. (1990). *Book of Common Prayer: Burial Rites of the Episcopal Church's.* Oxford University Press. Pp. 491-492.

4. Benson, H., & Klipper, M. (2000). *The relaxation response* [reissue edition]. New York: HarperTorch.

5. Tagore, R. (1969). *Stray birds, XLIV.* In E. Kubler-Ross, *On death and dying.* New York: Tollier / MacMillan.

6. The Holy Bible (RSV). (1952). Matthew 19:14. New York: American Bible Society.

7. Enriching Our Worship 2: Ministry with the Sick and Dying. (2000). *Burial of a child.* New York: Church Publishing. P. 121.

8. Enriching Our Worship 2: Ministry with the Sick and Dying. (2000). *Burial of a child.* New York: Church Publishing. Pp.181-186.

Chapter 11

1. Beth Israel, Continuum Health Partners, Inc. Department of Pain Medicine and Palliative Care. *Definition of palliative care.* Retrieved December 4, 2001, from http://www. stoppain .org /caregivers/spiritual_needs.html/.

2. Brihadaranyaka Upanishada IV.5.15.

3. Death and Dying. *Hinduism today.* Retrieved December 11, 1997, from http:// www .hinduismtoday.com html.

4. Sivananda Saraswati. (2001). *Japa Yoga.* Shivanandnagar, India: Distt Tehri-Garhwal for the Divine Life Society. P. 52.

5. Ibid., p. 63.

6. Ibid., p. 44.

7. The Benefits of Meditation. Available from www.consciouschoice.com/health/ meditation1103.html.

8. Harvard Gazette Archives. (2002). Meditation changes temperature. *Harvard Gazette Archives.* Available from www.news.harvard.edu/gazette/2002/04.18/09-tummo.html.

Chapter 12

1. Yusef Abdullah, A. (Trans.). (1989). *The meaning of the Holy Qur'an.* Maryland: Amana Publications. Chapter 41, verse 44.

2. Ibid., Chapter 12, verses 27-28.

3. Ibid., Chapter 26, verse 80.

4. Siddiq, H. A. (Trans.). (1977). Muslim, Imam. *Sahih Muslim.* Kitab Bhavan, India. Volume 2, Hadith 5435.

5. Yusef, Abdullah A. (Trans.). (1989). *The meaning of the Holy Qur'an.* Maryland: Amana Publications. Chapter 50, verses 15.

6. Siddiq, H. A. (Trans.). (1977). Muslim, Imam. *Sahih Muslim.* Kitab Bhavan, India. Volumes 3 and 4. Chapter 7, Saying 1,958.

7. Yusef, Abdullah A. (Trans.). (1989). *The meaning of the Holy Qur'an*. Maryland: Amana Publications. Chapter 7, verse 34.
8. Ibid., Chapter 4, verse 22.
9. Ibid., Chapter 52, verse 21.
10. Ibid., Chapter 7, verse 34.
11. Siddiq, H. A. (Trans.). (1977). Muslim, Imam. *Sahih Muslim*. Kitab Bhavan, India. Volume 7, Saying 575.

Chapter 13

1. Genesis 1:1-2; 2:7. Authors' translation.
2. Jewish Publication Society of America. (1985). *Tanakh—The new translation of the Holy Scriptures* (New JPS Translation); Isaiah 32:15. Philadelphia.
3. Joel 3:1 [2:28].
4. Numbers 27:16.
5. Numbers 27:18.
6. Rosman, S. M. (1994). *Spiritual parenting: A sourcebook for parents and teachers*. Wheaton, IL: Theosophical Publishing House. P. 6.
7. According to the Kabbalistic tradition, there are five soul-dimensions; the first three are named in the Bible. In ascending order toward God, they are: *Nefesh, Ruah, Neshamah, Hayah*, and *Yehidah*.
8. Ariel, D. S. (1998). *The mystic quest: An introduction to Jewish mysticism*. New York: Schocken. P. 123.
9. Wolf, L. (1999). *Practical Kabbalah*. New York: Three Rivers. Pp. 35-37.
10. Labowitz, S. (1996). *Miraculous living: A guided journey in Kabbalah through the ten gates of the tree of life*. New York: Simon & Schuster. P. 21.
11. Ibid., p. 196.
12. The Hebrew word for angels is *malakhim*. *Malakhim* refers to messengers of God, who may be partially divine or totally human.
13. Labowitz, S. P. 21.
14. Based on a prayer by Rabbi Bonita E. Taylor.
15. Eric Cassell is a clinical professor of public health at Weill Medical College of Cornell University and an attending physician at New York Presbyterian Hospital.
16. Cassell, E. J. (1991). *The nature of suffering and the goals of medicine*. New York: Oxford University Press. P. 33.
17. Lamentations 3:38.
18. Jeremiah 13:22.
19. Weiss-Rosmarin, T. (1947). *Judaism and Christianity*. New York: Jewish Book Club. P. 54.
20. Ezekiel 18.
21. Jeremiah 31:29-30.
22. Deuteronomy 24:16.
23. See Schwarzchild, S. S., s.v. "Suffering." *Encyclopedia Judaica, 15*, 485-486.
24. The Hebrew Bible is also known as the *Tanakh* or the Hebrew Scriptures. It contains the Five Books of Moses, the Prophets, and the Writings, including Psalms. Note: Christians often refer to the Bible as composed of two sacred documents; the Hebrew Bible, which they term the Old Testament, and the New Testament. While Jews recognize that the Christian

Scriptures are sacred to Christians, only those books that Christians term the Old Testament are sacred for Jews.

25. The Talmud is the important Jewish postbiblical commentary on leading a religious/moral life. More specifically, it is the vast compendium of Jewish thought developed by the rabbis in the postbiblical world between c. 200 BCE and 500 CE. There are two Talmuds—the Babylonian Talmud, which is the more authoritative, and the Jerusalem Talmud.

26. The Midrash is a collection of rabbinic sermons and interpretations of the Bible and Jewish law, compiled between c. 400-1550 CE.

27. Babylonian Talmud *Berakhot* 5a, citing Proverbs 3:12.

28. Ibid., *Berakhot* 5b. See also David C. Kraemer (1995), *Responses to suffering in classical rabbinic literature*. New York: Oxford University Press.

29. Zucker, D. J. (1995). Suffering. In L. Klenicki & G. Wigoder (Eds.), *A dictionary of the Jewish-Christian dialogue, expanded edition* (p. 206). A Stimulus Book. New York: Paulist.

30. Kushner, H. (1983). *When bad things happen to good people*. New York: Avon. P. 134.

31. Isaac Luria (1534-1572) continues to be known as one of the more outstanding masters of Kabbalah.

32. *Midrash Exodus Rabbah* 15.16; 15.12.

33. Genesis 1:27.

34. Kleinman, M. S. (1963). *Or Yesharim*. In L. I. Newman (Ed.), *The Hasidic anthology* (p. 67). New York: Schocken.

35. Ellenson, D. H. (1995). How to draw guidance from a heritage: Jewish approaches to mortal choices. In E. N. Dorff and L. E. Newman (Eds.), *Contemporary Jewish ethics and morality: A reader* (p. 133). New York: Oxford University Press.

36. Newman, L. E. (1995). Woodchoppers and respirators: The problem of interpretation in contemporary Jewish ethics. In E. N. Dorff & L. E. Newman (Eds.), *Contemporary Jewish ethics and morality: A reader* (pp. 144-147). New York: Oxford University Press.

37. A suggested list of books and articles dealing with Jewish ethics and morality is found in E. N. Dorff and L. E. Newman (Eds.). (1995). *Contemporary Jewish ethics and morality: A reader*. New York: Oxford University Press. Pp. 467-468.

38. Segal, S. (2002). Pain and suffering. *Beḥoref Hayamim—In the winter of life*. Wyncote, PA: Reconstructionist Rabbinical College (Center for Jewish Ethics). Pp. 87-88.

39. Lamm, M. (1969). *The Jewish way in death and mourning*. New York: Jonathan David. Pp. 5-6.

40. Genesis 3:19.

41. Klein, I. (1975). *A guide to Jewish religious practice*. New York: Jewish Theological Seminary of America. P. 275 f.

42. Heschel, A. J. (1991). *I asked for wonder*. New York: Crossroad. P. 88.

43. Exodus 24:7.

44. Frankel, E., & Teutsch, B. P. (1992). *The encyclopedia of Jewish symbols*. Northvale, NJ: Jason Aronson. Pp. 149-150.

45. Ibid., p. 176.

46. *Zohar, Terumah*, 3.141b ff.

47. Jacobs, L. (1973). *What does Judaism say about . . . ?* Jerusalem: Keter. P. 128.

48. Babylonian Talmud *Ketubot* 104a.

49. *Yalkut Shimoni*, Proverbs #943.

50. Jacobs, L. Pp. 128-129.

51. Newman, L. I. (Ed.). (1945). *The Talmudic anthology*. New York: Behrman House. Pp. 338-339, *Tosefta, Berakhot* 7.

52. Sonsino, R., & Syme, D. (1990). *What happens after I die?* New York: Union of American Hebrew Congregations. P. 3.

53. Psalm 23 speaks about life and about God protecting us, but on another level it says that even in death, God will be there with us. Psalm 16:10 says this even more clearly: "for you [God] will not abandon me to death [literally, *Sheol*], nor let your faithful one see destruction [literally, the pit]." According to Jewish tradition, God is with us at all times, in joy as in sorrow, in light as in darkness, in life as in death.

54. Numbers 27: 13; Numbers 31:2; 2 Samuel 12:23.

55. The root of the word *Sheol* may mean something like "hollow place." In its early formulation *Sheol*, the underworld, is the place to which the dead go. In the early biblical world, there is no concept of an individual soul. Rather, a person is a *nefesh haya* (a living *nefesh*), a living being (Genesis 2:7); when you die you become a *nefesh met* (a dead *nefesh*), a being that has died (Leviticus 21:11; Numbers 6:6). See Raphael, S. P. (1994). *Jewish views of the afterlife*. Northvale, NJ: Jason Aronson. P. 56; Gilman, N. (2000). *The death of death*. Woodstock, VT: Jewish Lights.

56. Psalms 88, 115:17; Ecclesiastes 9:10.

57. Segal, E. Judaism. In H. Coward (Ed.), *Life after death in world religions* (pp. 13-16). Maryknoll, NY: Orbis; Raphael, p. 43.

58. Babylonian Talmud *Berakhot* 8a. *Midrash Psalms* 11.6.

59. *Pesikta Rabbati* 44.8.

60. Judaism has a very rich tradition dealing with the Afterlife, one aspect of which is termed the World to Come, the *Olam ha-ba*.

61. *Mishna Avot* 4.17.

62. Babylonian Talmud *Berakhot* 17a.

63. Babylonian Talmud *Baba Batra* 58a.

64. Babylonian Talmud *Eruvin* 19a.

65. Babylonian Talmud *Taanit* 5a. *Midrash Proverbs* 6.1.

66. Babylonian Talmud *Rosh Hashanah* 17a.

67. Babylonian Talmud *Berakhot* 19a.

68. *Pesikta Rabbati* 50.1.

69. Babylonian Talmud *Nedarim* 40a.

70. Babylonian Talmud *Rosh Hashanah* 17a; *Shabbat* 33b.

71. Babylonian Talmud *Rosh Hashanah* 17a.

72. *Midrash Exodus Rabbah* 2.2.

73. Cf. *Midrash Numbers Rabbah* 13.2.

74. Moore, G. F. (1971). *Judaism in the first centuries of the Christian era* (Vol. 2.). New York: Schocken. P. 295.

75. Raphael, p. 157.

76. Orthodox Judaism today continues to assert this underlying philosophy of the Talmudic rabbis.

77. Cohen, N. J. (2000). *The way into Torah*. Woodstock, VT: Jewish Lights. Pp. 54-55.

78. *Midrash Genesis Rabbah* 8.6; Babylonian Talmud *Ketubot* 111a.

79. Babylonian Talmud *Taanit* 7a.

80. *Mishna Avot* 4.22.

81. *Mishneh Torah*, The Book of Knowledge, 90a. Raphael, p. 253.

82. *Mishneh Torah*, The Book of Knowledge, 91a. Raphael, p. 253. See Sonsino and Syme, p. 40 ff.

83. Cf. Babylonian Talmud *Taanit* 11a. *Zohar, Vayehi*, 2.221b; Raphael, p. 372.

84. Raphael, p. 382.

85. During this time our personalities are purified and the consequences of our emo-tional lives are brought to completion. Here, we are required to encounter all of the unex-pressed fear, sadness, pain, desire, grief, suffering, anger, and guilt—everything in the realm of relationships that we did not resolve during life. This stage corresponds with what we call *Gehenna*. This stage is finite; it can take up to a year, but whether that is in "human" time or "God" time is unclear.

86. As we journey through Lower and Upper *Gan Eden* we play out the last vestiges of our personal lives. Here, we are connected to the spiritual dimensions of existence and led to a spiritual repose for our souls.

87. Sonsino and Syme, p. 55-63.

88. Babylonian Talmud *Berakhot* 5b.

89. Babylonian Talmud *Shabbat* 127a.

90. Babylonian Talmud *Nedarim* 40a.

91. Ganzfried, S. (1961). *Code of Jewish law/Kitzur* Shulḥan Arukh (Rev. ed., Vol. 4, 193.1). New York: Hebrew Publishing. The Code of Jewish Law/Kitzur Shulḥan Arukh (abridged *Shulḥan Arukh*) is a handbook that lists standard Jewish practices from a traditional viewpoint.

92. Babylonian Talmud *Nedarim* 39b.

93. Ganzfried, S. (1961). *Code of Jewish law/Kitzur* Shulḥan Arukh (Rev. ed., Vol. 4, 193.3). New York: Hebrew Publishing.

94. Klotz, M. (2002). End of life care. *Beḥoref Hayamim—In the winter of life.* Wyncote, PA: Reconstructionist Rabbinical College (Center for Jewish Ethics). P. 109.

95. Ganzfried, S., vol. 4, 193.5.

96. Ibid., vol. 4, 193.3.

97. Townsend, J. T. (1989). *Midrash Tanhuma*, vol. 1, 3.5. (S. Buber Recension) (*Lekh Lekha*) Genesis 12:1 ff. Part V. Hoboken, NJ: Ktav.

98. Zucker, D. J. (1998). *American rabbis: Facts and fiction.* Northvale, NJ: Jason Aronson. P. 277.

99. Ganzfried, S., vol. 4, 193.4.

100. *Zohar, Vayigash*, 2.168b.

101. Taylor, B. E. (2005). The power of custom-made prayers. In Dayle A. Friedman (Ed.), *Jewish pastoral care: A practical handbook* (2nd ed., revised and expanded). Woodstock, VT: Jewish Lights.

102. Levy, N. (2002). *Talking to God.* New York: Knopf. P. 4.

103. Numbers 12:13. For a musical rendition of these words, see: Deborah Lynn Friedman (1995), EL NA R'FA NA LA, (ASCAP; lyrics from Numbers 12:13). On: *Renewal of Spirit*, Debbie Friedman. For information contact: Sounds Write Productions, Inc., 1-800/9-SOUND-9 (800-976-8639).

104. Taylor, B. E. (2006). The Muse of chanting. In Jack H Bloom (Ed.), *Jewish relational care, a-z: We are our other's keeper.* Binghamton, NY: Haworth.

105. MI SHEBEIRACH, (1988). Deborah Lynn Friedman. On: *Renewal of Spirit:* .

Mi she bei rach avoteinu	Mi she bei rach imoteinu
M'kor habracha l'imoteinu	M'kor habracha l'avoteinu
May the source of strength	Bless those in need of healing
Who blessed the ones before us	With r'fua shleima
Help us find the courage	The renewal of body
To make our lives a blessing	The renewal of spirit
And let us say, Amen	And let us say, Amen.

106. Deuteronomy 6:4.

107. Genesis 18:1ff.

108. As professional chaplains, we are engaged in learning how best to treat those who are compromised in our own and in each other's denominations or faiths. This extensive education is known as CPE (Clinical Pastoral Education) and is under the auspices of the Association for Clinical Pastoral Education—www.acpe.edu. This education, which can take from 1 to 4 years to complete, can lead to Board Certification by the Association of Professional Chaplains (APC) www.professionalchaplains.org, the Canadian Association for Pastoral Practice and Education/ Association canadienne pour la pratique et l'éducation pastorales (CAPPE/ACPEP) www.cappe.org, the National Association of Catholic Chaplains (NACC) www.nacc.org, and the National Association of Jewish Chaplains (NAJC) www.najc.org.

109. Genesis 12:1-3.

Chapter 15

1. Puchalski, C. M., & Larson, D. B. (1998). Developing curricula in spirituality and medicine. *Academic Medicine, 73*, 970. Association of American Medical Colleges. (1999). *Report III—Contemporary issues in medicine: Communication in medicine, Medical School Objectives Project (MSOP III)*. Washington, DC: Association of American Medical Colleges. P. 25.

2. Association of American Medical Colleges. (1998). *Report I—Learning objectives for medical student education: Guidelines for medical schools (MSOP I)*. Washington, DC: Association of American Medical Colleges.

3. Lo, B., Quill, T. E., & Tulsky, J. (1998). End of life care consensus panel: Discussion palliative care with patients. *Annals of Internal Medicine, 130*, 744-749.

4. Ibid.

5. Puchalski, C. M. (2002). Spirituality and end-of-life care: A time for listening and caring. *Journal of Palliative Medicine, 5*, 289-294. Post, S. G., Puchalski, C. M., & Larson, D. B. (2004). Physicians and patient spirituality: Professional boundaries, competency, and ethics. *Annals of Internal Medicine, 132*, 578-583. Astrow, A. B., Puchalski, C. M., & Sulmasy, D. P. (2001). Religion, spirituality, and healthcare: Social, ethical, and practical considerations. *American Journal of Medicine, 110*, 283-287.

6. Association of American Medical Colleges. (1998). *Report I—Learning objectives for medical student education: Guidelines for medical schools (MSOP I)*. Washington, DC: Association of American Medical Colleges.

7. Engles, G. L. (1977). The need for new medical model: A challenge for biomedicine. *Science, 196*, 129-136. Puchalski, C. M., & Larson, D. B. (1998). Developing curricula in spirituality and medicine. *Academic Medicine, 73*, 970-974. Sulmasy, D. P. (2002). A biopsychosocial-spiritual model for the care of patients at the end of life. *The Gerontologist, 42*(Suppl 3), 24-33.

8. Puchalski, C. M., & Romer, A. L. (2000). Taking a spiritual history allows clinicians to understand patients more fully. *Journal of Palliative Medicine, 3*, 129-137. Puchalski, C. M. (2002). Spirituality. In A. Berger, R. Portenoy, & D. Weissmann (Eds.), *Principles and practices of palliative care and supportive oncology* (2nd ed., pp. 800-812). Philadelphia: Lippincott Williams & Wilkins. Astrow, A. B., Puchalski, C. M., & Sulmasy, D. P. (2001). Religion, spirituality, and healthcare: Social, ethical, and practical considerations. *American Journal of Medicine, 110*, 283-287.

9. Lo, B., Ruston, D., Kates, L. W., Arnold, R., Faber-Langendoen, K., Puchalski, C. M., et al. (2002). Discussing religious and spiritual issues at the end of life: A practical guide for physi-

cians. *Journal of the American Medical Association, 287*, 749-754. Post, S. G., Puchalski, C. M., & Larson, D. B. (2004). Physicians and patient spirituality: Professional boundaries, competency, and ethics. *Annals of Internal Medicine, 132*, 578-583. Astrow, A. B., Puchalski, C. M., & Sulmasy, D. P. (2001). Religion, spirituality, and healthcare: Social, ethical, and practical considerations. *American Journal of Medicine, 110*, 283-287.

10. Kagawa-Singer, M. (1994). *Diverse cultural beliefs and practices about death and dying in the elderly, cultural diversity and geriatrics care: Challenges to the health professions.* Binghamton, NY: Haworth. Pp. 101-116.

11. Lo, B., Ruston, D., Kates, L. W., Arnold, R., Faber-Langendoen, K., Puchalski, C. M., et al. (2002). Discussing religious and spiritual issues at the end of life: A practical guide for physicians. *Journal of the American Medical Association, 287*, 749-754.

12. Weintraub, S. (1994). *Healing of soul, healing of body: Spiritual leaders unfold the strength and solace in Psalms.* Woodstock, VT: Jewish Lights.

13. Sloan, R. P., Bagiella, E., VandeCreek, L., Hover, M., Casalone C., Hirsch T. J., et al. (2000). Should physicians prescribe religious activities? *New England Journal of Medicine, 22*, 1913-1916.

14. Brett, A. S., & Jersild, P. (2003). "Inappropriate" treatment near the end of life: Conflict between religious convictions and clinical judgment. *Archives of Internal Medicine, 163*, 1645-1649.

15. Haughk, K. C., & McKay, W. J. (1994). *Christian caregiving: A way of life: Leader's guide.* Minneapolis, MN: Augsburg Fortress.

Chapter 16

1. Bruner, J. (1986). *Actual minds, possible worlds.* Cambridge, MA: Harvard University Press. Bruner, J. (1990). *Acts of meaning.* Cambridge, MA: Harvard University Press. Bruner, J. (2002). *Making stories: Law, literature, life.* New York: Farrar, Straus, and Giroux.

2. All names in the reported stories have been changed to protect people's identity.

3. We recognize that the distinction between *story* and *narrative* has received lively discussion among academics, but, for our purposes in this chapter, we will follow the growing convention of using these two terms interchangeably.

4. Kleinman, A. (1988). *The illness narratives: Suffering, healing and the human condition.* New York: Basic Books.

5. Mattingly, C. (1998). *Healing dramas and clinical plots: The narrative structure of experience.* New York: Cambridge University Press.

6. Mattingly, C., & Garro, L. C. (2000). *Narrative and the cultural construction of illness and healing.* Berkeley, CA: University of California Press.

7. Mishler, E. G. (1984). *The discourse of medicine: Dialectics of medical interviews.* NJ: Ablex; Mishler, E. G. (1999). *Storylines: Craftartists' narratives of identity.* Cambridge, MA: Harvard University Press, Cambridge, MA.

8. Mishler, E. G. (1999). *Storylines: Craftartists' narratives of identity.* Cambridge, MA: Harvard University Press.

9. Bruner, J. (2002). *Making stories: Law, literature, life.* New York: Farrar, Straus, and Giroux.

10. Barnard, D., Towers, A., Boston, P., & Lambrinidou, Y. (2000). *Crossing over: Narratives of palliative care.* New York: Oxford University Press.

11. Donnelly, W. J. (1988). Righting the medical record: Transforming chronicle into story. *Journal of the American Medical Association, 260*, 823-825.

12. Ibid.

13. Coles, R. (1989). *The call of stories: Teaching and the moral imagination.* Boston: Houghton Mifflin.

14. Ibid.

15. Sobel, R. J. (2000). Eva's stories: Recognizing the poverty of the medical case history. *Academic Medicine, 75*, 85-89.

16. Bruner, J. (1986). *Actual minds, possible worlds.* Cambridge, MA: Harvard University Press.

17. Engel, J. D., & Jones, D. L. (1995). Medicine as humanities. In S. K. Majumdar, L. M. Resenfield, D. B. Nash, & A. M. Audet (Eds.), *Medicine and health care into the twenty-first century* (pp. 409-443). Easton, PA: The Pennsylvania Academy of Science.

18. Charon, R. (1986). To render the lives of patients. *Literature and Medicine, 5*, 58-74.

19. Ways, P., Engel, J. D., & Finkelstein, P. (2000). *Clinical clerkships: The heart of professional development.* Thousand Oaks, CA: Sage.

20. Bruner, J. (1986). *Actual minds, possible worlds.* Cambridge, MA: Harvard University Press. Bruner, J. (1990). *Acts of meaning.* Cambridge, MA: Harvard University Press.

21. Frank, A. W. (1995). *The wounded storyteller: Body, illness and ethics.* Chicago: University of Chicago Press.

Chapter 17

1. Brady, M. J., Peterman, A. H., Fitchett, G., Mo, M., & Cella, D. (1999). A case of including spirituality in quality of life measurement in oncology. *Psycho-oncology, 8*, 417-428. Rousseau, P. (2000). Spirituality and the dying patient. *Journal of Clinical Oncology, 18*, 2000-2002. Chin-A-Loy, S. S., & Fernsler, J. I. (1998). Self-Transcendence in older men attending a prostate cancer support group. *Cancer Nursing, 21*, 358-363. Puchalski, C. M., & Romer, A. L. (2000). Taking a spiritual history allows clinicians to understand patients more fully. *Journal of Palliative Medicine 3*, 129-137.

2. Frankl, V. F. (1959/1992). *Man's search for meaning* (4th ed.). Boston: Beacon Press.

3. Ibid.

4. Kissane, D., Clarke, D. M., & Street, A. F. (2001). Demoralization syndrome: A relevant psychiatric diagnosis for palliative care. *Journal of Palliative Care, 17*, 12-21.

5. Frankl, V. F. (1959/1992). *Man's search for meaning* (4th ed.). Boston: Beacon Press.

6. Kies, D. *Making meaning. Composition.* Retrieved December 23, 2003, from http://papyr.com/hypertextbooks/engl_101/thesis3.html.

7. Beck, A. T. (1976). *Cognitive therapy and emotional disorders.* New York: International Universities Press.

8. Koenig, H. G., George, L. K., & Peterson, B. L. (1998). Religiosity and remission of depression in medically ill older patients. *American Journal of Psychiatry, 155*, 536-542.

9. Baider, L., Russak, S. M., Perry, S., et al. (1999). The role of religious and spiritual beliefs in coping with malignant melanoma: An Israeli sample. *Psycho-oncology, 8*, 27-35.

10. Park, C., & Folkman, S. (1997). Meaning in the context of stress and coping. *Review of General Psychology, 1*, 115-144.

11. Andrykowski, M. A., Brady, M. J., & Hunt, J. W. (1993). Positive psychosocial adjustment in potential bone marrow transplant recipients: Cancer as a psychosocial transition. *Psycho-oncology, 2,* 261-276.

12. Taylor, S. E. (1983). Adjustment to threatening events: A theory of cognitive adaptation. *American Psychologist, 38,* 1161-1173. Davis, C. G., Nolen-Hoeksma, S., & Larson, J. (1998). Making sense of loss and benefiting from the experience: Two construals of meaning. *Journal of Personality and Social Psychology, 75,* 561-574. Lazarus, R. S., & Folkman, S. (1984). *Stress, appraisal and coping.* New York: Springer. Brady, M. J., Peterman, A. H., Fitchett, G., Mo, M., & Cella, D. (1999). A case of including spirituality in quality of life measurement in oncology. *Psycho-oncology, 8,* 417-428.

13. Puchalski, C., & Romer, A. L. (2000). Taking a spiritual history allows clinicians to understand patients more fully. *Journal of Palliative Medicine, 3,* 129-137.

14. Karasu, B. T. (1999). Spiritual psychotherapy. *American Journal of Psychotherapy, 53,* 143-162.

15. Brady, M. J., Peterman, A. H., Fitchett, G., Mo, M., & Cella, D. (1999). A case of including spirituality in quality of life measurement in oncology. *Psycho-oncology, 8,* 417-428.

16. Ibid.

17. Breitbart, W., Chochinov, H. M., & Passik, S. D. (1998). Psychiatric aspects of palliative care. In D. Doyle, G. W. Hanks, & N. MacDonald (Eds.), *Oxford textbook of palliative medicine* (2nd ed., pp. 216-247). New York: Oxford University Press. Nelson, C., Rosenfeld, B., Breitbart, W., & Galietta, M. (2001). *Spirituality, depression and religion in the terminally-ill.* Manuscript submitted for publication.

18. Rousseau, P. (2000). Spirituality and the dying patient. *Journal of Clinical Oncology, 18,* 2000-2002.

19. Ibid.

20. Fawzy, F. I., & Fawzy, N. W. (1998). Group therapy in the cancer setting. *Journal of Psychosomatic Research, 45,* 191-200. Spiegel, D., Stein, S. L., Earhart, T. Z., & Diamond, S. (2000). Group psychotherapy and the terminally-ill. In H. Chochinov & W. Breitbart (Eds.), *The handbook of psychiatry in palliative medicine* (pp. 241-251). New York: Oxford University Press.

21. Yalom, I. D., & Greaves, C. (1977). Group therapy with the terminally-ill. *American Journal of Psychiatry, 134,* 396-400. Spiegel, D., Bloom, J., & Yalom, I. D. (1981). Group support for patients with metastatic breast cancer. *Archives of General Psychiatry, 38,* 527-533. Spiegel, D., Bloom, J., Kraemer, H., & Gottheil, E. (1989). Effects of psychosocial treatment on survival of patients with metastatic breast cancer. *Lancet, 340,* 888-891. Spiegel, D., Bloom, J., Kraemer, H., & Gottheil, E. (1989). The beneficial effect of psychosocial treatment on survival of metastatic breast cancer patients: A randomized prospective outcome study. *Lancet, 340,* 888-891. Spiegel, D., & Yalom, I. D. (1978). A support group for dying patients. *International Journal of Group Psychotherapy, 28,* 233-245. Spiegel, D., & Glafkides, M. C. (1983). Effects of group confrontation with death and dying. *International Journal of Group Psychotherapy, 4,* 433-447. Spiegel, D., Bloom, J. R., & Gottheil, E. (1983). Family environment of patients with metastatic carcinoma. *Journal of Psychosocial Oncology, 1,* 33-44. Ferlic, M., Goldman, A., & Kennedy, B. J. (1979). Group counseling in adult patients with advanced cancer. *Cancer, 43,* 760-766. Forester, B., Kornfeld, D. S., & Fleiss, J. L. (1985). Psychotherapy during radiotherapy: Effects on emotional and physical distress. *American Journal of Psychiatry, 142,* 22-27. Goodwin, P. J., Leszcz, M., Koopmans, J., et al. (1996). Randomized trial of group psychosocial support in metastatic breast cancer: The BEST (Breast-Expressive Supportive Therapy) study. *Cancer Treatment Review, 22,* 91-99.

Linn, M. W., Linn, B. S., & Harris, R. (1982). Effects of counseling for late stage cancer patients. *Cancer, 49*, 1048-1055. Edmonds, C. V. I., Lockwood, G. A., & Cunningham, A. J. (1999). Psychological response to long-term group therapy: A randomized trial with metastatic breast cancer patients. *Psycho-oncology, 8*, 74-91. Spiegel, D., Stein, S. L., Earhart, T. Z., & Diamond, S. (2000). Group psychotherapy and the terminally-ill. In H. Chochinov & W. Breitbart (Eds.), *The handbook of psychiatry in palliative medicine* (pp. 241-251). New York: Oxford University Press.

22. Cain, E. N., Kohorn, E. I., Quinlan, D. M., et al. (1986). Psychosocial benefits of a cancer support group. *Cancer, 57*, 183-189. Yalom, I. D. (1980). *Existential psychotherapy.* New York: Basic Books. Cella, D., & Yellen, S. (1993). Cancer support groups: The state of the art. *Cancer Practice, 1*, 56-61. Coward, D., & Reed, P. (1996). Self-transcendence: A resource for healing at the end of life. *Issues in Mental Health Nursing, 17*, 275-288.

23. Fawzy, F. I., & Fawzy, N. W. (1989). Group therapy in the cancer setting. *Journal of Psychosomatic Research, 45*, 191-200.

24. Hiatt, J. F. (1986). Spirituality, medicine, and healing. *Southern Medical Journal, 79*, 736-743. Coward, D. D. (1998). Facilitation of self-transcendence in a breast cancer support group. *Oncology Nursing Forum, 25*, 75-84. Chin-A-Loy, S. S., & Fernsler, J. I. (1998). Self-transcendence in older men attending a prostate cancer support group. *Cancer Nursing, 21*, 358-363.

25. Lazer, E. (1984). Logotherapeutic support groups for cardiac patients. *The International Forum for Logotherapy, 7*, 85-88. Quirk, J. M. (1979). Finding meaning everyday. *The International Forum for Logotherapy, 2*, 15-22. Zuehlke, T. E., & Watkins, J. T. (1975). The use of psychotherapy with dying patients: An exploratory study. *Journal of Clinical Psychology, 31*, 729-732.

26. Frankl, V. F. (1969/1988). *The will to meaning: Foundations and applications of logotherapy* (expanded edition). New York: Penguin Books.

27. Reed, P. (1991). Self-transcendence and mental health in oldest-old adults. *Nursing Research, 40*, 1-7.

28. Frankl, V. F. (1969/1988). *The will to meaning: Foundations and applications of logotherapy* (expanded edition). New York: Penguin Books.

29. Reed, P. (1991). Self-transcendence and mental health in oldest-old adults. *Nursing Research, 40*, 1-7. Chin-A-Loy, S. S., & Fernsler, J. I. (1998). Self-transcendence in older men attending a prostate cancer support group. *Cancer Nursing, 21*, 358-363.

30. Breitbart, W., Chochinov, H. M., & Passik, S. D. (1998). Psychiatric aspects of palliative care. In D. Doyle, G. W. Hanks, & N. MacDonald (Eds.), *Oxford textbook of palliative medicine* (2nd ed., pp. 216-247). New York: Oxford University Press.

31. Rosenfeld, B., Breitbart, W., Galietta, M., Kaim, M., Funesti-Esch, J., Pessin, H., et al. (2000). Schedule of attitudes toward hastened death: Measuring desire for death among terminally-ill cancer patients. *Cancer, 88*, 2868-2875.

32. Frankl, V. F. (1959/1992). *Man's search for meaning* (4th ed.). Boston: Beacon Press.

Chapter 18

1. Flinders, C. L. (1993). *Enduring grace: Living portraits of seven women mystics.* San Francisco: Harper. P. 129.

2. Roseman, J. L. 2005 Permission by author. From *Dance was Her Religion: The Spiritual Choreography of Isadora Duncan, Ruth St. Denis and Martha Graham.* (For further information see www.hohmpress.com.)

3. From personal electronic correspondence, January, 2003. Laird, R. (2001). *Grain of truth: The ancient lessons of craft.* New York: Walker. Laird, R. (2003). *A stone's throw: The enduring nature of myth.* Toronto, Ontario: Macfarlane Walter & Ross.

4. From personal electronic correspondence with Dr. Ross Laird, January 2003.

5. Stewart I: Sacred Woman, Sacred Dance. Inner Traditions, Vermont, 2000, p. 214.

6. From personal electronic correspondence with Beverly Lomar, February 2002.

7. Roseman, J. L. 2005. Permission by author. From *Dance was Her Religion: The Spiritual Choreography of Isadora Duncan, Ruth St. Denis and Martha Graham.* (For further information see www.hohmpress.com.)

8. *Parabola, XI*, No.3, 1986, 49-50.

9. From personal electronic correspondence with Vicki S. Burns, founding Program Director for The Wellness Community of Southeast Florida, January 2003.

10. From personal electronic correspondence with Nikki Todd, September 2002.

11. From personal electronic correspondence with Dr. Ross Laird, January 2003.

12. Kasayka, R. E., & Hatfield, K. (1994). *A Comparison of sedative vs. palliative music in treatment of persons in end-stage Alzheimer's disease.* Retrieved January 5, 2003, from http://www.heatherhill.org/music research 02.html.

13. From personal electronic correspondence with Beverly Lomar, February 2003.

14. Campbell, D. (1992). *Musical-Sacramental-Midwifery; The use of music in death and dying in music and miracles.* Wheaton, IL: Quest Books. P. 21.

15. Ibid., p. 19.

16. From personal electronic correspondence with Emily Spahr, January 2003.

17. Halpern, S. (1985). *Sound health: The music and sound that makes us whole.* San Francisco: Harper & Row. P. 38.

18. Goldman, J. (1992). *Healing sounds.* Boston: Element. P. 43.

19. From a personal interview with Dr. John Upledger, February 2003.

20. Morgenstern, S. (1958/1996). *Composers on music.* New York: Knopf.

21. This is incorrect information, since the use of music, chant, and vocals have a long and rich history in all cultures around the world.

22. Andrews, T. (2001). *Sacred sounds: Transformation through music and word.* St. Paul, MN: Llewellyn. P. 9.

23. Boucher, S. (1999). *Discovering Kwan Yin: Buddhist goddess of compassion.* Boston: Beacon Press. Pp. 102-105. This wonderful book explores the link between healing and the goddess, and is an insightful treatise on healing and goddess imagery.

24. From personal electronic correspondence with Dr. Joy Berger, February 2003. For additional information on Dr. Joy Berger's work, see www.hospiceinstitute.org.

25. From personal conversation with Theodora Roseman, January 2003.

26. From personal conversation with Jeri Howe. Jeri Howe is a music thanatologist in Seattle, Washington. Her company, Sacred Harmonies, works with various hospice hospitals. For further information, contact sacredharmony@earthlink.net or consult the music thanatology web page at www.music_thanatology.com.

27. Ibid.

28. Adapted by permission of Dr. Joy Berger, February, 2003. For the complete program of CORE VALUES; see http://www.musicofthesoul.com/griefguides.htm.

29. Durckheim, G. V., & Fried, K. (1986). Healing power and gesture. *Parabola, 30.*

Chapter 19

1. Morton, W. T., & Warren, J. C. (1846). London: People's Journal.
2. Seelaus, V. (1988). Fragmentation and divine transformation: Meditation on the compost heap. *THE WAY: A Review of Contemporary Christian Spirituality, 28,* 301.
3. Personal conversation with Karen McLennan.
4. Ibid.

Chapter 20

1. Gaynor, Mitchell L. (1999). *Sounds of healing: A physician reveals the therapeutic power of sound and music.* New York: Broadway Books.
2. Adapted from *What is music thanatology?* Available from: http://www .music-thanatologyassociation.com
3. Halstead, M. T., & Roscoe, S. T. (2002). Music as an intervention for oncology nurses. *Clinical Journal of Oncology Nursing, 6,* 332.
4. Barber, D.W. (2003). *The music lover's quotation book.* Toronto, Canada: Sound & Vision.
5. Ibid.
6. Bullfinch, T. (1998). *The Story of Orpheus & Eurydice,* in *Bullfinch's Mythology.* Available from http://www.bullfinch.org.
7. Barber, D.W. (2003). *The music lover's quotation book.* Toronto, Canada: Sound & Vision.
8. Stillwater, M., & Malkin, G. (2003). *Graceful passages: A companion for living and dying.* Novato, CA: New World Library. P. 31.
9. Ortiz, J. M. (1997). *The tao of music: Sound psychology, using music to change your life.* York Beach, ME: Samuel Weiser.
10. Malkin, G. (2004). *Unspeakable grace: The music of graceful passages.* Novato, CA: Wisdom of the World.
11. Gfeller, Kate E. et al. (1998). *An introduction to music therapy: Theory and practice.* Columbus, OH: McGraw Hill College Division.
12. *Care for the journey: Sustaining the heart of healthcare,* a program for practitioner renewal available at www.careforthejourney.net.
13. Kramer, K. (1988). *The sacred art of dying: How world religions understand death.* Mahwah, NJ: Paulist Press. P. 77.
14. Stillwater, M., & Malkin, G. (2005). *The heart of healing,* by Jeremy Geffen, from *Care for the journey: Messages and music for sustaining the heart of healthcare,* www.careforthejourney.net

Chapter 21

1. Worden, J. W. (1991). *Grief counseling and grief therapy: A handbook for the mental health practitioner* (2nd ed.). New York: Springer.

2. Doka, K. J., & Morgan, J. D. (Eds.). (1993). *Death and spirituality*. Amityville, NY: Baywood. P. 190.

3. Ibid., p. 191.

Chapter 22

1. Frankl, V. (1985). *Man's search for meaning*. New York: Washington Square Press.

Chapter 24

1. Stein, E. (2000). *Knowledge and faith* (W. Redmond, Trans.). Washington, DC: ICS Publications.

Index